DEMYSTIFYING INTEGRATED CARE

A Handbook for Practice

DEMYSTIFYING INTEGRATED CARE

A Handbook for Practice

DR KIRSTY MARSHALL

Professional Doctorate – Health and Social Care,
MSc Specialist Nursing Practice (District Nurse),
PGCert, Academic Practice, BSc Nursing Practice,
DipNursing, Queens Nurse
Senior Lecturer/Research Fellow (NCA)/Senior
Research Leader (NIHR), and Senior Associate (IFIC)
University of Salford, Northern Care Alliance NHS
Foundation Trust (NCA), National Institute for Health
Research (NHIR), International Foundation for
Integrated Care (IFIC)
University of Salford

DR HAYLEY BAMBER

Professional Doctorate in Health and Social Care,
MSc Advanced Occupational Therapy, BSc (Hons)
Occupational Therapy, PGCert Higher Education
Lecturer
University of Central Lancashire

DR RUTH GARBUTT

PhD, MA, PGDip, BA (Hons), PGCLTHE, PGCEE, MA,
SFHEA
Head of Social Work and Integrated Practice
Allerton Building
University of Salford

CHRIS EASTON

BA (Hons)
Director of Strategy and Impact at NHS Charities
Together
NHS Charities

ELSEVIER

Notices

Practitioners and researchers must always rely on their own experience and knowledge in evaluating and using any information, methods, compounds or experiments described herein. Because of rapid advances in the medical sciences, in particular, independent verification of diagnoses and drug dosages should be made. To the fullest extent of the law, no responsibility is assumed by Elsevier, authors, editors or contributors for any injury and/or damage to persons or property as a matter of products liability, negligence or otherwise, or from any use or operation of any methods, products, instructions, or ideas contained in the material herein.

ISBN: 978-0-323-93075-8

Content Strategist: Robert Edwards
Content Project Manager: Taranpreet Kaur/Suthichana Tharmapalan
Design: Patrick Ferguson
Marketing Manager: Deborah Watkins

Printed in India

Last digit is the print number: 9   8   7   6   5   4   3   2   1

Working together
to grow libraries in
developing countries

www.elsevier.com • www.bookaid.org

CONTENTS

PREFACE

Welcome to this book on integrated care. The Editors of this book have worked for many years in the practice and academic study of integrated care. They are all passionate that through its application there is the means to improve the health outcomes across populations and reduce the health inequalities that plague societies. I was delighted to have the opportunity to bring together the collective knowledge of the contributors to support the demystification of this complex but essential area of development in health and social care.

This book is based on many years of experience for the contributors and spans health, social care, and the wider community. For integrated care to reach its potential it needs to not just be a structural change that focuses on moving the chess pieces of health and social care around or providing more joined up services (although there is a need for significant structural change), it must focus on the development of a new culture that places people and communities at the heart of how services are designed and delivered, recognising that health comes from having healthy communities that foster opportunity, health, and wellbeing. Large statutory organisations, governments and policy makers need to yield the power that they hold and listen to the wider voices in the community to truly understand and learn new ways of being partners in health and social care and develop new and innovative ways of working with people and communities.

This book views integrated care through the lens of the World Health Organization's (2016) principles of integrated care. We did not set out to provide a 'one size fits all' interpretation of integrated care, but rather, reflect the complex nature of the topic and its many applications in practice.

Who is this book for?
This book is useful for students, practitioners, and academics who are interested in the development of integrated care. The book provides practical examples and academic analysis for the development of integrated care in several settings. To illuminate the topic, we have used real-life case studies that reflect the many areas in which integrated care can be applied. Through this approach, we aimed to make the book accessible to a wide range of people and demystify this complex and emergent model of health and social care.

Structure of the book
The book is delivered in five parts, taking the reader from the theoretical underpinning of integrated care, through systems, organisational, and practitioner levels to reflect the macro, meso, and micro levels of integrated care. Part V provides a wide range of examples of integrated care application to enlighten the reader to the opportunities and potential of integrated care.

Dr Kirsty Marshall

Kirsty has over 20 years of health care experience, starting her career as a health care support worker. She is now a senior academic specialising in Integrated Care. Kirsty worked as a district nurse and NHS service manager across Greater London and Greater Manchester. These experiences developed her belief that to support populations to be healthy, happy, and prosperous is the very foundation of how health services should be viewed, planned, and delivered and this needs to be revolutionised to put community and people at the centre of all we do. Since commencing her academic career she has taught, presented (nationally and internationally), and published on a range of integrated care topics. She completed her professional doctorate in 2020 researching the experiences of teams adopting neighbourhood working.

Dr Hayley Bamber

Hayley has over 20 years of health care experience, starting her career as a health care support worker in low and medium secure learning disability setting. She worked as an NHS Occupational Therapist throughout secondary community mental health services for the majority of her professional career, with a substantial period of time in integrated team management within East Lancashire. These experiences of integrated management illustrated the complex nature of integrating services and the significant need for co-production to support the process. She currently works as an academic and has delivered, taught, presented (nationally and internationally), and published on co-production. She completed her professional

doctorate in 2020 on developing an understanding of co-production and how this can be used as a vehicle to support organisational culture and change.

Dr Ruth Garbutt

Ruth is presently Head of Social Work and Integrated Practice at the University of Salford and has a background in Social Work and Social Policy. Her PhD research looked at the citizenship rights of people with disabilities and she also undertook a post-doctoral research fellowship looking at the views and experiences of young people with learning disabilities around relationships and sexuality. She has specialised in co-production and participatory research methods, and she has also led on interprofessional education initiatives in the Social Science Directorate at Salford University. She has a practice background working with people with learning disabilities, where an integrated approach has always been vitally important in order that people with learning disabilities get the best outcomes and live a valued and empowered life.

Chris Easton

Chris is Director of Strategy and Impact at NHS Charities Together, the national charity supporting the NHS through the NHS charity sector. Prior to joining the charity Chris spent 10 years in the NHS, initially working in national policy at NHS England and then subsequently within one of the ten boroughs of Greater Manchester, focusing on personalised care, integrated care, the social determinants of health, and integration.

Miriam Davies, PG Certificate in Higher Education, MSc SCPHN (HV), PGDip Specialist Community Public Health Nursing [SCPHN] (Health Visiting [HV]), Bachelor of Nursing degree
Adult Nursing Lecturer, Associate
    Fellowship HE
University of Salford

Claire Webber
Digital Wellbeing Project Manager
    for Tameside and Glossop (no
    longer in this role)

Sara Handley, RN, BSc, CSP/CPT-DN, PGCT, NMP, Fellow HEA, Queens Nurse
Assistant Director of Nursing
Adult Community Services
Royton, England

Dr Tracey Williamson, PhD, MSc, RGN
Consultant Nurse for Dementia and
    Hon Professor of Patient and
    Family Engagement
University of Worcester

Dr Elaine Ball, PhD, MA, RN PGCHE, Cert Ed
Senior Lecturer
University of Salford

Helen Kilgannon, Nye Bevan Executive Healthcare Leadership award, ILM 7 Executive Coaching, Charted MCIPD, PGDip Healthcare Management, BSc Hons
Associate Director
Advancing Quality Alliance (AQUA)
Warrington, England

Steve Kay, MA (Ethics), PGDip Youth & Community (JNC) BA (Hons) Post 16 Education
Assistant Director, Education and
    Early Help
Rochdale Borough Council

Charlotte Michell, PGDip Health Service Leadership (MA Level), National Professional Qualification in Integrated Leadership (MA Level), PGDip in Child and Adolescent Mental Health (MA Level)
Assistant Director for Integration and
    Health
Children's Services
Rochdale Council

Jason Gravestock, BSc RMN
Matron for Professional Standards
Tameside and Glossop NHS
    Integrated Care Trust

Dave Wilson, MA, DipSW
Team Manager, Adult Social Care,
Tameside Metropolitan Borough
    Council

Paula Bell, BSc Community Health
District Nurse Team Lead
Tameside and Glossop NHS
    Integrated Care Foundation Trust

Joanne Finnerty, BA (Hons) Social Studies, Chartered MCIPD
Programme Manager (Social Care
    Workforce)
NHS Greater Manchester Integrated
    Care

Dr Michelle Howarth, PhD, MSc, PGCHE, RGN
Senior Engagement Fellow
Edge Hill University

Dr Michaela Rogers, PhD, MA Social Work, PGCAP, BA (Hons) Social Policy
Senior Lecturer in Social Work
Department of Sociological Studies
University of Sheffield

Lynne Bowers
Director
The Health Creation Alliance
Birmingham, West Midlands

Dr Naomi Sharples, RNLD, RMN, BA Hons Ling, MBA, PGCert, SFHEA, DProf
Associate Dean Academic
    Development and International
University of Salford

Samantha Pywell, MSc Allied Health Practice, PGCAP, Academic Practice, BSc Occupational Therapy
Principal Lecturer – Social Prescribing
    Unit Coordinator
University of Central Lancashire

Linda Vernon, PGDip Digital Health Leadership, PGCert Digital Health, MSc Neuromusculoskeletal Healthcare, DipHE Aromatic Medicine, B. Physiotherapy
Digital Culture and Transformation
    Clinical Lead
Lancashire & South Cumbria
    Integrated Care Board

Dr Sarah Kate Smith, BSc Psychology (Hons), PhD
Health Services Research Fellow
Sheffield Hallam University

Chris Sewards, BA (Hons), MSc Advanced Practice in Dementia
Dementia and Older Persons
    Wellness Lead
Aspire for Intelligent Care and
    Support CIC
Manchester, England

Professor Julian Manley, PhD, MA, MSc, Dip HE, BA, FRSA
Professor
University of Central Lancashire

Lydia Hubbard, BA (Hons) Fashion Management, MSc Sustainability
PhD Candidate
Lancaster University

Dr Amanda Miller, PhD, PGCert HEPR, BSc (Hons), Dip HE Child Nursing
Head of Simulation and Skills
    Education
Edge Hill University

Dr Melanie Stephens, PhD, MA, PGCAP, BSc (Hons), DipN
Reader/Associate Professor in Adult
    Nursing
University of Salford

Dr Lorna Chesterton, PhD, MSc, BSc (Hons), DN, RGN, QN
Research Associate
Manchester Metropolitan University

Siobhán Kelly, BSc (Hons) Sociology and Criminology
PhD Candidate and Research
    Assistant
University of Salford

Professor Andrew Clark, BA (Hons), PhD
Professor
University of Salford

Professor Anya Ahmed, BA (Hons), PGCert (H&E), MSc, PhD
Professor of Wellbeing and
    Communities
Manchester Metropolitan
    University

Shirley Fisher, BSc Community Health Care Nursing
Quality Matron
University of Salford

Jamie Potts
Lived Experience Lead
University of Central Lancashire

Sushma Majithia
Lived Experience Lead
University of Central Lancashire

James Brooks
Lived Experience Lead
University of Central Lancashire

Erin O'Neill
Lived Experience Lead
University of Central Lancashire

Joseph Crammond
Lived Experience Lead
University of Central Lancashire

Katie Cairns
BSc (Hons) Occupational Therapy
Student
University of Central Lancashire

Dr Julie Alexandra Lawrence Doctor of Philosophy (Social Work)
Research Associate in Mental Health
    & Learning Disabilities
Manchester Metropolitan University

Dr Claire Brown, PhD Social Work, MSc Professional Practice in Health and Social Care, MA Social Work, PGCert Learning and Teaching in Higher Education, BSc (Hons) Psychology
Senior Lecturer
Teesside University

Cindy-Leigh Fallows
Specialist Nurse Learning Disability
Childrens' Community Learning
    Disability Team
Stepping Hill Hospital Stockport

Lucy Power
Learning Disability Nurse
Tameside & Glossop Learning
    Disability Hub

Georgia Thorpe
Social Worker
Stockport Metropolitan Borough
    Council

Kim Powell
Lived Experience Lead
University of Salford

Lisa Lewis
SEN Parent/Carer and Teaching
    Assistant in an SEN provision

Dr Evangelia Petropoulou, PhD, FHEA, MSc, PGCert, BA (Hons)
Lecturer
Edinburgh Napier University

Dr Lisa O'Leary, BA in Applied Social Studies (Social Care), MA in Sociology (Applied Social Research), PhD, PGCert
Lecturer/Programme Lead for MSc
    in Research Methods for Health
    and Social Care Practice
Edinburgh Napier University

Rachel Price, RMN, MSc, BSc, Specialist Practitioner (CMH) FHEA
Senior Lecturer
Manchester Metropolitan University

Miriam Collett, Professional doctorate candidate, RN Child, BSc (Hons) SCPHN – School Nursing, MSc, PGCAP, FHEA
Professional Doctorate Candidate
Lecturer and Lead for Specialist
    Community Public Health Nursing
University of Salford

ACKNOWLEDGEMENTS

There are so many people to thank in the development of this book. Firstly, all the authors who took time to contribute and share their expertise. Their academic, professional and practical experience provide the backbone of this book, providing a wide range of examples to support the reader to unpick the complex world of integrated care. We would like to express our thanks to our organisations (The University of Salford, The University of Central Lancashire, Tameside and Glossop Integrated Care NHS Foundation Trust, and the Northern Care Alliance NHS Foundation Trust) and those wider organisations that have supported us in developing the book and shared their journeys and experiences with us. We also need to give special thanks to our friends and families who have provided endless support, guidance, and care which enables us to have the time and space to dedicate to developing this book. I would like to thank all those at Elsevier who have provided support, knowledge, and expertise; starting a book is challenging and their support and guidance have been invaluable. Finally, I would personally like to thank my fellow editors who have read and edited hours of documents and chapters and provided me with amazing support and good humour throughout the book's development. I am eternally grateful for their hard work and dedication.

Thanks
Kirsty Marshall

PART I

Theory and Concepts of Integrated Care: Rhetoric and Reality

1

Population Health—People, Community, and Place

Dr Kirsty Marshall and Chris Easton

KEY CONCEPTS

- Redefining how we think about health and populations
- Defining population health
- Why population health is vital to supporting people
- How population health is supported by integrated care
- Expanding the scope of integrated care beyond health and care services to address the social determinants of health in the processes of care
- Population health management

INTRODUCTION TO POPULATION HEALTH

In this first chapter, we introduce population health as a cornerstone of integrated care. The chapter will move through the background to population health, definitions of both individual and population health, through to models and applications linking the relationships between systems, organisations, and the health of a population. This chapter emphasises a central proposition that integrated care cannot reach its potential without the adoption of a population health approach. The chapter takes influence from the work of Kindig (2007) but also draws on the wider sphere of literature from the field, including the work of the influential Michael Marmot in outlining the linkages between the social circumstances in which people live and their health outcomes. Population health management is not covered within this introductory chapter; the 'Further Reading' section provides useful resources on population health management strategies.

Considering the current position of health, there have been considerable developments and improvements in life expectancy over the last century, meaning that people are living longer and healthier lives in many counties (Buck et al., 2018). However, these improvements in health are not equally experienced or enjoyed, with the wider determinants of health and health inequalities remaining as significant influences on the health of individuals and communities (Warnecke et al., 2008). The 2020 Marmot review *'Health Equity in England: The Marmot Review 10 Years On'* concluded that a person's health and wellbeing is linked to the conditions in which they are born, grow, live, work, and age and inequities in power, money, and resources—the social determinants of health have a direct and real impact on the health of individuals and populations. Of course, this is not new thinking; health inequalities have been documented as a significant problem in many countries since the 1980s (Crombie et al., 2005). Warnecke et al. (2008) explain that when considering population health, it is important first to understand that there is a discrete difference between population health determinants and individual determinants. Population-level determinants include poverty, education levels, gender, and racial/ethnic distributions. These are normally expressed as averages, rates, and population characteristics. Meanwhile, individuals have risk factors including income, behaviour, genes, and educational attainment. It is important to recognise that population characteristics affect health outcomes independently of those at an individual level. Therefore, before the complex world of integrated care can be explored, there needs to be an understanding of the context and conditions that have led to a greater focus on population health and subsequently the rise in integrated care (in its many forms).

BACKGROUND

Health systems worldwide have been facing increasing challenges from growing numbers of people living with long-term conditions or complex comorbidity. The situation has been exacerbated by a failure to address the social determinants of health that influence individual health and the health of whole populations (Farmanova et al., 2019; Marmot et al., 2010, 2020). The UK provides an example of these challenges. The UK has an ageing population, and is moving towards having more of its population over the age of 65 years than under 15 (Office for National Statistics, 2017). Although most people in this society are living longer and are healthier than in the past, there are inequalities that have plagued the nation's health. There are an estimated 15 million people in England with one or more long-term conditions, including diabetes, coronary heart disease, and chronic obstructive pulmonary disease (Department of Health, 2012; Public Health England, 2018). An example of the impact of the wider determinants of health and how they shape health outcomes in the UK can be seen in mortality rates: deaths were 1.76 times higher for men and 1.77 times higher for women per 100,000 in the most deprived areas compared to the least deprived areas in 2019. The COVID-19 pandemic has further widened this divide.

A system that focuses not just on episodic care but also aims to reduce wider health inequalities is vital if the health of whole populations is to be improved (Marmot et al., 2020). It has been stated that only 20% of health outcomes are influenced by a person having access to high-quality healthcare, stressing that 80% of health outcomes can be attributed to other factors such as health behaviours (30%), social and economic models (40%), and physical environment (10%) (Remington et al., 2015). Therefore, population health requires a wide range of interventions across a system, including not just health and social care, but also bodies such as housing, criminal justice, sustainability, education, and transport. Importantly, population health activity should be co-produced with the population.

Population Health and Integrated Care Development

Population health is a central feature of integrated care development, but prior to exploring how the two concepts interplay, it is important to explore how placing population health at the centre of integration requires a fundamentally different mindset. Population health is a far broader term than 'public health' and it aims to engage a wider set of stakeholders, creating a collective sense of responsibility across multiple organisations and individuals (Buck et al., 2018).

What is Health to an Individual?

Before diving into the concept of population health, it is worthwhile considering how health has been constructed as a concept and how this might influence the services that aim to support the health of individuals and communities. One of the most well-known and enduring definitions of health is that health is *'a state of complete physical,* *mental and social wellbeing and not merely the absence of disease or infirmity'* (World Health Organization [WHO], 1946). At the time, this definition was a significant step forward, as it placed health as a positive paradigm rather than *'merely the absence of disease'*. However, in recent years this definition has come into question. For example, Huber et al. (2011) argue that inclusion of the word 'complete' unintentionally contributes to the medicalisation of society. After all, how often can anyone claim a sense of a complete state of *physical, mental, social wellbeing*, and therefore, are we all unhealthy? It is worth noting that the WHO added further qualifications on its definition in 1986, stating that health was *'a resource for everyday life, not the objective of living. Health is a positive concept emphasizing social and personal resources, as well as physical capacities'* (WHO, 1986).

In recent years, there has been a greater recognition that health needs to be viewed through a wider lens. These changes including reconceptualising health on a continuum rather than as a static state, a growing acknowledgement that health requires adaptations, and understanding that a person's health is influenced by social, personal, and environmental factors (Krahn et al., 2021). In view of these wider dimensions, Krahn et al. (2021) suggested a new definition of health:

> 'Health is the dynamic balance of physical, mental, social, and existential wellbeing in adapting to conditions of life and the environment'.

Krahn et al. (2021) and Huber et al. (2011) aim to present health in a more inclusive way, seeing good health as requiring adaptation and coping with the stress and influence of social, personal, and environmental factors rather than a place of completeness. These views of health link strongly with the seminal work of Antonovsky (1979) who introduced the concept of salutogenesis, which states that a person with a strong sense of coherence is more able to mobilise resources and assets to cope with stressors. This mobilisation influences a person's movement on the health Ease/Dis-ease continuum (Mittelmark & Bauer, 2017).

When health is viewed through these wider lenses, the complexity of the enablers and disenablers to health can seem vast. Kindig (2007), for example, draws attention to health being influenced by social, economic, biological, and environmental factors. As a 2009 *Lancet* editorial states, 'the fact is that one cannot be healthy in an unhealthy society' (Books, 2009). Kronenfeld (2008) adds that, with many disciplines involved in population health, there will be different agendas and lenses that will influence its development. With the current climate of person-centred care and personalisation of care, it is also important to consider how people understand their role in population health and how population health links to individual health creation.

What is Population Health?

As previously stated, a person's health and wellbeing is linked to the conditions in which they are born, grow, live, work, and age (Marmot et al., 2020). Arah (2009) further states that individual and population health cannot be defined without informative contextualisation with the other, as they are intrinsically linked to one another and impact each other. Therefore, it is important to consider individual concepts of health when defining population health.

Population health, as the name suggests, looks at entire populations and is an approach that aims to prevent ill health, improve physical and mental health outcomes, and promote wellbeing by reducing health inequalities (Buck et al., 2018). Shahzad et al. (2019) echo this, stating that population-based approaches move beyond the traditional biomedical model, acknowledging the impact of the wider determinants of health (Chapter 2) and how these determinants impact on individuals, subgroups, and whole populations. Nash (2012) outlines the broader nature of population health, explaining that approaches need to address the distribution of health outcomes through a wide spectrum of activities spanning a large field of actors and organisations, including health promotion and wellbeing (across the life span), chronic disease management, provision of care, and actions on factors effecting health. Nash (2012) goes on to explain that there are four pillars on which population health sits:

- Health policy
- Public health
- Chronic disease management
- Quality and safety

Populations are often geographically located (nations, regions, and neighbourhoods), but can also be defined in different ways: for example, employees, ethnic groups, and subpopulations in locations (Kindig et al., 2008). The term 'population health' has its origins in Canadian health research, and an earlier definition was proposed by Kindig and Stoddart (2003) who stated that population health is *'the health outcomes of a group of individuals, including the distribution of such outcomes within the group'*. This definition centred on the proposition that health includes both health outcomes and patterns of health determinants in a population and should take account of the policies and interventions that link the two. Nash (2012) explains that the goals of population health approaches are better coordination of required care, increased emphasis

on prevention and wellbeing, eradication of disparities in health outcomes, and increased transparency and accountability.

Where individual health interventions focus on supporting an individual's health journey, population health interventions are directed at large groups or populations, including implementation of policies that could impact on entire communities. Importantly, population health interventions focus on sociocultural factors and environmental conditions (Hawe & Potvin, 2009). The Greater Manchester Combined Authority (GMCA) provides some examples of the adoption of population health approaches. As a geographical area, the 10 boroughs of Greater Manchester have some of the worst health outcomes in the UK, with considerable variations in health outcomes between the most and least deprived (Walshe et al., 2018). One example from this region was a cross-organisation project to prevent food insecurity during the pandemic. The project used several data sources to identify areas that had poor accessibility to food shops that were accepting Free School Meal replacement vouchers. This evidence was then used to support the council and voluntary sector organisations to better target areas of highest need and where they would have the greatest impact (GMCA, 2022). This project represents an intersection between population health and integrated care approaches as the intervention aimed to maintain the health of the population through targeted food distribution and used a network of organisations integrating their practice to make greater use of resources and work together to provide an ethical and equitable solution.

Population Health and Rethinking Approaches to Health and Social Care

Having discussed individual and population concepts of health, let us now consider how professionals' predetermined ideas and concepts of health and wellbeing influence the adoption of population health. A challenge for population health is how to enable organisations and professionals to engage in activities that transcend traditional approaches to health and social care and support health and wellbeing of populations as well as individuals (Buck et al., 2018). Kindig (2007) states that professionals tend to view health at an individual level: for example, a nurse within a clinical environment assessing a patient with end-stage heart failure will be considering that episode of care and the needs of the person at that time. However, as previously stated, the determinants that lead to that episode of care are complex and early intervention and population-level activities could have dramatically changed that person's health outcomes. As Goodwin et al.

(2013) state, the core of a population health approach to integrated care is a shift in how we work with people. This view was further developed by Struijs et al. (2015) who state that, to provide truly population-centred services that improve the health of populations impacted by social determinants, the scope of integrated care needs to be expanded to bridge the gaps not only within the health systems but also between the health and social systems and the wider system. To conclude, there needs to be a shift in how organisations and professionals view their roles and relationships with each other and the communities and individuals they work with. This must include investment in a public health workforce, upskilling of health and social care professionals, blending and introducing new roles, and engaging with the community as partners in population health (Buck et al., 2018). Considering the example of end-of-life care, people live longer today than in the past and have more complex conditions, frailty, and multimorbidity. If a population-based rather than episodic approach was adopted in end-of-life care, it would require strategic proactive planning, emphasising early identification; whole-system thinking, including community; and an inclusive approach that builds on existing best practice from a wide range of partners. Importantly, the approach needs to be underpinned by population-based outcome metrics that aim to inspire and spread excellence (Thomas & Grey, 2018). An example of a population-based approach can be seen in the Dying Matters campaigns that open up and encourage community awareness and conversations (Hospice UK, 2023).

Models of Population Health

When applying population health approaches, the use of models may support engagement and understanding of the concepts. Friedman and Starfield (2003) note that the design and models used in population health have several variables, including:

- Different categories of factors affecting population health, with different emphasis on categories (wider determinants)
- Different depictions of causal relationships in population health
- Different presentations of interactions in population health
- Different presentations of factors as actually determining population health
- Different emphases on the distinction between population health and individual health

The diversity in emphasis will steer and direct the development of population health differently, which will in turn influence how integrated care develops and how resources are distributed within a system (Goodwin et al., 2013).

The King's Fund (Buck et al., 2018), an influential UK think tank, suggests that there are four pillars to a model of population health:

- The wider determinants of health
- Our health behaviours and lifestyle
- An integrated healthcare system
- The places and communities we live in and with

These pillars differ in emphasis to the pillars presented previously by Nash (2012) (health policy, public health, chronic disease management, and quality and safety). This change may be reflective of the greater emphasis on the development of integrated systems that are inclusive of a wide group of partners. The King's Fund (2019) model goes further in explicitly highlighting the role of the overlaps between the pillars (Fig. 1.1)—these are not siloed activities but rather dynamic and moveable influences on the health of a population, which are described together as a population health system.

The system proposed by the The King's Fund (Buck et al., 2018) acknowledges the interplay between pillars and presents integrated care as a mechanism and enabler for the development of population health.

Population Health and the Economy

McCartney et al. (2019) found that countries with social democratic regimes, higher public spending, and lower income inequalities have populations with better health and they concluded that politics, economics, and public policy are important determinants of population health. It was acknowledged within their review that there were varying levels of evidence, but one of the best-quality pieces of evidence presented was the link between income inequality and self-rated health and mortality. These findings are reflected in wider studies in the UK: for example, the Marmot reports (Marmot et al., 2010, 2020) demonstrated links between deprivation and health and between geographical location and health. Another notable report was from the WHO's evidence brief into the impact of COVID-19 (WHO, 2021), which demonstrated that deprivation and poverty were associated with a higher incidence of infections, hospitalisation, and mortality in several different countries. This is important when considering integrated care as a driver for population health, as systems need to be designed in a way that stretches further than traditional organisation boundaries and embraces working with a full range of partners.

A shift in the economy in recent years that has led to an emerging social determinant of health is the rise of alternative and precarious employment practices, particularly the rise of the 'gig' economy. While there is no agreed overarching definition of the gig economy, a report by the UK Department of Business, Energy and Industrial Strategy

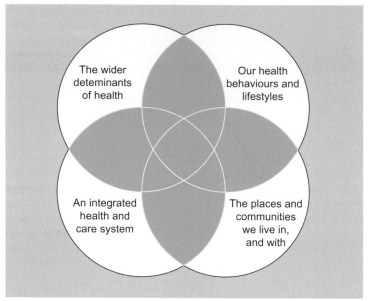

Fig. 1.1 A population health system.

(DBEIS) in consultation with the Institute for Employment Studies suggests the following working definition:

> 'The gig economy involves the exchange of labour for money between individuals or companies via digital platforms that actively facilitate matching between providers and customers, on a short-term and payment by task basis'.
>
> ***(DBEIS, 2018:4)***

The link between precarious employment and worsening health outcomes is already established (van der Noordt et al., 2014). However, in response to its increased prevalence, Gray et al. (2020) conducted a systematic review to explore the links between health and precarious employment in young people, migrants, and women. They found that subgroups were unequally exposed to these practices, and that these practices lead to poorer health outcomes in mental health and wellbeing. For men, exposure to precarious employment put them at greater risk of mortality and premature mortality. However, they acknowledged that there was a need for further research to address gaps in knowledge around young people and migrants. Gray et al. (2020) demonstrated the dynamic nature of health inequalities and how established inequalities are changed and worsened by developments in the nature of work.

CONCLUSION

Population-level health determinants have a significant impact on the health outcomes of populations and individuals within those populations. Therefore, if we are to move to integrated systems, it is important that professionals, communities, and citizens are engaged in improving the health of a population and emergent integrated systems embed population health at their heart. This approach is not without challenges, as it involves bringing together the community with traditional and non-traditional partners to innovate and find new solutions that tackle some of the most difficult challenges to people's health and wellbeing.

References

Antonovsky, A. (1979). *Health, stress, and coping*. San Francisco: Jossey-Bass.

Arah, O. A. (2009). On the relationship between individual and population health. *Medicine, Health Care and Philosophy, 12*(3), 235–244. https://doi.org/10.1007/s11019-008-9173-8

Books, Z. (2009). What is health? The ability to adapt. *The Lancet, 373*(9666), 781. https://doi.org/10.1016/s0140-6736(09)60456-6

Buck, D., Baylis, A., Dougall, D., & Robertson, R. (2018). *What is population health?* King's Fund. https://www.kingsfund.org.uk/audio-video/population-health-animation?

Crombie, I. K., Irvine, L., Elliott, L., Wallace, H., & World Health Organization. (2005). *Closing the health inequalities gap: an international perspective (No. EUR/05/5048925)*. Copenhagen: WHO Regional Office for Europe.

Department for Business, Energy & Industrial Strategy. (2018). *The characteristics of those in the gig economy*. London: DBEIS.

Department of Health. (2012). *Long term conditions compendium of information*. Third edition. https://www.gov.uk/government/publications/long-term-conditions-compendium-of-information-third-edition

Farmanova, E., Baker, G. R., & Cohen, D. (2019). Combining integration of care and a population health approach: a scoping review of redesign strategies and interventions, and their impact. *International Journal of Integrated Care, 19*(2), 5. https://doi.org/10.5334/ijic.4197

Friedman, D. J., & Starfield, B. (2003). Models of population health: their value for US public health practice, policy, and research. *American Journal of Public Health, 93*(3), 366-369

Gray, B. J., Grey, C., Hookway, A., Homolova, L., & Davies, A. R. (2020). Differences in the impact of precarious employment on health across population subgroups: a scoping review. *Perspectives in Public Health, 141*(1), 37–49. https://doi.org/10.1177/1757913920971333

Greater Manchester Combined Authority. (2022). *Research: Health*. https://www.greatermanchester-ca.gov.uk/what-we-do/research/research-health/

Goodwin, N., Sonola, L., Thiel, V., & Kodner, D. L. (2013). Co-ordinated care for people with complex chronic conditions: *Key lessons and markers for success*. London: King's Fund.

Hawe, P., & Potvin, L. (2009). What is population health intervention research? *Canadian Journal of Public Health, 100*(1), 8–14. https://doi.org/10.1007/bf03405503

Hospice U.K. (2023). *Dying Matters*. https://www.hospiceuk.org/our-campaigns/dying-matters/dying-matters-awareness-week

Huber, M., Knottnerus, J. A., Green, L., Van Der Horst, H., Jadad, R., Kromhout, D., Leonard, B., Lorig, K., Loureiro, M. I., Van Der Meer, J. W., & Schnabel, P. (2011). How should we define health? *British Medical Journal*, 26;343.

Kindig, D. (2007). Understanding population health terminology. *The Milbank Quarterly, 85*(1), 139–161. https://doi.org/10.1111/j.1468-0009.2007.00479.x

Kindig, D. A., Asada, Y., & Booske, B. (2008). A population health framework for setting national and state health goals. *Journal of the American Medical Association, 299*(17), 2081–2083. https://doi.org/10.1001/jama.299.17.2081

Kindig, D., & Stoddart, G. (2003). What is population health? *American Journal of Public Health, 93*(3), 380–383. https://doi.org/10.2105/AJPH.93.3.380

Krahn, G. L., Robinson, A., Murray, A. J., Havercamp, S. M., Havercamp, S., Andridge, R., ... & Witwer, A. (2021). It's time to reconsider how we define health: Perspective from disability and chronic condition. *Disability and health journal*, 14(4), 101129.

Kronenfeld, J. J. (2008). *Care for major health problems and population health concerns. Impacts on patients, providers and policy (Research in the Sociology of Health Care, Vol. 26)*. Bingley: Emerald Group Publishing.

Marmot, M., Allen, J., Goldblatt, P., Boyce, T., McNeish, D., Grady, M., & Geddes, I. (2010). *Fair society, healthy lives: The Marmot review*. London: Strategic Review of Health Inequalities in England Post-2010.

Marmot, M., Allen, J., Boyce, T., Goldblatt, P., & Morrison, J. (2020). *Health equity in England: The Marmot review 10 years on*. London: Institute of Health Equity.

McCartney, G., Hearty, W., Arnot, J., Popham, F., Cumbers, A., & McMaster, R. (2019). Impact of political economy on population health: a systematic review of reviews. *American Journal of Public Health, 109*(6), e1–e12. https://doi.org/10.2105/ajph.2019.305001

Mittelmark, M. B., & Bauer, G. F. (2017). The meanings of salutogenesis. In M. B. Mittelmark, S. Sagy, M. Eriksson, G. F. Bauer, J. M. Pelikan, B. Lindström, & G. A. Espnes (Eds.), *The Handbook of Salutogenesis* (pp. 7–13). Springer.

Nash, D. B. (2012). *The Population Health Mandate – A Broader Approach to Care Delivery*. San Diego: Jefferson School of Population Health, Thomas Jefferson University. The Governance Institute.

Office for National Statistics. (2017). https://www.ons.gov.uk/aboutus/transparencyandgovernance/freedomofinformationfoi/ukpopulation2017

Public Health England. (2018). Health profile for England: 2018. https://www.gov.uk/government/publications/health-profile-for-england-2018

Remington, P. L., Catlin, B. B., & Gennuso, K. P. (2015). The county health rankings: rationale and methods. *Population Health Metrics, 13*(1), 1-12.

Shahzad, M., Upshur, R., Donnelly, P., Bahrmal, A., Wei, X., Feng, P., & Brown, A. D. (2019). A population-based approach to integrated healthcare delivery: a scoping review of clinical care and public health collaboration. *BMC Public Health, 19*(1), 708. https://doi.org/10.1186/s12889-019-7002-z

Struijs, J. N., Drewes, H. W., & Stein, K. V. (2015). Beyond integrated care: challenges on the way towards population health management. *International Journal of Integrated Care, 15*, e043. https://doi.org/10.5334/ijic.2424

Thomas, K., & Gray, S. M. (2018). Population-based, person-centred end-of-life care: time for a rethink. *British Journal of General Practice, 68*(668), 116–117. https://doi.org/10.3399/bjgp18X694925

van der Noordt, M., IJzelenberg, H., Droomers, M., & Proper, K. I. (2014). Health effects of employment: a systematic review of prospective studies. *Occupational and Environmental Medicine, 71*(10), 730–736. https://doi.org/10.1136/oemed-2013-101891

Walshe, K., Lorne, C., McDonald, R., Coleman, A., & Turner, A. (2018). *Devolving health and social care: learning from Greater Manchester*. Manchester: University of Manchester.

Warnecke, R. B., Oh, A., Breen, N., Gehlert, S., Paskett, E., Tucker, K. L., et al. (2008). Approaching health disparities from a population perspective: the National Institutes of

Health Centers for Population Health and Health Disparities. *American Journal of Public health, 98*(9), 1608–1615. https://doi.org/10.2105/ajph.2006.102525

World Health Organization (WHO). (1946). *Constitution of the World Health Organization*. Basic Documents, Geneva: World Health Organization.

World Health Organization (WHO). (1986). *The 1st international conference on health promotion*. http://www.who.int/healthpromotion/conferences/previous/ottawa/en/

World Health Organisation. (2021, 6 December). *COVID-19 and the social determinants of health and health equity: evidence brief*. https://www.who.int/publications/i/item/9789240038387

Further Reading

Reports

Buck, D., Baylis, A., Dougall, D., & Robertson, R. (2018). *What is population health?* King's Fund. https://www.kingsfund.org.uk/audio-video/population-health-animation?
A UK perspective and vision for population health development.

Foot, J. (2012). *What makes us healthy? The asset approach in practice: evidence, action, evaluation*. http://janefoot.com/downloads/files/healthy%20FINAL%20FINAL.pdf
While this document is older, it has some really good insights into how asset-based healthcare can support population health.

Website

Institute of Health Equity
https://www.instituteofhealthequity.org/home

Really useful reports and resources focused on reducing health inequalities internationally.

2

Wider Determinants of Health— Inequalities and Equity

Miriam Davies

KEY CONCEPTS

- Wider determinants of health
- Social gradient
- Health equity
- Population health

INTRODUCTION

As we move from the concept of population health as a core component of integrated care, it is important that we consider the driving forces that have motivated health and social care systems across the world to move to more integrated ways of working. It is important to develop an understanding of how the wider determinants of health can inform and support integration at all levels of a system, from partnerships and strategic development to how therapeutic relationships are built on an individual level. In an integrated care system, the links between health and wellbeing, housing, transportation, health literacy, physical environment, food, digital access, and environment need to be transparent so that everyone from the home-care worker to the chair of partnership boards can more effectively support individuals to have lasting and positive outcomes (Chamberland, 2018).

Within this chapter, the wide-reaching factors affecting health and wellbeing will be explored. A case study will be used to demonstrate how an integrated approach to care can help to deliver multifaceted services in a more streamlined way that meets the needs of service users more effectively.

THE IMPACT OF SOCIAL AND ECONOMIC FACTORS ON HEALTH AND WELLBEING

Social and economic factors have a significant influence on how we live and age. These factors also affect our health, our attitude to our own health, and how we use services (NHS England, 2019). Dahlgren and Whitehead (1991) developed a model to help identify these factors which are also known as wider or social determinants of health (Fig. 2.1).

These influences on health include our personal characteristics, lifestyle choices, social networks and opportunities, living and working conditions, and wider environmental and socioeconomic factors (Public Health England [PHE], 2017). Kickbusch et al. (2021) identified the need to consider digital literacy and technological resources within the wider determinants of health due to the growing impact digital transformation can have on health outcomes. The response to the COVID-19 pandemic uncovered inequalities in health due to disparities in access to digital resources and health services as well as varying ability to share health data (Marmot et al., 2020b; Pickett et al., 2021). Chapter 3 provides an example on how a community-led integrated approach can be used to address the inequalities caused by digital access.

Social determinants will vary depending on the individual, the community, and the population. For instance, Canada has developed its own social determinants of health for their population, including indigenous peoples status, race, gender, education, early life, disability, and social exclusion, amongst others, acknowledging the influence these factors have on the health of their population (Raphael, 2009). These models recognise the biopsychosocial resources we all require to live well and reach our potential (Raphael, 2009). Social determinants can be viewed as stepping stones in achieving Maslow's (1943) hierarchy of needs (Fig. 2.2), which is a hierarchy that requires each human need to be met to reach our full potential, or self-actualisation. When considering individuals with complex needs in Doncaster, if someone does not have their basic needs met, such as a safe place to live and regular supply of food and water, how are they able to meet their health needs and remain healthy?

CASE STUDY

Doncaster is a town in South Yorkshire in England with a Complex Lives Alliance that has developed a 'whole system approach' to address the complex needs experienced within their community. The Complex Lives Alliance was designed to break the negative spiral between homelessness, poor physical and mental health, and offending, while acknowledging the impact that wider determinants of health such as childhood trauma, learning disabilities, substance misuse, and poor mental health can have on health inequalities. It was felt that a multiagency approach, including the NHS, local government, housing, and voluntary sector, was needed to address local needs.

A review of services, including a homelessness review (Doncaster Council, 2019a), identified that around £50 million was being spent on public services to address local issues, and yet people with complex problems still had unmet needs and service provision was failing to make sustainable changes within the community.

To provide some context, the health profile of Doncaster is below the national average for life expectancy and rates of hospital admission due to violence, alcohol, and self-harm related incidents are higher than the average in England (Office for Health Improvement & Disparities, 2022). Alcohol-related admissions in 2018 were 25% higher than national averages, according to Doncaster's Joint Strategic Needs Assessment (JSNA) (Doncaster Council, 2021). Childhood poverty, unemployment levels, and levels of contact with mental health services were also found to be higher than national averages (Doncaster Council, 2021). As part of their review of services, Doncaster Council (2019a) identified that 72% of the homeless population had support needs, most commonly due to mental health issues. It was deemed the only way to address these issues effectively was by using a collaborative, integrated, place-based approach. In line with the NHS Long Term Plan (NHS England, 2019), services were reconfigured to enable a 'whole systems' approach, drawing on multiagency collaboration and collective action to address the public health challenges within the local area in a sustainable way (Doncaster Council, 2019b).

In developing the alliance, several factors had to be considered. The impact of wider determinants were acknowledged and formed part of their action plan. A root cause analysis determined that professionals were not working together or communicating effectively, there was a lack of consistency, service users were not being listened to, and simple practicalities were not in place. For instance, inadequate data-sharing methods and services/information were not tailored to meet service users' needs (Doncaster Council, 2019a).

One of the strengths of this project was that the team explored the vulnerabilities and complex needs of this group closely, listened to them, and worked in partnership with them to reconfigure services to meet their multifaceted needs, working collectively as a team. Ethnographic profiles of clients were developed to better understand cultural norms and get their perspective and insight. This meant that they were able to address a variety of needs such as housing, drug addiction, substance misuse, and mental health more effectively. An asset-building approach which draws on the strengths of the local community and collectively builds resources to support and meet local needs was employed to help individuals integrate into the local community and become more self-sufficient (Doncaster Council, 2019a, 2019b).

The team found that they were able to work more efficiently by working collaboratively. As services were communicating more and working in partnership, they no longer duplicated work, which in turn increased engagement as processes were more streamlined with greater continuity of care (Doncaster Council, 2019a). The changes they have made since forming a multiprofessional alliance have been found to improve homelessness by 70%, meaning that they can focus on more upstream approaches to local issues and grow the programme further. As part of the evolving collaboration, they now have a nurse and general practitioner drop-in clinic to improve access to health services, which was identified as a problem for this client group. More upstream approaches have been promoted by greater tailoring of services, such as through Personal Housing Plans that unpick the causes of homelessness, delivering services where they are needed and accessible rather than solely in the city centre, as well as embedding good practice from other areas, such as Oldham's autism strategy to improve services and access for people with autism and increase awareness and training amongst professionals (Doncaster Council, 2019a; Oldham Council, 2017).

This case study is an example of how wider factors that affect health have to be considered in order to successfully meet patients' needs. A crucial part of this is exploring and learning what these influences on population health are so they can be effectively addressed. It also highlights the necessity of integrated, collaborative working to meet the multidimensional needs that exist within populations which are most often connected (King's Fund, 2021).

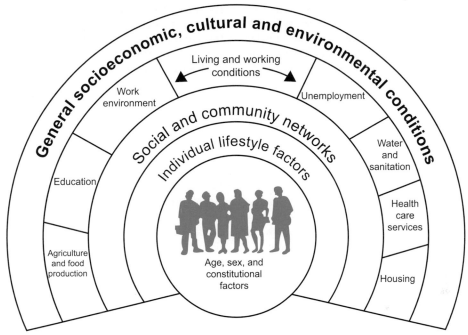

Fig. 2.1 Social determinants of health. (Dahlgren & Whitehead, 1991)

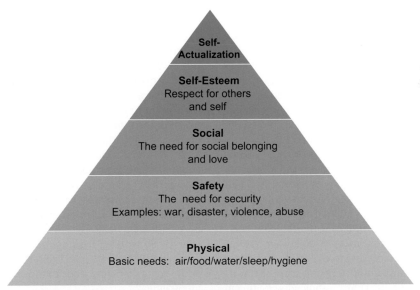

Fig. 2.2 Hierarchy of needs. (Maslow 1943)

How Easy Is it to be Healthy?

The case study above demonstrates how several social and economic factors have been influencing the health of the population in Doncaster. Housing, unemployment, substance misuse, crime, and mental health were all identified as having a detrimental effect on the health of the community. Furthermore, these factors can exacerbate and compound each other, increasing the complexity of service users' needs (PHE, 2021a). Doncaster Council's review (Doncaster Council, 2019a) acknowledged that homelessness in their constituency was most triggered by substance misuse or mental health issues. Health systems can on occasion make the situation worse; for instance, homeless individuals have historically been excluded from being seen by a GP as they do not have the required ID. Although there are now campaigns and schemes such as Doncaster Complex Alliance to change this, this highlights how these wider determinants can compound to negatively impact on health (NHS England, n.d.). Those that are the most vulnerable are often the least likely to access health services, even though they need them the most. Hart (1971) identified back in 1971 that an inverse care law exists, with those with a higher burden of disease being most likely to have the poorest access and delivery of services, whereas those in good health have access to the best-quality care (Mercer et al., 2021). This phenomenon is still a problem today and the COVID-19 pandemic has accentuated inequalities in health both locally and internationally (King's Fund, 2021; Marmot et al., 2020b). Health inequities develop because of the wider social and economic influences on health and they therefore need to be addressed to reduce inequalities in health (King's Fund, 2021).

Health inequalities and equity. Unfortunately, the distribution of wealth, power, and resources is not equal, which leads to inequalities in health (Donkin et al., 2018), costing the NHS around £4.8 billion each year (PHE, 2021a). If the determinants of health are not distributed fairly, it causes disparities in health status (King's Fund, 2020; Marmot et al., 2020a; PHE, 2021a). Individuals with good social networks, education, and employment have better health outcomes, leading to a social gradient of health. This social gradient is most noticeable when comparing the correlation between poverty and life expectancy, with the most deprived areas having the lowest life expectancy and the most affluent areas having the highest (PHE, 2021a). This leads to regional and geographical disparities in health on a local, national, and international level (King's Fund, 2020). Individuals with protected characteristics, such as age, sex, race, disability, or groups that are marginalised or excluded from society, may be at higher risk of health inequalities. A recent cross-sectional study (Watkinson et al., 2021) into ethnic inequalities in England identified that health-related quality of life was worse in 88% of ethnic minority groups within its survey when compared to the White population. Inequalities were highest in the Romani and Irish Traveller communities, followed by Bangladeshi and Pakistani communities. These inequalities were associated with a higher prevalence of long-term conditions and comorbidities as well as

lower confidence levels in self-managing these conditions, which was noted to be more pronounced in women within the age bracket of 55–75 years. Furthermore, 9 out of 17 ethnic minority groups involved in the study had negative experiences of primary care services, which was highest in the Asian metagroup (Watkinson et al., 2021). This demonstrates the inequity of health status across the population and emphasises the need to address these avoidable and preventable health inequalities. To improve health outcomes, we must reduce health inequalities and rebalance the playing field (NHS England, n.d.).

The Five Year Forward view (NHS, 2014), The Long Term Plan (NHS England, 2019), and the Marmot Reviews (Marmot et al., 2010, 2020a, 2020b) all acknowledge the widening health gap between the richest and poorest individuals in society and the need for this to be addressed. However, the Marmot Review 10 years on (Marmot et al., 2020a) and the COVID-19 response *'Build Back Fairer'* (Marmot et al., 2020b) are stark reminders that we have not improved since Marmot's first review. In fact, since 2010, life expectancy has stalled and the gap between rich and poor has widened (Iacobucci, 2019; Marmot et al., 2020a, 2020b). This means that the richest in society are estimated to have over 9 years of life and up to 19 more healthy years than those in the most deprived areas (ONS, 2019). This inequity within society means there are growing disparities in quality of life between the richest and poorest, which are influenced by these wider determinants and the social gradient these factors create (PHE, 2021a).

For services to reduce health inequalities and the inverse care law (people who most need healthcare are least likely to receive it), they need to meet the specific needs of the population. This means addressing the social gradient by ensuring those with the highest burden of disease and those who are most vulnerable and at risk are supported and their needs are addressed.

Doncaster Complex Alliance is an example of a local community addressing population health by identifying the diverse needs of the population and the wider influences affecting health which were preventing sustainable change. By working together as a collective with greater resources, knowledge, and skills, they can more effectively address the complex needs of those at most risk of health inequalities.

The NHS Long Term Plan identifies the need for greater focus on addressing population health. One way in which these four aspects will be promoted is through the development of integrated care systems (ICSs) (NHS England, 2019), enabling services across different sectors such as local council, NHS, and the voluntary sector to work more collaboratively. In this way, resources can be shared to address needs within the local area as well as improve the transition between primary and secondary care (NHS England, 2019). With the support of local government and multisector involvement, it is hoped that wider determinants of health can be addressed more effectively, enabling more preventative healthcare responses (King's Fund, 2021). There have been concerns that the transition from clinically-led commissioning groups to ICSs have potential to cause significant disruption, reduce the clinical voice, and/or may be difficult to implement in light of local government cuts, particularly if there is not adequate leadership in place to enable true collaboration (British Medical Association, 2021; The Health Foundation, 2021). However, it is acknowledged that there are numerous benefits to bringing service providers and commissioners together to work more closely together, such as increased productivity, flexibility and efficiency of services, and a more person-centred approach to care, by drawing on shared resources and expertise to tackle the wider influences and factors affecting health (NHS England, n.d.; Stansfield et al., 2019). Doncaster Complex Lives Alliance is a good example of this.

Tackling wider determinants and health inequalities. Health inequalities are preventable and they must be addressed as a matter of social justice (Marmot et al., 2020a). However, the inequity is caused by a complex web of influences, making it challenging to address. Health bodies in Britain have had legislative responsibilities to reduce health inequalities since the Health and Social Care Act came into place in 2012; however, we actually have wider inequalities in health now than we did in 2012 (Marmot et al., 2020a).

In Marmot's first review (Marmot et al., 2010), he identified the need to focus on the following six aspects to address the social gradient in health: to ensure all children have the best start in life, are able to reach their full potential, have equal opportunities for employment, have a healthy standard of living, a clean and healthy place to live, and have access to public health services. Ten years on, these aspects remain equally important, but to ensure those that need these opportunities the most access them, proportionate universalism is needed. This means that everyone is entitled to a basic level of care which can be increased depending on the needs of individuals and communities. This addresses the inverse care law and actively tackles health inequalities by increasing the package of care for the most vulnerable and at risk, evening out the playing field (Marmot et al., 2020a, 2020b). A good example of this model in practice is the service delivery of 0–19 services covered by health visitors and school nurses. Services are delivered at different levels depending on the needs of the child or family. This starts as a universal service for all, with targeted support for those assessed as requiring a greater level of intervention and specialist services for those at most risk (PHE, 2021b). This model is designed to include a greater range of professionals, interventions, and support to those most in need, drawing on the collective skills and resources of different professionals and agencies working together.

A central focus of this service is to give children the best start in life and promote their health and development, which also promotes health equity (Marmot et al., 2010). Addressing needs in early childhood can break the cycle of health inequalities through the life course and reduce the burden of ill health later on in life (Marmot et al., 2020a).

The case study in Doncaster also highlights effective ways in which we can address wider determinants of health and health inequalities. It acknowledges the importance of collaborating with stakeholders (most importantly the client group), listening to them, and exploring their personal challenges and individual needs to be able to successfully address them. Stansfield et al. (2019) claim that including community members and stakeholders in all aspects of a community project, including the planning, development, and evaluation, as they have done at Doncaster Complex Lives, can increase engagement with services as well as empower those individuals involved (Stansfield et al., 2019).

By identifying the wider influences on health in their specific population and how these factors influence each other, professionals have been able to put in place more preventative approaches such as increasing client independence, promoting stability, and reaching out to vulnerable individuals such as those about to leave prison or care (Team Doncaster, 2021). This has helped to promote more sustainable changes in health amongst the client group. Community engagement and commitment is crucial to address population health. This can be achieved through drawing on asset-building, strength-based approaches to empower and enable people (Stansfield et al., 2019).

On a global level, the World Health Organization (2020) have developed the United Nations' Sustainable Development Goals (SDGs) to tackle health inequalities and wider determinants of health on an international scale. There are 17 SDGs which include goals such as no poverty, no hunger, quality education, good health and wellbeing, and gender equality. The action plan to address these 17 goals by 2030 requires community engagement, accurate health data and better digital health, action on wider determinants of health, research, improved primary care services, and sustained financing to support these changes (WHO, 2020).

CONCLUSION

Health is affected by a complex array of factors, the most influential being social and economic aspects. The unequal balance of resources at the local, national, and international levels leads to a social gradient in health, where the most affluent areas have the best health outcomes and the most deprived have the worst. We have a social duty to address this widening gap of health inequalities. Ways in which this can be achieved is through levelling up and targeting support to those most in need as well as strengthening health prevention strategies. Identifying the wider determinants that impact on health will help us understand some of the challenges individuals and communities face in being and staying healthy. Due to the complexity of multiple factors impacting on health, there is a need for a multiagency, collective approach, drawing on a wide range of skills and resources to meet the complex needs of individuals, communities, and populations at highest risk of health inequalities. Therefore, to be effective, collaboration needs to happen at the individual, community, and system levels (NHS England, n.d.).

References

British Medical Association. (2022, November 14). *Integrated care systems (ICSs)*. https://www.bma.org.uk/advice-and-support/nhs-delivery-and-workforce/integration/integrated-care-systems-icss

Chamberland, L. (2018). Leveraging social determinants in integrated care solutions. *International Journal of Integrated Care*, *18*(s2), 232. https://doi.org/10.5334/ijic.s2232

Dahlgren, G., & Whitehead, M. (1991). *Policies and strategies to promote social equity in health [White paper]*. Institute for Futures Studies.

Doncaster Council. (2019a). *Homelessness review*. https://dmbcwebstolive01.blob.core.windows.net/media/Default/Housing/Homelessness%20Review%202019.pdf

Doncaster Council. (2019b). *Doncaster Homelessness and Rough Sleeping Strategy 2019-2024*. https://dmbcwebstolive01.blob.core.windows.net/media/Default/Housing/Documents/Homelessness%20and%20Rough%20Sleeping%20Strategy%202019%20to%202024%20Final%20web%20version%201.pdf

Doncaster Council, (2021). Joint Strategic Needs Assessment (JSNA). https://www.teamdoncaster.org.uk

Donkin, A., Goldblatt, P., Allen, J., Nathanson, V., & Marmot, M. (2018). Global action on the social determinants of health. *BMJ Global Health*, *3*, e000603. https://doi.org/10.1136/bmjgh-2017-000603

Hart J. T. (1971). The inverse care law. *Lancet (London, England)*, *1*(7696), 405–412

Iacobucci, G. (2019). Life expectancy gap between rich and poor in England widens. *British Medical Journal*, *364*, l1492. https://doi.org/10.1136/bmj.l1492

Kickbusch, I., Piselli, D., Agrawal, A., Balicer, R., Banner, O., Adelhardt, M., et al. (2021). The Lancet and Financial Times Commission on governing health futures 2030: growing up in a digital age. *The Lancet, 398*(10312), 1727–1776. https://doi.org/10.1016/S0140-6736(21)01824-9

Marmot, M., Allen, J., Goldblatt, P., Boyce, T., McNeish, D., Grady, M., & Geddes, I. (2010). *Fair society, healthy lives: The Marmot review*. London: Institute of Health Equity.

Marmot, M., Allen, J., Boyce, T., Goldblatt, P., & Morrison, J. (2020a). *Health equity in England: The Marmot review 10 years on*. London: Institute of Health Equity.

Marmot, M., Allen, J., Goldblatt, P., Herd, E., & Morrison, J. (2020b). *Build back fairer: The COVID-19 Marmot review. The pandemic, socioeconomic and health inequalities in England*. London: Institute of Health Equity.

Maslow, A., H. (1943). A theory of human motivation. *Psychological Review, 50*(4), 370–396. https://doi.org/10.1037/h0054346

Mercer, S. W., Patterson, J., Robson, J. P., Smith, S. M., Walton, E., & Watt, G. (2021). The inverse care law and the potential of primary care in deprived areas. *The Lancet, 397*(10276), 775–776. https://doi.org/10.1016/s0140-6736(21)00317-2

NHS. (2014). *Five year forward view*. https://www.england.nhs.uk/wp-content/uploads/2014/10/5yfv-web.pdf

NHS England. (2019). *The long term plan*. https://www.longtermplan.nhs.uk/wp-content/uploads/2019/08/nhs-long-term-plan-version-1.2.pdf

NHS England (n.d.). *Integrated care in action*. https://www.england.nhs.uk/integratedcare/resources/case-studies/integrated-care-in-action-health-inequalities/

Office for Health Improvement & Disparities. (2022). *Local Authority health profiles: Fingertips public health data*. https://fingertips.phe.org.uk/profile/health-profiles/data#page/1/gid/1938132695/pat/6/par/E12000003/ati/201/are/E08000017/yrr/1/cid/4/tbm/1

Office for National Statistics. (2019). *Health state life expectancies by national deprivation deciles, England and Wales: 2015-2017*. https://www.ons.gov.uk/peoplepopulationandcommunity/healthandsocialcare/healthinequalities/bulletins/healthstatelifeexpectanciesbyindexofmultiplede privationimd/2015to2017

Oldham Council. (2017). *Oldham's Autism Strategy (2017-2021)*. https://www.oldham.gov.uk/info/200373/learning_disabilities/1747/oldham_s_autism_strategy

Pickett, K., Taylor-Robinson, D., et al. (2021). *The child of the North: Building a fairer future after COVID-19*. The Northern Health Science Alliance and N8 Research Partnership. https://www.thenhsa.co.uk/app/uploads/2022/01/Child-of-the-North-Report-FINAL-1.pdf

Public Health England. (2017). *Chapter 6: social determinants of health*. https://www.gov.uk/government/publications/health-profile-for-england/chapter-6-social-determinants-of-health

Public Health England. (2021a). *Place-based approaches for reducing health inequalities: main report*. https://www.gov.

uk/government/publications/health-inequalities-place-based-approaches-to-reduce-inequalities/place-based-approaches-for-reducing-health-inequalities-main-report

Public Health England. (2021b). *Health visiting and school nursing service delivery model.* https://www.gov.uk/government/publications/commissioning-of-public-health-services-for-children/health-visiting-and-school-nursing-service-delivery-model

Raphael, D. (2009). *Social determinants of health: the Canadian perspectives.* (2nd edition). Toronto: Canadian Scholars' Press.

Stansfield, J., South, J., & Mapplethorpe, T. (2019). What are the elements of a whole system approach to community-centred public health? A qualitative study with public health leaders in England's local authority areas. *British Medical Journal Open, 10*, e036044. https://doi.org/10.1136/bmjopen-2019-036044

Team Doncaster. (2021). *Joint strategic needs assessment.* https://www.teamdoncaster.org.uk/jsna

The Health Foundation. (2021). *Integrating care: Next steps to building strong and effective integrated care systems across England.* https://www.health.org.uk/news-and-comment/consultation-responses/integrating-care%253A-next-steps-to-building-strong-and-effectiv

The King's Fund. (2020). *What are health inequalities?* https://www.kingsfund.org.uk/publications/what-are-health-inequalities

The King's Fund. (2021). *Integrated care systems explained: making sense of systems, places and neighbourhoods.* https://www.kingsfund.org.uk/publications/integrated-care-systems-explained

Watkinson, R., Sutton, M., & Turner, A. (2021). Ethnic inequalities in health-related quality of life among older people in England: secondary analysis of a national cross-sectional survey. *The Lancet Public Health, 6*(3), 145–154. https://doi.org/10.1016/S2468-2667(20)30287-5

World Health Organisation. (2020). *Health data: A critical element to meet the SDGs.* https://www.who.int/data/stories/health-data-a-critical-element-to-meet-the-sdgs

Further Reading and Activities

Office for Health Improvement & Disparities (formerly PHE) Fingertips Public Health Data

https://fingertips.phe.org.uk/
Look up the public health profile in your local area or your area of work using the Fingertips database. This will allow you to compare statistics for wider determinants of health such as air pollution, overcrowding, and percentage of population in employment with the national average as well as check the health status within this population and how it compares to other areas in the UK.

Index of Multiple Deprivation (IMD)

https://assets.publishing.service.gov.uk/government/uploads/system/uploads/attachment_data/file/835115/IoD2019_Statistical_Release.pdf
The IMD is the official measure for deprivation in England. It considers the following determinants within the score: income, employment, health deprivation and disability, education, crime, living environment, and housing.

Life Path Project

https://www.lifepathproject.eu/
Life Path Project is a European research cooperative based in Geneva that has been researching the socioeconomic imprint on our health to inform policymakers and policies.

GM Health and Social Care Partnership

https://www.gmhsc.org.uk/news/greater-manchester-gp-practices-leading-the-way-on-black-health-improvement/
The GM Health and Social Care Partnership offers training programmes for GP practices to increase cultural competencies, targeted services, and interventions to help reduce inequalities and reach those that need support the most. The Black Health Improvement Programme was commissioned by the Caribbean & African Health Network, which is designed to improve access to health services for this ethnic group.

3

The Role of People and Community and the Revolutionising of Health and Wellbeing

Dr Kirsty Marshall and Claire Webber

KEY CONCEPTS

- Health creation
- Collaboration in health and social care
- Voluntary sector
- Person-centred approaches
- More than medicine

INTRODUCTION

The Health Creation Alliance (HCA) describes health creation as the process through which a sense of purpose, hope, mastery, and control is gained by individuals and communities resulting in enhanced health and wellbeing (HCA, 2022). This chapter will introduce some of the key concepts and underpinning principles of health creation and explore its impact through a case study. The chapter aims illuminate discussion on how communities are the heart of revolutionising health and wellbeing and how professionals, organisations, and the system can support environments for healthy communities.

In this chapter we build on the concepts on population health discussed in Chapter 1 to explore how professionals, organisations, and the system can engage with population health and linking system activity and community activities to enhance both population and individual health. Health creation is important if integrated care is to truly impact on the health of populations. As integrated care developments must stretch further than merely a redesign or restructure of health and care services, it requires a rethinking of how we approach health and how we view the complexity of people's lives (Crisp, 2020). The integrated care movement across the world is an opportunity to radically rethink the lens we view health through and the culture of organisations that strive to support health and social care. If integrated care is embraced fully, it should aim for a seismic shift in the relationships between people, communities, places, and the organisations which aim to serve them. There is the potential for health and social care to move to a position where they sit within the neighbourhoods with people proactively creating environments for health creation as well as being there for people in times of need.

Nigel Crisp, in his excellent book *Health Is Made at Home and Hospitals Are for Repair* (2020), calls for health professionals to give up NHS (healthcare) thinking and to look at health in a completely different way. This chapter aims to support that journey by demonstrating how health is generated and created by communities and individuals and how engaging and working with communities on creating environments that support healthy lives has the potential to transform health outcomes for people throughout the life course. The chapter will outline some of the key theories and thinking in health creation, the background to its development, and its potential to support practitioners when working with people and communities. To support the learning in this chapter, an excellent case study will be used to demonstrate key principles of health creation, the role that healthcare organisations can play in supporting communities, and the role of the practitioner.

A report for the Good Things Foundation by Cebr, an independent economics and business research consultancy, suggests that seven million British adults in the UK are digitally excluded and this will have a significant reduction in the value and potential of technology (Good Things Foundation, 2018). However, digital exclusion is not simply a UK issue; the United Nations estimate that almost half the world's population (3.7 billion people) remains disconnected (UN, 2021). Exclusion has a dramatic impact on a person's health, wellbeing, education, and social engagement, both acting as a health inequality and exacerbating other inequalities; for example, the impact on people with long-term and enduring mental health issues (Serafino, 2019; Spanakis et al., 2021). Technological change means that digital skills are increasingly important for connecting with others, accessing information and services, and meeting the changing demands of the workplace and economy. The 'digital divide' is a new and emerging health inequality between those who engage with the online world and those who do not, which has given rise to disparities in access to opportunities, knowledge, services, and goods (Spanakis et al., 2021).

CASE STUDY

The Greater Manchester Combined Authority (2020) suggested that as many as 1.2 million residents in Greater Manchester may be digitally excluded. In an increasingly digital age, those who are not engaging effectively with the digital world are at risk of being left behind.

Empowering an individual with digital skills has a huge impact on improving their independent living, such as by accessing internet banking, ordering groceries and repeat prescriptions, online appointment booking, and using a search engine. This is in addition to the wider social and mental health impacts of having more resources to remain in touch with friends and loved ones, reducing loneliness through increased connection with the community, learning new skills, and accessing support in innovative ways. The result is a huge increase in the person's overall health and wellbeing (Gann, 2019; Serafino, 2019; Spanakis et al., 2021).

The case study here tells the journey of a simple idea discussed over coffee to what became a thriving, established NHS-funded programme which has successfully improved digital literacy across Tameside and Glossop.

In 2018, a casual conversation took place between the participant of a 'Life Skills' support group and a mentor about how difficult modern life must be for those who were digitally excluded. As part of his own development towards increased wellbeing, his mentor encouraged him to act, and a basic plan was developed. The concept was to recruit members of the community who had information technology (IT) skills but who were struggling to overcome personal challenges and obstacles, preventing them from fully engaging with society. These volunteers would refurbish unwanted IT equipment which would be donated via requests made to local businesses and the wider community, and which could then be given to those without the means to access technology. The service would give a sense of fulfilment and purpose to the volunteers and provide IT equipment to those in need.

The idea immediately gained traction and a newly recruited hands-on team of trustees developed the concept into 'PCrefurb', an official Glossop-based charity which quickly attracted the attention of the local community, causing equipment donations to increase. A bid to the National Lottery Fund was successful and a manager was recruited. The team of refurbishing volunteers grew and they began to work together once a week at a community venue, further helping them to build their social skills and confidence. Through word-of-mouth, members of the public began popping in with their digital skills questions, and informal training would often also take place alongside the hardware repairs.

During the COVID-19 lockdown in March 2020, PCrefurb donated 150 tablets to care homes and hospices to help residents keep in touch with their loved ones, an initiative which attracted the attention of the local NHS. In June 2020, the charity was approached and asked if could they both increase their provision of equipment and provide formal digital skills training, as the NHS England (2019) is committed to making a more concerted and systematic approach to address digital exclusion. It had been identified that there is a close correlation between digital inequality and health and social disadvantages, including less access to care and support, a lower life expectancy, below average income, decreased education and employment opportunities, poorer housing, and a lack of voice and visibility in a modern world.

The service was commissioned, a project manager was appointed, and in September 2020 the 'Digital Wellbeing Project' was launched. The objective was to create a team of 'Digital Champion' volunteers, who would support community members to grow their basic digital skills and confidence, and in turn enhance their overall health and wellbeing. The Project established several official referral pathways, such as the Social Prescribing Service, Neighbourhood Mental Health Services, social housing providers, and other local charities, and provided a device and/or digital skills training as necessary. Many of the original refurbishing volunteers still work together at a weekly workshop to repair donated equipment, whilst other funding streams allow new equipment to be purchased. All devices (smartphones, tablets, laptops, and desktop machines) are given on a 3-month rolling loan, which can be extended long-term if necessary, and

(Continued)

CASE STUDY—cont'd

any donated equipment that is beyond economical use or repair is stripped down and recycled via an external agency, with all costs accrued added back into the charity to benefit the Project.

The training provided is person-centred, at a beginner level, and can be carried out at a client's home if required due to health issues or in a local community venue such as a library. 'Digital Cafe' group training sessions are held at various venues across Tameside and Glossop, with the further aim of addressing social isolation. As a charity, it is not possible to provide data for those without a connection to the internet; however, the Project informs people about the most cost-effective options available to them and guides them through the application process if required.

Despite the frustrating challenges of the COVID-19 restrictions at the start of the Project, which meant that training could not be carried out in-person until July 2021, by March 2022 the Digital Wellbeing Project had received over 300 referrals, 187 devices had been loaned, and 275 in-person training sessions had been delivered, with 19 community venues signed up to host a Digital Cafe. This is remarkable in such a short period of time, and all stemming from one casual conversation over coffee.

Clients referred into the Project (Fig. 3.1) are of various ages with differing backgrounds and needs.

Most clients report that the Project has improved their wellbeing and has 'changed their lives'. One such person was Mark:

Mark was referred into the Digital Wellbeing Project requiring all the 'three D's'—data, device, and digital skills. His referral form stated that he had a disability and was feeling isolated and low as he lived alone without much interaction. The first thing provided was to guide Mark through the minefield of internet access

options available to him, and Mark chose to sign up for a low-cost monthly contract with a major provider which was available cheaply to those receiving benefits. As Mark had never used a device before, he was given a user-friendly tablet via the Project's Lending Library and matched with one of the Digital Champions, Jason.

Mark was especially worried about the issue of internet safety, and so at their first session, alongside showing him how to use his new tablet, Jason took Mark through an online education course. At the age of 56, Mark was also thrilled to set up his very first email address, saying '*I now feel part of society!*'

Jason then went on to introduce Mark to the limitless entertainment possibilities on YouTube and other online television channels and showed him how to shop safely online and use a search engine. Mark couldn't believe that all these resources were at his fingertips!

Mark's medical condition meant that he needed more control over his healthcare, and so Jason helped him to register on Patient Access. This gave Mark much more independence when booking appointments and ordering his prescriptions. Jason showed him how to access trusted medical advice via the NHS website and use a lifestyle app to further increase his wellbeing.

At their final training session, Mark was confident that he now had the information and skills to be able to continue to use his new device independently. He told Jason that the Digital Wellbeing Project had completely changed his life by opening his eyes to all the day-to-day tasks that he could do online, saying '*I never knew all of this was possible! I love connecting with others online and I'm getting quite addicted to it!*' His low mood had lifted, his general health had improved, and after making some acquaintances online, he felt positive about using digital means to further connect with his community.

Enid* (80): her husband has passed away and she wants to learn how to use Zoom to attend a bereavement support group	Ron* (90): wants to join in with his local seated exercise class and find out more about being healthy online	Susan* (49): her son has moved overseas and she wants to video chat with him as she is feeling very low about his absence	Ann* (51): wants to use the internet to search for a job and complete online education courses
David* (62): has had a stroke and wants to do his shopping and banking online now	Margaret* (75): wants to use the internet to explore her hobbies of art and history	Linda* (58): can no longer travel due to poor health and wants to continue to experience the world via online means instead	Mary* (65): wants to create digital art as part of her mental health support art therapy sessions

Fig. 3.1 Client examples from the Project. *Consent to use the clients' first names has been given.

SALUTOGENESIS AND THE FOUNDATIONS OF HEALTH CREATION

The founding principles from which current thinking on 'health creation' is based are often attributed to the seminal work of Aaron Antonovsky, a medical sociologist and the father of the theory of 'salutogenesis'. His philosophical approach was based on understanding the origins of health as opposed to merely searching for the disease causation (pathogenesis) (Lindström & Eriksson, 2005). Antonovsky (1979) introduced the concept 'salutogenesis', urging a move away from the pathogenic approach that remained dominant in Western medical thinking and that views people in a binary 'well/ill or healthy/diseased' paradigm, arguing that the complexity of health needed to be viewed as a continuum (healthy/disease).

Antonovsky (1996) makes the assertion that there is a bias towards downstream management of disease rather than prevention as he states 'the devotion of the disease care system to saving swimmers drowning downstream by heroic measures'. In this, he poses the questions of how people get to the point that they are 'drowning' and who and what pushes them to this point. This is an interesting place to start to understand Antonovsky's work, which asks us to consider salutary factors or factors that actively promote health rather than reduce risk.

A central tenant of the theory of salutogenesis is a sense of coherence (SoC). SoC is explained as an orientation to life that is viewed on a continuum, and that it is comprehensible, manageable, and meaningful. Antonovsky (1979) argues that the strength of a person's SoC is a significant factor in facilitating the movement toward health. Lindström & Eriksson (2005) explain an SoC as the ability to realise ones own resources and capacity to use resources and assets available to maintain one's own health.

Health as a Human Right

A powerful testimony from the case study was from one participant who stated that with the access and education to digital technology through the project he felt like now being part of society. The magnitude and impact of this simple statement required some unpicking. It is useful here to consider health in its wider context as a fundamental human right. The UN's Universal Declaration of Human Rights (1948) and 1966 International Covenant on Economic, Social and Cultural Rights place health as a fundamental human right. This right does not just equate to the right of access to hospitals and services; the right to health extends further, incorporating a wide range of factors enabling people to live a healthy life (safe drinking water, adequate sanitation, safe food, nutrition, housing, safe working and environmental conditions,

health-related education, and gender equality) (Office of the United Nations High Commissioner for Human Rights, 2008). The WHO (2017) state several ways that a rights-based approach is important to ensuring the health of populations, as follows.

- Creates a legal obligation on states.
- Requires health policy and programmes to prioritise creation of greater equity.
- Health must be experienced without discrimination on the grounds of race, age, ethnicity, or other status (including tackling discriminatory laws).
- Health should be considered in relation to its wider societal context.
- Should include meaningful participation, including non-state actors such as nongovernmental organisations, in all phases of programming: assessment, analysis, planning, implementation, monitoring, and evaluation.
- Include the right to control one's health and body (for example, sexual and reproductive rights).
- To be free from interference (free from torture and non-consensual medical treatment and experimentation).
- Health protection that gives everyone an equal opportunity to enjoy the highest attainable health.
  (WHO, 2017)

It is also important to recognise that the right to health is inseparable from other rights such as food, housing, work, education, information, and participation (WHO, 2017). Integrated care aims to embed principles of population health, and health creation at its core is underpinned by principles of fairness and equity (WHO, 2016). Therefore, we must consider the interdependency of health within its wider societal context. Individual attainment of this fundamental human right is dependent on the creation of healthy communities and reductions in health inequalities. Returning to the client statement, access to digital technology is something many take for granted. Shopping, entertainment, communicating, learning, welfare, and healthcare are all areas that have moved into a digital world (HCA, 2022). The statement at the start of this section demonstrates the magnitude of the impact of a lack of digital literacy and access to simple technology on an individual's sense of belonging in society and in social isolation. The impact of social isolation cannot be overstated, as seen in an English longitudinal study of ageing which found that loneliness and isolation are associated with poorer cognitive function among older adults (Shankar et al., 2013). In addition, a systematic review and meta-analysis of longitudinal observational studies linked deficiencies in social relationships with an increased risk of developing coronary heart disease and stroke (Valtorta et al., 2016). Health creation needs to be approached as an international and interconnected issue which requires traditional services not only to reset their focus and consider how integration and integrated care can assist in enhancing point-of-care services but also how population health and health creation can reduce downstream need.

Creating Health, Shifting Thinking

Let's start with a basic understanding that the community has not sat around waiting for health and social care to sweep in with this great idea to rescue people from themselves. The case study is only one of a vast array of community activities that are created and grown within communities. Educators, civil leaders, employers, community organisers, and households have been creating health for a long time (Crisp, 2021). However, the intersectional challenges of health inequalities and unequal societies has led to unacceptable imbalances in the health outcomes of people (Marmot et al., 2020) (discussed in Chapter 1). The HCA states that there are 3 Cs of health considerations (Table 3.1).

There is a rebalancing of the relationship between communities and the health and care (and wider) system. It is those within the system who need to address how organisations place themselves and their teams as part of the communities. How do we change to better connect with each other and support building healthy communities? A first step will be understanding community assets who innovate, build, and create health (Foot, 2012).

What is a Community Asset?

A community asset comes in many forms, and these are outlined in Table 3.2.

Furthering work by Foot and Hopkins (2010), a systematic scoping review by Cassetti et al. (2019) identified three key features of asset-based approaches: connecting assets, publishing available assets, and enabling assets to flourish. A system-wide approach is important to support community assets as this action cannot be taken in isolation (NHS, 2019). For example, mapping of community assets will enable gaps to be identified and guide resource allocation to meet community need and grow assets.

Here is an example of how the system and community can interact to create an environment for the growth of community assets. The Digital Wellbeing Project (outlined in the case study) was approached by Minds Matter (an NHS-commissioned service that provides resources in the community for those with mental health conditions) to look at collaborative activities (joining an NHS service and a community asset). The team at Mind Matters had recognised that the health inequalities caused by the digital divide impacted their clients and therefore wanted to address this. As with many projects, this was accelerated by COVID-19: many materials provided have been moved online which had created barriers for some clients. Spanakis et al. (2021) explain that the impact of digital exclusion during COVID-19 was magnified for those with mental health conditions. The teams worked together to

TABLE 3.1 The 3 Cs of Health Creation	
Contact	Contact with people and communities should be meaningful and constructive.
Confidence	Relationships should focus on increasing the confidence of individuals and communities.
Control	Leading to greater control over our lives and the determinants of our health. People also need an adequate income, a suitable home, an engaging occupation, and a meaningful future.

HCA (2022)

TABLE 3.2 What Are Assets?	
Practical Skills	**Residents' Skills, Knowledge, and Capacity**
Passions and interests	The motivation within local communities
Social capital within communities	Networks, connections, social infrastructure (formal and informal)
Community and voluntary associations	Vibrant community, voluntary, social enterprise, and faith sectors
Resources	Available resources within the community
Physical and economic resources	Physical/economic resources available to the community

Foot & Hopkins, (2010)

remove barriers by streamlining processes, training, and digital provision.

The following feedback was provided on the collaboration:

'Minds Matter are proud that during these difficult times the benefits of this collaboration with the Digital Wellbeing Project have lasted beyond the initial need. Together we have opened a new digital world for those managing a long-term condition and have given them the confidence to become more connected through accessing online coffee mornings and workshops, and also by connecting with the other local support services such as the Social Prescribing Team. This is an example of collaboration between partners who traditionally may not have worked together but through mutual goal and respectful working were able to increase access with a vulnerable group.'

RETHINKING RELATIONSHIPS

Simpson and Graham (2021) argue that it is important that frontline workers, healthcare leaders, strategic leads, and decision-makers also comprehend and engage in the processes that are involved in community health creation as this will enable them to explore ways that they might adapt their practice or adopt new practices.

How professions should adapt their practice or adopt new practices is not homogenous: each professional group within a neighbourhood will have a different history, values, and philosophical approaches. A study by Marshall (2020) into neighbourhood teams found that while teams may have worked in parallel for many years, they had to reconstruct their understanding of each other's role when brought together in a neighbourhood and manage long-held misconceptions about each profession to build a new understanding of how they could develop future practice. Ultimately, these teams gained meaning and understanding by reaching for their shared values and ethical underpinnings such as a sense of social justice (Chapter 16 discusses interprofessional education and transforming culture in greater depth). To truly gain benefit from an integrated approach, professionals need to blur established interprofessional boundaries to implement new roles and intraindividual boundaries that delineate the different roles occupied by one person (Zee, 2019). Importantly, these relationships need to stretch further into how professionals work with the community and individuals. Crisp (2020) states that key to the transformation is connecting with people on a human level, making connections between people and organisations, and underpinning these communications with mutual learning and codevelopment. This is supported by Charles (2022) who states that this interconnection will support community strengthening and efficient, coherent, integrated systems. Importantly, this should include support to develop social infrastructure. Within the case study, this interconnected working could be seen in in how the project team brought together a wide range of people from across the spectrum (Clinical Commissioning Group, the Person and Community Centred Approaches Team within Tameside and Glossop Integrated Care Foundation Trust, Tameside Council and volunteer groups). These groups came together as the Digital Wellbeing Programme Board. There were key principles used to underpin the board to ensure that everyone involved could use their knowledge and experience to play a part in codeveloping the Project. This ethos was vitally important as previous studies have demonstrated that smaller organisations, and especially the voluntary sector, can feel excluded, and that shared vision and purpose is vital (Beacon, 2015).

THE SYSTEM AND EMBEDDING OF HEALTH CREATION

As with all change that involves transforming political, cultural, and financial contexts, developing systems that embrace and enable community health creation will not be easy (Crisp, 2020). A key challenge will be finding ways to come together and measure value across a system, as sometimes the benefits of action taken in one sector are reaped by another, but all should ultimately be guided toward improved population health (Lovell & Bibby, 2018).

The systems and structures in which we live, work, and are educated all contribute to building beliefs about health and illness. These underlying beliefs subsequently impact discussions on funding, resourcing, and allocation of activity. Frenk and Gómez-Dantés (2017) describe how health is strongly influenced by the dichotomies in which it is framed, which has a detrimental impact on innovation and advancement of health. For example, health services tend to think in terms of prevention versus treatment, vertical versus horizontal, primary versus specialised care, infections versus noncommunicable diseases (NCDs), and knowledge versus action. As a result of this binary thinking, there is a disconnect between determinants of health and healthcare itself, rather than recognition of the interdependency. DeSalvo et al. (2021) explain that reductions in the mortality burden from infectious diseases such as typhoid and cholera could not have been achieved without improvements in sanitation. The challenge of this is that it runs counter to the concept outlined in the earlier section that health is a human right and it is interdependent on a range of wider contextual issues.

Frenk and Gómez-Dantés (2011) state that we face a triple burden of disease globally through common infections, NCDs, and long-term conditions, and this triple burden is compounded by problems related to globalisation, like pandemics and the health consequences of climate change. The COVID-19 pandemic brought the interdependency of health and determinants of health into stark focus. The pandemic exacerbated existing challenges, revealing pervasive racial and socioeconomic inequities in healthcare access, quality, and outcomes (DeSalvo et al., 2021). The long-term impacts of the pandemic on mental and physical health, economy, and society are yet to be fully revealed; however, the lessons from the pandemic present an opportunity to address population health needs in a way that recognises the interconnection of life and health rather than holding to the old ways that see health, wellbeing, and illness split and fragmented (Crisp, 2021; Frenk & Gómez-Dantés, 2017).

The case study presents an example of how communities drive innovation and how the system, organisations, and professionals can all aid in the creation of an environment that enables this innovation to flourish. The initial conversations were not based on policy or government objectives; they were driven by the recognition of a need in the community by members of that community—the charity founders recognised that there were multiple benefits that could be had, reflecting theories discussed earlier in this chapter. For example, there are clear and well-documented benefits to enabling greater access to digital technologies, like reduction in social isolation and greater access to services and education (Serafino, 2019; Spanakis et al., 2021). However, the benefits to those refurbishing the devices were just as important, as they could draw meaning and purpose from the activity and contribute to their community through becoming Digital Champion volunteers, volunteer drivers, and refurbishing volunteers. A literature review conducted for the Institute for Volunteering Research (Paylor, 2011) found that there were several positive impacts of volunteering including wellbeing of volunteers, increased feelings of self-esteem, a sense of belonging, and building a network of support (Paylor, 2011). This research is supported in a wider body of evidence on volunteering that states being a volunteer can improve physical and mental health and has intrinsic societal benefits for the wider community (Southby et al., 2019). In the case of the Digital Champion volunteer who supported Mark, he himself had been suffering with social anxiety. However, the newfound confidence which he gained through his volunteering meant that he felt able to apply for a job in a similar role, using the Digital Wellbeing Project Manager as a reference, and was successful in gaining employment. Another volunteer attributes her role as being a key factor in improving her mental health, saying:

> 'At the beginning of the pandemic I suffered massively with my mental health. It's taken a while due to everything going on but I'm loving this journey I am on now. I'm feeling more positive and happier every day, so this is benefiting me just as much as the people I'm helping. It's an amazing feeling to be able to make such a difference to someone's life.'

The role of the system within this example was to create opportunities for funding, growth, and development, thereby creating an environment for communities to flourish and grow. *Asset-based places: A model for development*, proposed by the Social Care Institute for Excellence (SCIE) states that organisations can support asset creation through:

- Reframing the narrative—from a focus on people's needs to people's and communities' assets
- Building a dynamic picture of personal and community assets
- Connecting people, assets, and each other
- Growing and becoming mobile—creating the right environment for an asset-based approach to succeed
- Monitoring impact and learning from evidence (SCIE, 2017)

Previously, the role of the system was that of supporter and cheerleader to the community rather than controller. This is an important distinction, as a range of international studies have found that the voluntary sector often feel that they do not have an equal voice at the table when working with large statutory bodies, as they do not have the capacity or resources to match the larger partners. The inequity in power and resources between organisations can lead to disengagement of the very organisations that should be at the heart of these community projects and health creation. In the case study example, the project grew from the community: it was the community members who recognised the complex biopsychosocial needs within the local population, and the community that had the solution and skills to bring about change. Where the integrated system came in was with the ability to provide resources and support for growth and sustainability of the project.

Asset-Based Commissioning

Asset-based commissioning is vital to creating environments where communities can flourish. Asset-based commissioning involves enabling people to become equal cocommissioners and coproducers to make the best complementary use of all assets to improve life and community outcomes. Asset-based commissioning is discussed in detail in Chapter 11, where the strategic approach needed will be introduced. However, reflecting on the case study here shows an example of how the commissioning of a community asset can provide value and resources to improve people's health outcomes.

Impact on People

If we are to tackle the health inequalities within society and improve outcomes, we must not just treat people as they become unwell but look to create health within our communities. Both systems and people have a role to play in rebalancing our approach to our health. The case study clearly demonstrated the impact of this on an individual, especially in terms of both their mental and physical health. If we map the case against the 3 Cs of health creation, the project here developed meaningful contacts, built confidence for volunteers and users of the service, and enabled all involved to gain greater control over their lives. As a result, there were improvements in the mental health of those who engaged with the project. However, there are many projects, charities, and community groups in every community which impact on population and individual health. Communities are galvanised by local issues and are often best placed to identify opportunities for health creation. This was clearly demonstrated through multiple community responses during the COVID-19 pandemic (McGregor-Paterson, 2021).

CONCLUSION

Health creation has its roots in the work of Aaron Antonovsky and aims to increase the years people live in good health across all communities. It should not be viewed as an individual, community, or system responsibility but rather a shared responsibility where all have a role to play in developing an environment that enables people to live healthy and happy lives. The case study here demonstrated how health creation can be generated through an integrated care approach, where a community project was supported by the system to grow and flourish.

References

Antonovsky, A. (1979). *Health, stress, and coping*. San Francisco: Jossey-Bass.

Antonovsky, A. (1996). The salutogenic model as a theory to guide health promotion. *Health Promotion International*, *11*(1), 11–18. https://doi.org/10.1093/heapro/11.1.11

Beacon, A. (2015). Practice-integrated care teams–learning for a better future. *Journal of Integrated Care*, *23*(2), 74–87. https://doi.org/10.1108/JICA-01-2015-0005

Cassetti, V., Powell, K., Barnes, A., & Sanders, T. (2020). A systematic scoping review of asset-based approaches to promote health in communities: development of a framework. Global health promotion, 27(3), 15–23.

Charles, A. (2022, August 19). *Integrated care systems explained: making sense of systems, places, and neighbourhoods*. King's Fund. https://www.kingsfund.org.uk/publications/integrated-care-systems-explained

Crisp, N. (2020). *Health is made at home, hospitals are for repair*. Billericay: SALUS.

Crisp, N. (2021). Human flourishing in a health-creating society. *The Lancet*, *397*(10279), 1054–1055. https://doi.org/10.1016/S0140-6736(21)00585-7

DeSalvo, K., Hughes, B., Bassett, M., Benjamin, G., Fraser, M., Galea, S. et al. (2021). Public health COVID-19 impact assessment: lessons learned and compelling needs. *NAM Perspectives*, *2021*. https://doi.org/10.31478/202104c. 10.31478/202104c.

Foot, J. (2012). *What makes us healthy? The asset approach in practice: evidence, action, evaluation*. http://janefoot.com/downloads/files/healthy%20FINAL%20FINAL.pdf

Foot, J., & Hopkins, T. (2010). *A glass half-full: how an asset approach can improve community health and well-being*. Improvement and Development Agency. https://www.local.gov.uk/sites/default/files/documents/glass-half-full-how-asset-3db.pdf

Foot, J. & Hopkins, T. (2010) *A glass half-Full, how an asset approach can improve community health and well-being I&DeA*, Retrieved from https://www.local.gov.uk/publications/glass-half-full-10-years-review

Frenk, J., & Gomez-Dantes, O. (2011). The triple burden: disease in developing nations. *Harvard International Review*, *33*(3), 36–40.

Frenk, J., & Gómez-Dantés, O. (2017). False dichotomies in global health: the need for integrative thinking. *The Lancet*, *389*(10069), 667–670. http://dx.doi.org.salford.idm.oclc.org/10.1016/S0140-6736(16)30181-7

Gann, B. (2019). Transforming lives: combating digital health inequality. *IFLA Journal*, *45*(3), 187–198. https://doi.org/10.1177/0340035219845013

Good Things Foundation. (2018). *The economic impact of digital inclusion in the UK: A report for Good Things Foundation*. https://www.goodthingsfoundation.org/insights/the-economic-impact-of-digital-inclusion-in-the-uk/

Greater Manchester combined authority. (2020). Addressing the digital divide across greater. Manchester. https://www.greatermanchester-ca.gov.uk/what-we-do/digital/digital-inclusion-agenda/

Health Creation Alliance. (2022). *Health creation: addressing national health inequalities priorities by taking a health creating approach*. https://thehealthcreationalliance.org/

Lindström, B., & Eriksson, M. (2005). Professor Aaron Antonovsky (1923–1994): the father of the salutogenesis. *Journal of Epidemiology & Community Health*, *59*(6). 511-511.

Lovell, N., & Bibby, J. (2018). *What makes us healthy?*. London: Health Foundation.

Marmot, M., Allen, J., Boyce, T., Goldblatt, P., Morrison, J. (2020). Health inequality in England: The Marmot review 10 years on. London: Institute of Health Equity.

Marshall, K. (2020). An exploration of neighbourhood team members experiences of the transition from traditional health and social care teams to integrated care systems, within a defined health and social care economy. (Publication No. 59618) (Ph.D. thesis, University of Salford, UK).

McGregor-Paterson, N. (2021). *Learning from the community response to COVID-19; how the NHS can support communities to keep people well*. The Health Creation Alliance. https://thehealthcreationalliance.org/wp-content/uploads/2021/04/THCA-Report_Community-response-to-COVID-19_NHS-learning-FINAL_-April-2021.pdf

NHS England (2019) The NHS long term plan. https://www.longtermplan.nhs.uk/

Office of the United Nations High Commissioner for Human Rights, (2008). *The right to health, fact sheet 31*. Geneva: United Nations.

Paylor, J. (2011). *Volunteering and health: evidence of impact and implications for policy and practice*. London: Institute for Volunteering Research.

Serafino, P. (2019). *Exploring the UK's digital divide: the scale of digital exclusion in the UK; those who aren't currently using the internet, how digital skills vary for different groups of the population and some of the barriers to digital inclusion*. Office of National Statistics. https://www.ons.gov.uk/peoplepopulationandcommunity/householdcharacteristics/homeinternetandsocialmediausage/articles/exploringtheuksdigitaldivide/2019-03-04

Shankar, A., Hamer, M., McMunn, A., & Steptoe, A. (2013). Social isolation, and loneliness: relationships with cognitive function during 4 years of follow-up in the English Longitudinal Study of Ageing. *Psychosomatic Medicine, 75*(2), 161–170. https://doi.org/10.1097/psy.0b013e31827f09cd

Simpson and Graham. (2021). Digging deeper, going further: creating health in communities. https://thehealthcreationalliance.org/wp-content/uploads/2021/03/THCA-report-_-Digging-deeper-going-further_-creating-health-in-communities-Final-March-2021.pdf

Social Care institute for excellence. (2017). Asset-based places: a model for development https://www.scie.org.uk/future-of-care/asset-based-places

Southby, K., South, J., & Bagnall, A. (2019). A rapid review of barriers to volunteering for potentially disadvantaged groups and implications for health inequalities. *VOLUNTAS: International Journal of Voluntary and Nonprofit Organizations, 30*(5), 907–920. https://doi.org/10.1007/s11266-019-00119-2

Spanakis, P., Peckham, E., Mathers, A., Shiers, D., & Gilbody, S. (2021). The digital divide: amplifying health inequalities for people with severe mental illness in the time of COVID-19. *British Journal of Psychiatry, 219*(4), 529–531. https://doi.org/10.1192/bjp.2021.56

UN General Assembly, Universal Declaration of Human Rights, 10 December 1948, 217 A (III), available at: https://www.refworld.org/docid/3ae6b3712c.html

United Nations. (2021, April 27). *With almost half of world's population still offline, digital divide risks becoming 'new face of inequality', Deputy Secretary-General warns General Assembly*. https://www.un.org/press/en/2021/dsgsm1579.doc.htm

Valtorta, N. K., Kanaan, M., Gilbody, S., Ronzi, S., & Hanratty, B. (2016). Loneliness and social isolation as risk factors for coronary heart disease and stroke: systematic review and meta-analysis of longitudinal observational studies. *Heart, 102*(13), 1009–1016. https://doi.org/10.1136/heartjnl-2015-308790

World Health Organization. (2016). *Integrated care models: an overview*. https://www.euro.who.int/__data/assets/pdf_file/0005/322475/Integrated-care-models-overview.pdf

World Health Organization. (2017). *Human rights and health*. https://www.who.int/news-room/fact-sheets/detail/human-rights-and-health

Zee, K.V. D. (2019). *Professional boundaries and new role adoption in a multidisciplinary healthcare team* [Doctoral dissertation]. University of Groningen.

Further Reading

Book

Crisp, N. (2020). *Health is made at home, hospitals are for repair*. Billericay: SALUS.
Nigel Crisp's book reflects on a wide range of projects that support health creation.

Website

The Health Creation Alliance https://thehealthcreationalliance.org/health-creation/
Multiple resources and reports relating to health creation.

4

Living with Long-Term Conditions or Multiple Comorbidities—Changing Demographic and Epidemiology

Miriam Davies

KEY CONCEPTS

- Ageing population
- Comorbidities
- Polypharmacy
- Personalised care planning
- Self-management

INTRODUCTION

In 2016, Lafond, Charlesworth, and Roberts's health foundation report described the current UK health and care system as a perfect storm of financial pressure and increased demand (Lafond et al., 2016). An ageing population, changing demographics, and epidemiological shifts had led services to a breaking point. This situation has only been exacerbated during the COVID-19 pandemic, which laid bare the cracks in health and care systems across the world (Lewis & Ehrenberg, 2020; Lewis et al., 2020). Within this chapter, a case study will be used to explore how the changing demographic and epidemiological nature of many countries has led to radical rethinking of health and social care with many policymakers looking to integrated care as a solution to the challenges presented.

CHANGING DEMOGRAPHICS AND EPIDEMIOLOGY

It is an established phenomenon that people are living longer. Life expectancy has increased by almost 30 years in this century alone (Department of Health & Social Care [DHSC], 2021). This demographic shift is happening nationally and globally and has led to population ageing (Charles, 2021; Eurostat, 2021a, 2021b; United Nations,

2019). In the UK, projections for the next decade indicate that this trend is set to continue with the population of people over 65 growing from 18%–21% by 2028 (Office for National Statistics [ONS], 2019). One-fifth of the European population is already over 65 (Eurostat, 2021b). By 2050, 17% of the global population will be over 65 years old (United Nations, 2019). However, these extra years of life are associated with increased morbidity and disability (NHS England, 2019a), which can consequently impact on quality of life (Eurostat, 2021b) and increase the burden on health services (Global Burden of Disease Study [GBD], 2020). As discussed in the 'wider determinants of health' (chapter 2), inequalities exist in relation to healthy years of life depending on socioeconomic status (DHSC, 2021). On average, people living in deprived areas can expect 18 more years living in ill health in comparison to those from affluent areas (ONS, 2019). Therefore, the demographic trend of population ageing has profound implications for health and social care services (Kingston et al., 2018). The impact this has on an individual level is highlighted in the Marmot Review (2010) which asserts *'inequalities are a matter of life and death, of health and sickness, of wellbeing and misery'*.

The greatest risks globally on the burden of disease include pollution, obesity, and substance misuse, particularly as we are now seeing declines in smoking across the world (GBD, 2020). This highlights the impact lifestyle factors have on health, healthy years of life, and consequently on current health trends. According to McGinnis et al. (2002), lifestyle factors are either a contributor or cause of mortality 40% of the time. This is pertinent when considering that noncommunicable diseases such as cardiovascular disease, chronic respiratory disease, diabetes, and cancer are the biggest causes of mortality globally (WHO, 2017). There are lifestyle risk

CASE STUDY

There are 20 million people in the UK currently affected by musculoskeletal conditions (Global Burden of Disease Study [GBD], 2020) and over 30% of the UK population suffer with chronic pain (Versus Arthritis, 2021). The wider implications of this also have a significant impact on health and wellbeing. In Europe, chronic pain is estimated to effect 25–35% of adults and 1 in 5 have lost their job because of this (Breivik et al., 2013). In addition, depression is four times more likely in an individual suffering with pain (Mills et al., 2019).

The Integrated Pain and Spinal Service (IPASS) was developed by Berkshire West NHS Trust to address these needs more effectively in their local area. It has joined together the specialist spinal service and community pain team to provide specialist assessments from a range of different professionals for patients suffering with chronic pain (NHS Berkshire Foundation Trust, 2021). A holistic approach is used, exploring the impact of the pain on activities of daily living. Further assessments and examinations are performed so that services can be tailored to the patient's needs. An individualised programme is developed for each patient that may include a range of services such as physiotherapy, education sessions to understand more about their pain, psychotherapy, and pharmacological and nonpharmacological treatment options (NHS Berkshire Foundation Trust, 2021). This is an example of a personalised, holistic programme that draws on the wider knowledge and expertise of the multi-professional team to address the multifaceted nature of pain. Furthermore, it focuses on patient education and peer support to empower individuals and promote greater self-management, which is key to living well with chronic illness (Smith et al., 2021).

The aims of the programme were to develop better continuity between primary and secondary care. This was to reduce duplication and provide a more streamlined service to improve patient experience and reduce waiting lists (NHS Berkshire Foundation Trust, 2021). In addition, a better choice of treatment options was needed for patients, particularly for those with poorly managed symptoms. Strategies to support self-management of pain were also needed. It was hoped that these changes would help prevent readmissions to hospital and enable cost savings. In West Berkshire alone, readmissions over 5 years were costing over 2 million pounds (NICE, 2018).

Key stakeholders met regularly to inform and co-develop the programme. Training was delivered by secondary care providers, in line with the best available evidence, and services were aligned with NICE (2016) clinical guidelines for back pain to ensure consistency and to promote evidence-based service delivery. To enable better continuity of care between services and professionals, the process for referring patients was changed. A strong focus around self-management and education was embedded from the start (NHS Berkshire Foundation Trust, 2021; NICE, 2018).

This integrated and collaborative approach to redesign the service has paid off; since the initiation of IPASS, waiting lists have reduced from 9 months to 4 weeks (NICE, 2018). This has meant patients are able to seek treatment closer to home and tackle their pain early on, in some cases preventing the onset of chronic pain. Patient satisfaction has improved with 90% of patients rating the service as 'excellent'. Readmissions to hospital have also reduced with 62% of patients now being treated in the community instead, creating a saving of around £130,000 each year (NICE, 2018).

It was acknowledged that multidisciplinary collaboration was an essential ingredient to this project's success. Close working and communicating across sectors and with key stakeholders, including patients, was crucial in the development and successful running of the programme (NICE, 2018).

---

factors associated with each of these conditions including obesity, smoking, substance misuse, and inactivity (DHSC, 2021).

The leading causes of disability or morbidity in England are musculoskeletal disorders followed by mental health conditions: this equates to 40% of years spent with disability (DHSC, 2021). There is an established correlation between mental ill health and having long-term physical health issues, with over 30% of people with a long-term condition having a mental health issue as well (NHS England, 2019a). Risk factors for mental health disorders such as alcohol, substance misuse, and physical inactivity are also risk factors for some of the most common long-term conditions such as cardiovascular disease, diabetes, chronic respiratory diseases, and cancer (WHO, 2017). Chronic conditions can negatively impact on emotional health; furthermore, mental health disorders can also exacerbate long-term conditions and can affect patients' ability to self-manage (WHO, 2017). This highlights the need for innovative, collaborative projects such as IPASS to address multifaceted clinical needs and complexities in a holistic and sustainable way.

Comorbidity can be defined as having one or more conditions that occur concurrently with a primary illness (WHO, 2017). The prevalence of comorbidity increases with age, consequently there are growing numbers of the population living with multiple long-term conditions because of our ageing population (Coulter et al., 2015). Multimorbidity refers to individuals with more than two long-term health conditions: this can include mental health disorders, substance misuse, learning disabilities, chronic pain, or frailty (NICE, 2016). It is anticipated that by 2025 around 3 million people will have two or more long-term conditions and by 2035 there will be double the number of older people with four or more conditions (NHS England, 2019a). By 2035, one in three people are expected to have a mental illness (Kingston et al., 2018).

This demonstrates the value of an integrated approach to care delivery such as IPASS, where health needs are not addressed in isolation and wider social and psychological factors are included in a personalised package of care that meets complex needs. Health cannot be addressed in isolation as social, psychological, and physical health are inextricably linked, commonly exacerbating each other (Public Health England [PHE], 2021). Services need to be adaptable and tailored to individuals and they must join together to accomplish this (NHS, 2021). Therefore, a shift is needed, moving away from the predominantly acute-focused reactive delivery of care to a system redesign where prevention and integrated systems work together in a proactive way to address the changing needs of our population (NHS England 2021; NHS, 2021).

Challenges with Long-term Conditions

There are a range of complexities when caring for patients with multimorbidities, particularly if age and frailty are also a factor (Kingston et al., 2018). As identified earlier, multiple conditions can exacerbate each other and compound, leading to a range of symptoms that can significantly impact on both physical and mental health.

Medication for these conditions also becomes increasingly complex. As the number of medications rise, so too does the risk of side effects, interactions, and contraindications (NICE, 2018). According to Kingston et al. (2018), an individual with five conditions will be on at least 11 different medications. Polypharmacy can be problematic in that it can lead to certain medication no longer having a therapeutic effect for a patient, the risks may start to outweigh the benefits, interactions of different medications may become harmful to the patient, or the volume of medication may become unmanageable and problematic (Royal Pharmaceutical Society, n.d.). These issues can also lead to greater need for health services and support, making it harder for patients to self-manage autonomously (NICE, 2018). According to a national GP survey, patients between 2012 and 2018 have reported that support for long-term conditions has worsened in recent years, and support was identified as better for certain conditions such as cancer than others such as autism (Quality Watch, 2018).

The more conditions an individual has, the more health services they are likely to require. A higher burden of disease is associated with a need for a greater range of professionals to be involved. Half of all GP appointments are for chronic and long-term conditions, and they use 70% of primary and secondary care budgets (NHS England, 2019b). Information sharing and digital access to health information within the NHS is often lacking and this has been a barrier to collaborative working in the past (DHSC, 2021; Coulter et al., 2015). The lack of digital integration between health settings can cause breakdown in communication and less continuity of care. This can cause frustration for patients as service delivery is less effective and efficient, therefore service user needs are not adequately met. This can also lead to more reactive as opposed to proactive approaches to care (DHSC, 2019).

The complexities and challenges of coordinating care for long-term conditions demand an integrated approach; however, it is acknowledged that systems and clinical infrastructure have not always been in place to enable this to happen (Coulter et al., 2015; NHS England, n.d.). There has been a culture of services working in silos, focusing on one condition with a lack of consideration for wider factors affecting patients' health and wellbeing (NHS England, n.d.). These challenges need to be overcome to adequately meet the health needs of our current and future population.

Solutions and Next Steps

Personalised care and self-management are key tools in supporting patients to live well with their long-term conditions. Patients who are engaged with their plan of care and 'activated' are more likely to be successful in behaviour change and concordant with treatment, have less admissions to hospital, and have improved health outcomes

---

CASE STUDY

Theory-Practice Reflection Point
Consider the current needs of patients in your clinical area. What conditions are most prevalent and why? Consider which approaches are going to be most effective in addressing some of these community needs.

(Coulter et al., 2015). Patient activation refers to a person's understanding, competence, and confidence in managing their health condition (Hibbard et al, 2015). For self-management to be effective, care must be led by the patient and tailored to their needs. The patient must be an active part of their treatment plan and personalised care planning is needed, in line with the Comprehensive Model of Personalised Care (DHSC, 2019; Coulter et al., 2015; NHS England, 2019b). This allows shared decision-making and creates an ongoing dialogue between clinicians and the patient to tailor support to their needs and help them set and achieve their own goals and priorities (NICE, 2016). Personalised care planning has been found to improve a range of health outcomes including lung function, HbA1c levels, quality of life, and self-management skills such as patient activation and empowerment (Coulter et al., 2015; NICE, 2016). These improved outcomes were associated with greater concordance with treatment and levels of self-care, with strongest results when there was consistency and when the personalised care planning process was embedded as part of routine care (Coulter et al., 2015). However, it was acknowledged that for this to be achieved, reconfiguration of primary care organisations would be needed to enable the delivery of integrated, coordinated services that address multiple clinical needs in a holistic, proactive, and consistent way. This highlights the system level changes that are necessary for these approaches to be successful. The current drive within policy and legislation for more integrated systems within the NHS is therefore a positive step forward (NHS England, 2019a; NHS, 2019; NHS, 2021). Success stories such as IPASS are proof that this way of working can make significant, sustainable changes to the health of a population (NHS Berkshire Foundation Trust, 2021; NICE, 2018).

Essential elements to optimise personalised care planning include setting achievable goals, providing a range of treatment options (both pharmacological and non-pharmacological) and having a designated coordinator as well as follow-up care (NICE, 2016). This is an approach that Norway has been using since 2001 when they introduced the Individual Care Plan, which utilises care coordinators to manage health and social care services for individuals (Romøren et al., 2011). The Comprehensive Model of Personalised Care draws on proportionate universalism, increasing the support package for those with more complex needs and targeting those who need it the most, drawing on specialist support from the multidisciplinary team (NHS England, 2019b). In doing so, this is also seeking to reduce inequalities in health (PHE, 2021).

An example of personalised care planning in practice is the Greater Manchester Community Pharmacy Care Plan service where pharmacists develop individualised care plans for patients with diabetes and cardiovascular disease to promote self-management. An evaluation of the service identified significant improvements to quality of life and patient activation, medicine concordance, and physical health improvements such as lower blood pressure, cholesterol levels, and body mass index. As identified earlier, long-term conditions and multimorbidity are associated with several challenges in relation to medicine management (NICE, 2018). This service draws on the expertise of pharmacists to optimise medicine use and tailor treatment to patients' needs which is crucial for safe and effective management in long-term conditions (NICE, 2016). This highlights the value in investing in personalised care plans and promoting self-management of long-term conditions.

This approach also enables more proactive, preventative care, encouraging people to take ownership of their own health and to live more independently (DHSC, 2021). By working in partnership and in a more integrated way, a wider range of services can be offered to patients (NHS England, 2019a). IPASS is a good example of this, particularly as the personalised approach and providing a wider range of services improved patient satisfaction. This was only possible through professionals working together and joining forces (NHS Berkshire Foundation Trust, 2021). Integrated care can also reduce hospitalisation and enable better preventative care (NHS England, 2019a). To promote healthy ageing and reduce years spent with disability, preventative strategies at primary, secondary, and tertiary stages are needed (Kingston et al., 2018; United Nations, 2019).

Self-management can also be promoted through peer support and education, which was another key focus in the development of IPASS (NHS Berkshire Foundation Trust, 2021). Education is a powerful tool in improving outcomes for patients with chronic pain, whether this be education around exercise, medication, rehabilitation, or self-management. By drawing on a multidisciplinary approach, a wider range of expertise and knowledge can be utilised (Breivik et al., 2013). Considering the ageing population, the need to educate and inform people how to promote their own health and wellbeing is becoming increasingly important (United Nations, 2019).

Joint care planning processes, where an individualised care plan is developed by multiple professionals, can streamline processes, promote integration, and enable holistic needs to be met (WHO, 2017). This enables the wider factors affecting health to be considered and for treatment to be tailored to the individual (WHO, 2017; DHSC, 2021). This is another strength of the IPASS service as a range of clinicians feed into the personalised management plan. The wider implications of pain on the individual and their ability to perform activities of daily living are considered by the different professionals and appropriate interventions are put in place to address these holistic needs.

One way in which we can meet holistic needs more effectively and tailor support to individuals and their community is through social prescribing, an approach that has been promoted within the NHS Long Term Plan as a way of strengthening communities and meeting wider health needs, as well as a key driver in the government's Universal Personalised Care agenda (NHS England, n.d.; NHS England, 2019a). Social prescribing uses community referrals to a wide range of local and nonclinical services to support wider social needs, including loneliness, sedentary behaviour, and stress, to build resilience. With the use of linked workers, wider factors influencing health can be addressed using a more biopsychosocial model of care (Buck & Ewbank, 2020). For instance, activities such as social interaction and physical exercise can positively impact both physical and emotional health (Gibson, 2012). Evaluations of social prescribing programmes have found statistically significant improvements in patients' mental health and wellbeing. It has also been found to reduce work-load pressures in primary care (NHS England, n.d.). More systematic research is needed in this area, but as the evidence base for this discipline grows it can be harnessed and utilised more (Buck & Ewbank, 2020).

The Long Term Plan has identified 'the need for integrated primary care and mental health services to meet patients' holistic needs more effectively. Social prescribing forms an important part of this integration, enabling wider social needs to be addressed alongside health conditions. It is hoped that the Long Term Plan's agenda to expand and strengthen mental health services can be achieved through the statutory integrated care systems (ICSs) that are being developed (DHSC, 2021).

Several exciting digital developments are coming to the fore which will allow health services to be more predictive, personalised, and focused on prevention (DHSC, 2021). Precision medicine tailors treatment more accurately to the individual by using genetic data to predict risk (UK Health Security Agency, 2018). By analysing our genetic makeup more closely, we can learn about rare diseases, identify unknown conditions, and pick up on risk factors before patients are symptomatic. Treatment can therefore be more proactive and upstream, as well as being tailored to individuals' levels of risk, targeting their needs more precisely and leading to more effective treatment options that reduce side effects and symptoms. Precision public heath, which refers to this approach at the population level, can use genomic sequencing to categorise populations according to risk (DHSC, 2019): for instance,

tailoring screening according to associated risks across an entire population rather than relying on national screening tools. We are living in an age where monitoring and tracking of data is becoming increasingly accepted. These capabilities need to be harnessed appropriately to promote and advance public and population health, ensuring public trust is maintained and data protection principles are guaranteed (DHSC, 2019). The UK Biobank is gathering a database of genetic and health information from over half a million UK participants to aid research and development in this area (DHSC, 2019).

Digital resources and interventions such as wearable devices, smart technology, and online programmes are being increasingly used to promote health and wellbeing, self-management, and health surveillance/monitoring (DHSC, 2019; Lagan et al., 2020). However, equity and access need to be carefully considered with digital health interventions to prevent further inequalities in health (Dagher et al., 2022; Western et al., 2021). Digital upskilling of staff is also required to embed digital health effectively and compassionately within health services (UK Health Security Agency, 2018). Although the pandemic has forced services to update and become more digital, systems are not joined up and there is a lack of established infrastructure (DHSC, 2019; DHSC, 2021). The UK government's white paper acknowledges some of these current barriers, claiming that statutory ICSs as well as legislating around data sharing will address some of these system-based issues and enable better collaboration so that integrated working can be embedded across health and social care services (DHSC, 2021). Although legislation can enable change, it will require a whole-systems approach and shift in ways of working to overcome the barriers that currently exist as well as substantial investment to provide the resources needed (Raus et al., 2020). Through pooling resources and budgets and sharing data more effectively, care can be more integrated, more effective, and transformative (DHSC, 2021).

CONCLUSION

The changing patterns in demographics and epidemiology are leading to a range of complexities in meeting population health needs. The ageing population and increase in chronic illnesses, exacerbated by the pandemic, has put increasing pressure on the NHS and social care services. Our systems must be updated and adapted to address these current health trends. The health service and the population it serves has changed irrefutably since the NHS was first developed. Single delivery services focused predominantly on acute care needs are no longer meeting the complexity of need that is currently enveloping our health service. To tackle these health and social issues at a local, national, and international level, a different approach is needed. Services must work more closely together as integrated teams to effectively address the multifaceted health issues that are becoming increasingly prevalent in our society. This will enable better continuity between primary and secondary care, provide a wider range of services to address complex issues, and enable more personalised care to meet individuals' diverse and holistic needs. Considering our ageing population, shifting to a more preventative approach to deliver care that empowers and promotes self-care is crucial. It is encouraging to see effective embodiments of this in practice, such as IPASS and community pharmacy care plans. It is hoped that policy and legislative changes being introduced will help embed the principles of integrated and personalised care into local areas in a more consistent way to help address the changing needs of our population.

References

Breivik, H., Eisenberg, E., & O'Brien, T. (2013). The individual and societal burden of chronic pain in Europe: the case for strategic prioritisation and action to improve knowledge and availability of appropriate care. *BMC Public Health*, 13, 1229. https://doi.org/10.1186/1471-2458-13-1229

Buck, D., & Ewbank, L. (2020). *What is social prescribing?* King's Fund. https://www.kingsfund.org.uk/publications/social-prescribing

Charles, A. (2021). *Integrated care systems explained: making sense of systems, places and neighbourhoods*. The King's Fund. https://www.kingsfund.org.uk/publications/integrated-care-systems-explained

Coulter, A., Entwistle, V. A., Eccles, A., Ryan, S., Shepperd, S., & Perera, R. (2015). Personalised care planning for adults with chronic or long-term health conditions. *Cochrane Database Systematic Review*, 3(3), CD010523. https://doi.org/10.1002/14651858.cd010523.pub2

Dagher, L., Nedunchezhian, S., Hadi El Hajjar, A., Zhang, Y., Deffer, O., et al. (2022). A cardiovascular clinic patients' survey to assess challenges and opportunities of digital health adoption during the COVID-19 pandemic. *Cardiovascular digital health journal*, 3(1), 31–39.

Department of Health & Social Care. (2019). *Advancing our health: prevention in the 2020s*. https://www.gov.uk/government/consultations/advancing-our-health-prevention-in-the-2020s/advancing-our-health-prevention-in-the-2020s-consultation-document

Department of Health & Social Care. (2021). *Integration and innovation: working together to improve health and social care for all*. https://www.gov.uk/government/publications/working-together-to-improve-health-and-social-care-for-all/integration-and-innovation-working-together-to-improve-health-and-social-care-for-all-html-version

EuroStat. (2021a). *Healthy life years statistics*. https://ec.europa.eu/eurostat/statistics-explained/index.php?title=Healthy_life_years_statistics#Healthy_life_years_at_birth

EuroStat. (2021b). *Population structure and ageing*. https://ec.europa.eu/eurostat/statistics-explained/index.php?title=Population_structure_and_ageing

Global Burden of Disease Collaborative Network. (2020). *Global Burden of Disease Study 2019 (GBD 2019) Results*. Seattle: Institute for Health Metrics and Evaluation (IHME).

Gibson, C.-A. (2012). Review of posttraumatic stress disorder and chronic pain: the path to integrated care. *Journal of Rehabilitation Research & Development*, 49(5), 753–776. https://doi.org/10.1682/jrrd.2011.09.0158

Hibbard, J. H., Greene, J., Shi, Y., Mittler, J., & Scanlon, D. (2015). Taking the long view: how well do patient activation scores predict outcomes four years later. *Medical Care Research and Review*, 72(3), 324–337. https://doi.org/10.1177/1077558715573871

Kingston, A., Robinson, L., Booth, H., Knapp, M., Jagger, C., & MODEM project. (2018). Projections of multi-morbidity in the older population in England to 2035: estimates from the Population Ageing and Care Simulation (PACSim) model. *Age and Ageing*, 47(3), 374–380. https://doi.org/10.1093/ageing/afx201

Lafond, S., Charlesworth, A., & Roberts, A. (2016). *A perfect storm: an impossible climate for NHS providers' finances?* London: Health Foundation.

Lagan, S., Aquino, P., Emerson, M. R., Fortuna, K., Walker, R., & Torous, J. (2020). Actionable health app evaluation: translating expert frameworks into objective metrics. *NPJ Digital Medicine*, 3, 100. https://doi.org/10.1038/s41746-020-00312-4

Lewis, L., & Ehrenberg, N. (2020). *Realising the true value of integrated care – Beyond COVID*. International Foundation for Integrated Care. https://integratedcarefoundation.org/publications/realising-the-true-value-of-integrated-care-beyond-covid-19-2

Lewis, R., Pereira, P., Thorlby, R., & Warburton, W. (2020). *Understanding and sustaining the health care service shifts accelerated by COVID-19*. The Health Foundation. https://www.health.org.uk/publications/long-reads/understanding-and-sustaining-the-health-care-service-shifts-accelerated-by-COVID-19

Marmot, M., 2010. Fair Society, Healthy Lives: the Marmot Review: strategic review of health inequalities in England post-2010

McGinnis, J. M., Williams-Russo, P., & Knickman, J. R. (2002). The case for more active policy attention to health promotion. *Health affairs*, 21(2), 78–93.

Mills, S., Nicolson, K., & Smith, B. (2019). Chronic pain: a review of its epidemiology and associated factors in population-based studies. *British Journal of Anaesthesia*, 123(2), 273–283. https://doi.org/10.1016/j.bja.2019.03.023

National Institute of Clinical Excellence. (2016). *Low back pain and sciatica in over 16s: assessment and management*. https://www.nice.org.uk/guidance/NG59

National Institute of Clinical Excellence. (2018). *The Integrated Pain and Spinal Service (IPASS): A unique, integrated and collaborative approach to persistent pain management.* https://www.nice.org.uk/sharedlearning/the-integrated-pain-and-spinal-service-ipass-a-unique-integrated-and-collaborative-approach-to-persistent-pain-management

NHS Berkshire Foundation Trust. (2021). *Integrated Pain & Spinal Service (IPASS).* https://www.berkshirehealthcare.nhs.uk/our-services/physical-and-community-healthcare/integrated-pain-and-spinal-service-ipass/

NHS. (2019). *Breaking down barriers to better health.* https://www.england.nhs.uk/wp-content/uploads/2019/04/breaking-down-barriers-to-better-health-and-care-march19.pdf

NHS. (2021). *Integrated care: next steps to building strong and effective integrated care systems across England.* https://www.england.nhs.uk/wp-content/uploads/2021/01/integrating-care-next-steps-to-building-strong-and-effective-integrated-care-systems.pdf

NHS England. (2019a). *The NHS long term plan.* https://www.longtermplan.nhs.uk/publication/nhs-long-term-plan/

NHS England. (2019b). *Comprehensive model of personalised care.* https://www.england.nhs.uk/personalisedcare/comprehensive-model-of-personalised-care/

NHS England. (2021). *The future of NHS human resources and organizational development Report.* https://www.england.nhs.uk/publication/the-future-of-nhs-human-resources-and-organisational-development-report/

NHS England. (n.d). *Social prescribing.* https://www.england.nhs.uk/personalisedcare/social-prescribing/

Office for National Statistics. (2019). *Health state life expectancies by national deprivation deciles, England and Wales: 2015 to 2017.* https://www.ons.gov.uk/peoplepopulationandcommunity/healthandsocialcare/healthinequalities/bulletins/healthstatelifeexpectanciesbyindexofmultipledeprivationimd/2015to2017

Public Health England. (2021). *Place-based approaches for reducing health inequalities: main report.* https://www.gov.uk/government/publications/health-inequalities-place-based-approaches-to-reduce-inequalities/place-based-approaches-for-reducing-health-inequalities-main-report

Quality Watch. (2018). Are patients benefitting from better integrated care? https://www.nuffieldtrust.org.uk/public/files/2019-01/integrated_care/index.html

Raus, K., Mortier, E., & Eeckloo, K. (2020). Challenges in turning a great idea into great health policy: the case of integrated care. *BMC Health Services Research*, 20(130), 130. https://doi.org/10.1186/s12913-020-4950-z

Romøren, T. I., Torjesen, D. O., & Landmark, B. (2011). Promoting coordination in Norwegian health care. *International Journal of Integrated Care*, 11(127), e127. https://doi.org/10.5334/ijic.581

Royal Pharmaceutical Society. (n.d). Polypharmacy:Getting your medication right retrived https://www.rpharms.com/recognition/setting-professional-standards/polypharmacy-getting-our-medicines-right

Smith, S., Wallace, E., O'Dowd, T., & Fontin, M. (2021). Interventions for improving outcomes in patients with multimorbidity in primary care and community services. *Cochrane Database of Systematic Reviews*, 1(1), CD006560. https://doi.org/10.1002/14651858.cd006560.pub4

United Nations. (2019). *World population ageing.* https://www.un.org/en/development/desa/population/publications/pdf/ageing/WPA2017_Highlights.pdf

Versus Arthritis. (2021). *The state of musculoskeletal health 2021. Arthritis and other musculoskeletal conditions in numbers.* https://www.versusarthritis.org/media/24238/state-of-msk-health-2021.pdf

UK Health Security Agency. (2018). *Predictive prevention and the drive for precision public health.* https://ukhsa.blog.gov.uk/2018/11/20/predictive-prevention-and-the-drive-for-precision-public-health/

Western, M. J., Armstrong, M. E. G., Islam, I., Morgan, K., Jones, U. F., & Kelson, M. J. (2021). The effectiveness of digital interventions for increasing physical activity in individuals of low socioeconomic status: a systematic review and meta-analysis. *International Journal Behavioural Nutrition and Physical Activities*, 18, 148.

World Health Organisation. (2017). *Addressing comorbidity between mental disorders and major noncommunicable diseases.* https://www.euro.who.int/__data/assets/pdf_file/0009/342297/Comorbidity-report_E-web.pdf

Further Reading and Resources

Royal Pharmaceutical Society – Medicine Optimisation
https://www.england.nhs.uk/personalisedcare/comprehensive-model-of-personalised-care/

Resources and information about how to promote safe medicine management.

Biobank
https://www.ukbiobank.ac.uk/learn-more-about-uk-biobank

Find out more about this British database of genetic and health information to aid research in this area.

5

What Is Integrated Care and Why Is it Different?

Dr Kirsty Marshall and Sara Handley

KEY CONCEPTS

- How integrated care is conceptualised
- The complexity of definition
- Rationale implementation
- The core concepts and building blocks of integrated care
- An understanding of macro, meso, and micro levels

INTRODUCTION

Previous chapters have sought to conceptualise the demographic, epidemiological, and political contexts that have led to an upsurge of interest in integrated care. This chapter aims to outline what is meant by the term 'integrated care' and will move from the complexity of definition to understanding the core principles and building blocks required to make integrated care a reality. An important feature of integrated care models is that they require a radical rethink of how we view health and the mechanisms that support people's health. Attempts to develop more integrated systems require a focus on populations, systems, organisations, professionals, and individuals. Therefore, this chapter will explore the 'macro', 'meso', and 'micro' levels of integrated care (Charles, 2020; WHO, 2016).

The case study used to support this chapter explores a meso-initiative in the northwest of England, which commenced during the COVID-19 pandemic. This case study was selected as an example of how the breaking down of traditional barriers can transform service delivery and improve wellbeing and health of residential home residents.

CASE STUDY   An Integrated Response to the Management of COVID-19 in Care Homes

The COVID-19 pandemic challenged traditional models of healthcare as it exposed cracks in health and social care systems and the broadening health inequalities in many communities (Marmot et al., 2021). The pandemic also drove forward innovation in integrated care, as systems galvanised to support each other in ways that months earlier would have seemed out of reach (Horton et al., 2021). The following case is one of many innovations during the pandemic which saw services come together to support integration of services and cross-boundary working to ensure that a safe level of care continued to be provided. The first wave of COVID-19 hit the residential home sector in the UK extremely hard as the highly contagious respiratory disease spread rapidly within the homes and had a devastatingly high mortality rate. COVID-19 had a disproportionate impact on people who worked in social care in the early waves of the pandemic (Office of National Statistics [ONS], 2020). This had a significant impact on residents and the staff attempting to manage relentless levels and intensity of care (Hinsliff-Smith et al., 2020). It is important to recognise that residential homes in England provide care such as washing, dressing, taking medicines, and support with activities of daily living. If nursing care is required within a residential care home, it is provided by the NHS community nursing teams and the primary care sector (general practice).

The case study is based on actions taken by the adult community nursing service to support their residential care home colleagues. Early in the pandemic, the team recognised that their traditional modes of care delivery

---

(responding to referrals) would not be sufficient to maintain care. This situation was exacerbated as care homes tried to manage the spread of infection by reducing the number of people (including professionals) coming into their homes.

Stakeholders came together from across the local system to use their collective knowledge to design a whole-system care home support strategy. Part of this strategy was the implementation of a small team with the core purpose to support care homes to provide, maintain, and ensure safe care. This team was called the STICH (Supporting Treatment in Care Homes) team.

The team worked alongside the existing Quality Assurance Officers to identify residential home providers who required significant support in their service delivery during the pandemic. A unique element of this team and where it broke down traditional barriers was that it did not form part of the regulatory supervision of residential homes. The team not only responded to incidents but aimed to provide early intervention by being invited by the homes to provide additional support. A unique feature

of the team was that, once they commenced working with a home, they used principles of integration to link to the wider system, ensuring a far wider and more holistic intervention. The team was also able to take referrals to support individuals from community and care homes, including same-day visits to homes and individuals. The aims of the team are outlined in Fig. 5.1.

By adopting an integrated approach, the team was able to share health expertise and resources with the homes to reduce the impact of the pandemic on residents. The team had several impacts, including a reduction of emergency admissions from care homes to hospital, reduction in total bed days, and the development of stronger working relationships between care homes and their health and social care colleagues. As the team moved from its pandemic role and became embedded into the wider system, this transition represented a strengthening of the integrated approach. The ongoing approach included developing data and intelligence sharing between commissioners of services, NHS providers, and primary care.

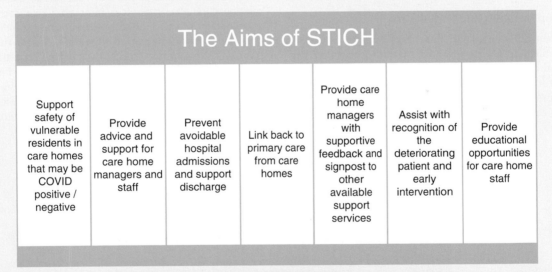

Fig. 5.1 Aims of STICH.

INTRODUCING INTEGRATED CARE

The following section aims to provide an outline of the many faces and facets of integrated care, providing an insight into the complexities of definition and the underpinning principles. While integration and integrated care have been the cornerstone of many health and social care policies across the world for over 40 years, the concept remains elusive and nebulous (RAND Europe, 2012). Goodwin (2016) explains that the variance in definitions has been driven by the many legitimate purposes, stakeholders, and requirements involved in integrated care. In short, integrated care can mean many things to many people, and the context in which integrated care happens will affect how integrated care is conceptualised (Marshall, 2020). Thorstensen-Woll et al. (2021) provide the following insight in their King's Fund paper: *'Integrated care aims to improve people's outcomes and experiences of care by bringing services together around people and communities'*. This is a useful starting point, as it highlights the change in thinking required to move from a system that privileges organisational requirement to one that is co-ordinated around people and communities and is centred on place rather than siloed structures (Ham & Curry, 2011).

Integration and Integrated Care

Before exploring the concept of integrated care, it is important to differentiate these two very interchangeable but different concepts. Shaw et al. (2011) highlight that these are significantly different concepts, explaining that integrated care is the organising principle that underpins care delivery and integration is a set of methods, processes, and models that are used to bring about integrated care. Fig. 5.2 demonstrates how this can be applied to the case study and Fig. 5.3 demonstrates a system-level example.

The figures demonstrate the interplay between integration and integrated care and how integration activities lead to the establishment of an integrated care approach.

Conceptualising Integrated Care

Goodwin (2016) explains that, at its essence, integrated care is a whole-system approach that brings together fragmented and episodic healthcare by coordinating delivery to better provide for communities. This view is supported by Thorstensen-Woll et al. (2021) who state that integrated care needs to address fragmentation and the lack of coordination that people experience when they enter health and social care systems. The case study demonstrates an example of the breaking down of traditional barriers and siloed working as the system came together to support a sector under incredible pressure from the pandemic. An interesting point here is that the project not only focused on health delivery but also galvanised the skills of the health sector to support care homes that are privately owned. In doing so, they placed care of people and communities at the centre of their actions.

An important challenge to consider when conceptualising integrated care is that it can be tempting to view the required transformation through the lens of government policy, economic drivers, and professional positioning, which could limit the potential as these only consider the structural or transactional changes (Marshall, 2020). After all, it seems common sense that if services talked to each other, had systems that share information, and had professionals who work flexibly across boundaries, care provision will improve. Solely considering structural change will provide only a part of the solution to integrated care without addressing the cultural changes required to change the relationship between services, people, and community. As explained by Marshall (2020), without understanding the core concepts of integration, there is a danger that systems will superimpose traditional thinking onto the new approaches and in doing so curtail the potential benefits. Therefore, the first step into understanding integrated care is to be open to new ways of thinking and unlearning previous knowledge. In their study into the development

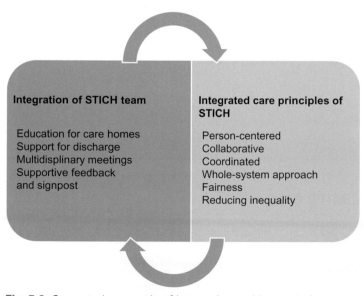

Fig. 5.2 Case study example of integration and integrated care.

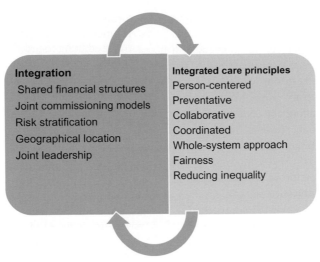

Integration
Shared financial structures
Joint commissioning models
Risk stratification
Geographical location
Joint leadership

Integrated care principles
Person-centered
Preventative
Collaborative
Coordinated
Whole-system approach
Fairness
Reducing inequality

Fig. 5.3 System example of integration and integrated care.

of home care services, Cegarra-Navarro et al. (2015) highlighted that for implementation to be successful there is a requirement to reorientate organisational values and norms through the changing of cognitive structures, mental models, dominant logic, and core assumptions that guide behaviour. Therefore, restructuring how you think about the concept of health and care should be the starting point to understanding integrated care. This need to reconceptualise care can be observed in the case study. Traditionally, support for residential homes was managed through regulatory control and inspection. The case study's scope was not to change these structures but rather to provide a collaborative early intervention that enabled the residential homes to access support from the wider system. The development of the new team sought to transgress this approach by adopting a collaborative cross-boundary approach where homes felt able to invite the wider system into their home to help improve care provision. This case study demonstrated on a small scale that there is a need to challenge underlying relationships when considering integration activities. The team enabled a different relationship to be fostered between the quality team, the wider system, and the care homes who needed a different level of support to meet the challenge presented by the pandemic. The team members and care homes were able to build on previous relationships to react to the changing environment. Cultural shifts in care are explored further at systemic and organisational levels within Chapter 21.

Complexity in Definition

The sheer volume of definitions and descriptions of integrated care can be overwhelming. In 2009, a review by

Suter et al., 2009 into health systems integration yielded approximately 175 definitions and concepts, and this number will have significantly increased in the following years due to the increased political and academic interest in the subject. However, the lack of an overarching agreed-upon definition is not unsurprising given that integrated care is by its very nature context-dependent and has been applied in multiple ways using multiple methods and tools over an extended period (Billing et al., 2003). Although it may not be possible or useful to have a single definition of integrated care, there are some significant definitions that provide an insight into a conceptual approach.

The World Health Organization (WHO) Regional Office for Europe defines integrated services as:

'an approach to strengthen people-centred health systems through the promotion of the comprehensive delivery of quality services across the life-course, designed according to the multidimensional needs of the population and the individual and delivered by a coordinated multidisciplinary team of providers working across settings and levels of care. It should be effectively managed to ensure optimal outcomes and the appropriate use of resources based on the best available evidence, with feedback loops to continuously improve performance and to tackle upstream causes of ill health and to promote wellbeing through intersectoral and multisectoral actions'

WHO Regional Office for Europe, 2016

Several core components of integrated care can be viewed in the WHO definition, including prevention, resource use, and person-centred approaches; however, it could be argued that this definition is for services and would be too complex for a layperson to understand. If integrated care is to challenge dynamics of health and social care, the definition needs to not only explain concepts to professionals but also place people at the heart of how integrated care is spoken about and understood. Shaw et al. (2011) also provide a valuable framing from which to enter an exploration of what integrated care aims for:

'… reflecting a concern to improve patient experience and achieve greater efficiency and value from health delivery systems. The aim is to address fragmentation in patient services, and enable better coordinated and more continuous care, frequently for an ageing population which has increasing incidence of chronic disease.'

While both the previous definitions provide an insight from a services perspective, an alternative and more person-centred definition of integrated care has been provided by National Voices (2013). National Voices is a coalition of charities that works towards people being in control of their health and care.

'I can plan my care with people who work together to understand me and my carer(s), allow me control, and bring together services to achieve the outcomes important to me.'

Framing integrated care from the perspective of people as the user of the service provides a different and important viewpoint that is less present in the first two definitions. While there are aspects common to all the definitions, including patient experience, fragmentation of delivery, and developing a person-centred approach, each one also misses characteristics of the wider concept of integrated care. Kodner (2009) explains that this lack of specificity and clarity in the definition has the potential to hinder systematic understanding and real-world application of integrated care. A question therefore needs to be considered: is it even possible to draw one all-encompassing definition for integrated care given that its application is so context-specific? An alternative could be to focus on the underpinning principles of integrated care to provide guidance on essential factors that influence care. The WHO Principles of Integrated Care (WHO, 2016) (Table 5.1) provide one such set of principles.

Applying these principles to context-specific integrated care programmes could support the design process while providing opportunity for self-determination within

TABLE 5.1   World Health Organization Core Principles of Integrated Care

Comprehensive	Care offered in a way that is responsive to the needs and aspirations of the populations and individuals
Equitable	Equity of access of care to all
Sustainable	Care should be provided in a way that promotes sustainability
Coordinated	Care should wrap around the person and be coordinated in a way that benefits the person
Continuous	Care should be provided across the life course
Holistic	All aspects of a person's life need to be considered
Preventative	Prevention and the social determinates of health and ill health need to be central
Empowerment	People should have control of their own health
Respectful	Care should consider and be sensitive to people's dignity, social situation, and culture
Collaborative	Delivering and planning care to include stakeholders
Co-produced	People are active partners at strategic, organisational, and individual levels
Governed through shared accountability	Between care providers and local people to ensure quality care and improved health outcomes
Evidence-informed	Best evidence based and assessed through measurable outcomes
Whole-systems thinking	Whole system rather than silos
Ethical	Risk-benefit ratio is considered for all interventions

(WHO, 2016)

individual settings. Another approach used to support integrated care development is in the application of the International Foundation for Integrated Care (IFIC) building blocks for integrated care. These blocks were redefined by Lewis and Ehrenberg (2020) to reflect the impact of the pandemic on planning for integration. The main building blocks are presented in Fig. 5.4 and applied in Fig. 5.5.

While the WHO Core Principles of Integrated Care (WHO, 2016) provide a useful guide to the underpinning ethical and cultural approach, the building blocks identified by the IFIC provide a very practical approach that enables planning, delivery, and evaluation. Fig. 5.5 demonstrates the application of the building blocks to the STICH project.

Application of these building blocks is also useful in evaluating integrated care projects. An example of this can be seen in the evaluation by Ehrenberg et al. (2020) of a transformation of a New Zealand health authority. In this evaluation, the use of the building blocks formed part of the evaluation logic model. One advantage of this approach was that the organisation was able to reflect on their past, current, and future state in integrated care and identify areas of strengths and improvements in each block. For example, a particular strength was the move to digital, which had provided agility and flexibility in delivery of primary health care. The building blocks can potentially provide focus while enabling flexibility for areas to develop their collected vision and definition.

Understanding Macro, Meso, and Micro Levels of Integrated Care

When progressing integrated care, the sheer scale of the transformation can feel daunting. So far in this chapter, there has been an exploration of the complexity of definition, moving towards understanding integrated care through its underpinning principles and the building blocks of development. In the final section, we will explore how integrated care can viewed through a conceptual model of primary care setting (Angus & Valentijn, 2018; Valentijn et al., 2013).

The Building Blocks of integrated Care

- Shared values and vision
- Population health and local context
- People as partners in care
- Resilient communities and new alliances
- Workforce capacity and capability
- System-wide governance and leadership
- Digital solutions
- Aligned payment systems
- Transparency of progress, results, and impact

Fig. 5.4 The building blocks of integration. (Lewis & Ehrenberg, 2020.)

Shared values and vision	Population health and local context	People as partners in care
• Bringing together stakeholders • Shared vison	• Identified vulnerable population	• COVID-19 response • Collaborative • Shared responsibility
Resilient communities and new alliances	Workforce capacity and capability	System-wide governance and leadership
• Development of a new relationship with care homes	• Upskilling of care home teams • New ways of working introduced	• Development of a system-wide strategy that brought together a wide range of stakeholders
Digital solutions	Aligned payment systems	Transparency of progress, results, and impact
• Core to the development—digital technology enabled ongoing support	• Not impacted at this stage	• Open evaluation and reporting through trust governance

Fig. 5.5 Building blocks applied to the STICH project.

The model firstly emphasises that integrated care must be person-focused and should reflect a biopsychosocial perspective of health, acknowledging that health problems should not merely be viewed in biological terms but have multiple causative factors, including the social determinants of health (Valentijn et al., 2013). The requirement to take a person-centred and population-health approach links the model and the Core Principles of Integrated Care (WHO, 2016) and reflects the premise that integrated care is not just about moving chess pieces on the board but is a far more radical and cultural approach to supporting people and communities.

Valentijn et al. (2013) viewed integrated care through macro, meso, and micro lenses. This approach enables the multifaceted phenomenon of integrated care to be viewed through a simplification of reality, enabling the complex interactions of integrated care to be examined and interventions to be planned, implemented, and evaluated at local and system levels.

Macro—system level. Macro-level integrated care has the potential to enhance efficiency, quality of care, quality of life, and consumer satisfaction (Suter et al., 2009). Ham and Curry (2011) add that macro-level integration includes a wide range of stakeholders across the system, including purchasers, providers, the voluntary sector, and the community. The importance of this level of integration is that it sets structures, processes, financing, and vison for the system as a whole. Integration at the macro level requires tailor-made changes to fit the needs of people and populations across the continuum of care and tackling the structural barriers to integrated care.

When planning integrated care implementation, it is also important to consider that integration can happen both vertically and horizontally (Table 5.2). These two types are interlinked and, at its most complex, integrated care solutions will involve both (Ham & Curry, 2011).

There have been several notable examples of macro-level integrated health and care systems. A commonly cited example is Kaiser Permanente (USA), which is the largest integrated care system in America and is considered an exemplar in the delivery of quality services that support patients in maintaining health and wellbeing (Curry & Ham, 2010; McHugh et al., 2016). Within the UK Devolution, Greater Manchester saw the development of Greater Manchester Strategic Partnership, consisting of 10 local authorities, 12 clinical commissioning groups, 15 NHS trusts and foundation trusts, and NHS England (McKenna & Dunn, 2015). April 2016 saw the legal transfer of power and budget, and an ambitious plan was commenced to reduce health inequalities and improve efficiencies through the expansion and rapid adoption of integrated care (Walshe et al., 2018).

TABLE 5.2 Vertical and Horizontal Integration in Integrated Care	
Vertical integration	A disease-focused approach; for example, integration of primary, secondary, and tertiary services—upstream/downstream approach
Horizontal integration	Bringing together the whole system to improve the overall health of people and populations; cross-sectional collaboration is a core component, and the aim is to improve overall health of a population with services across territories

(Ham & Curry 2011; Moisan et al., 2021; Valentijn et al., 2013)

Meso. The case study within this chapter is an example of a meso-level integration. Ham and Curry (2011) describe meso-integration as integrated care for groups of people with the same disease or conditions—for example, people living in residential homes, people with specific chronic disease, or people from disadvantaged groups. Valentijn et al. (2013) further describe two types of meso-integration: organisational and professional integration. Organisational integration refers to how integrated organisations are linked and the extent of interlinked production and delivery of services. An example of this is the pooling of skills and expertise of different organisations. In the case study, the team was developed as a cross-organisational approach to support a specific group, placing the needs of people in residential homes at the heart of the project. The aims of the team (Fig. 5.1) demonstrate an approach that linked several parts of the system, viewing the homes as part of a wider system with shared responsibility rather than a siloed organisation. The case study also provided an example of professional meso-integration, as the development of the STICH team enabled clinical, quality assurance, and residential home teams to develop new intra- and interorganisational relationships, shifting traditional roles to provide a comprehensive approach to supporting the homes. Emphasis was placed on building mutual respect and shared vision and goals between stakeholders and through a shared vision to improve care in a time of crisis.

Micro—clinical integration. Finally, micro-level integration is how individuals work with those accessing care. Micro-level integration or clinical integration refers to how a person's care services are coordinated across various professions, institutions, and boundaries (Valentijn et al., 2013). Valentijn et al. (2013) further explain that a significant challenge at this level is that processes often are designed to manage a disease pathway rather than being person-focused, leading to clinical integration being based on narrow, disease-oriented medical interventions rather than enabling a person's journey to be integrated across time, place, and discipline. Micro-level integration is vitally important as it is the point a person connects with services; how fragmented or integrated these services are will directly influence a person's outcomes and experiences (Curry & Ham, 2010). Within the case study, micro-level integration developed as the team progressed and a need was identified for individual support of at-risk residents. At this point, team members would work with care to coordinate support around the person, bringing in medical care and wider system support to wrap around the person.

IMPACT ON PEOPLE

When considering how integrated care impacts people, the contextual nature and diversity of integrated care needs to be considered. How integration impacts people will be influenced by who, how, and what is integrated and what levels of integrated care are included. Within the case study, there were several direct influences on different groups of people, including:

- The workforce within the STICH team
- The workforce within the residential homes
- The residents themselves

Internal evaluation identified improved links and relationships between care home providers and community health providers as a core benefit of adopting a more integrated approach. The experience of this team matches the findings in several previous studies, such as that by Mitchell et al. (2020) who found in their qualitative study of integration of community health and social care services that communication, shared purpose, and leadership were core to successful integration and that improved relationships between professionals had the potential to increase trust.

Other impacts reported from the implementation include:

- Prevention—The team's emphasis on preventative measures helped to avoid crisis, reduce the number of hospital admissions, and improve general health, outcomes, and patient experience.
- Patient safety—Focused multidisciplinary team management support for high-risk community patients and help to address issues that threaten patient safety and safeguarding issues.
- Staff morale/job satisfaction—The workstream had a positive impact on care workers, increasing their confidence and proficiency in caring for patients with complex needs.

CONCLUSION

When commencing the journey to understanding integrated care, it is important to start with people and this simple point: people do not live their lives in silos, and therefore services for people cannot deliver effectively in silos. Integrated care is highly contextual and influenced by a range of factors (political, economic, and conceptual). It is widely recognised that there is no 'one size fits all' definition. However, an understanding of the underpinning principles of integrated care will support the development of local visions and strategic development as well as guide perspectives, views, and expectations of various stakeholders in the system.

References

Angus, L., & Valentijn, P. P. (2018). From micro to macro: assessing implementation of integrated care in Australia. *Australian Journal of Primary Health*, *24*(1), 59–65. https://doi.org/10.1071/py17024

Billings, J. R., Coxon, K., & Alaszewski, A. (2003). *Empirical research methodology for 'Procare' research. Version 3*. Canterbury: Centre for Health Services Studies, University of Kent.

Cegarra-NavarroJ. G., Wensley, A. K., & Polo, M. T. S. (2015). A conceptual framework for unlearning in a homecare setting. In J. S. Edwards (Ed.), *The essentials of knowledge management* (pp. 153–174). Palgrave Macmillan.

Charles, A. (2020). *Integrated care systems explained: making sense of systems, places and neighbourhoods*. King's Fund. https://www.kingsfund.org.uk/publications/integrated-care-systems-explained

Curry, N., & Ham, C. (2010). *Clinical and service integration: The route to improve outcomes*. King's Fund. https://www.kingsfund.org.uk/publications/clinical-and-service-integration

Ehrenberg, N., Terris, A., & Marshall, K. (2020). *A rapid review of the health care home model in Capital And Coast District Health Board*. Oxford: International Foundation for Integrated Care. https://www.ccdhb.org.nz/about-us/integrated-care-collaborative-alliance/health-care-home/

Goodwin, N. (2016). Understanding integrated care. *International Journal of Integrated Care*, *16*(4), 6. https://doi.org/10.5334/ijic.2530

Ham, C., & Curry, N. (2011). *Integrated care: What is it? Does it work? What does it mean for the NHS?* London: King's Fund. https://www.kingsfund.org.uk/sites/default/files/field/field_publication_file/integrated-care-summary-chris-ham-sep11.pdf

Hinsliff-Smith, K., Gordon, A., Devi, R., & Goodman, C. (2020). The COVID-19 pandemic in UK care homes – revealing the cracks in the system. *Journal of Nursing Home Research*, *6*, 58–60. https://doi.org/10.14283/jnhrs.2020.17

Horton, T., Hardie, T., Mahadeva, S., & Warburton, W. (2021). *Securing a positive health care technology legacy from COVID-19*. London: Health Foundation. https://www.health.org.uk/publications/

long-reads/securing-a-positive-health-care-technology-legacy-from-covid-19

Kodner, D. L. (2009). All together now: a conceptual exploration of integrated care. *Healthcare Quarterly (Toronto, Ont.)*, *13*, 6–15. https://doi.org/10.12927/hcq.2009.21091

Lewis, L., & Ehrenberg, N. (2020). *Realising the true value of integrated care – Beyond COVID*. International Foundation for Integrated Care. Retrieved https://integratedcarefoundation.org/covid-19-knowledge/realising-the-true-value-of-integrated-care-beyond-covid-19?mc_cid=eec3e2883d&mc_eid=b6c2555b9d

Marmot, M., Allen, J., Goldblatt, P., Herd, E., & Morrison, J. (2021). *Build back fairer: The COVID-19 Marmot review: The pandemic, socioeconomic and health inequalities in England*. London: Institute of Health Equity. https://www.health.org.uk/publications/build-back-fairer-the-covid-19-marmot-review

Marshall, K. (2020). *An exploration of neighbourhood team members experiences of the transition from traditional health and social care teams to integrated care systems, within a defined health and social care economy* (Publication No. 59618) [Professional Doctorate thesis]. University of Salford.

McHugh, M. D., Aiken, L. H., Eckenhoff, M. E., & Burns, L. R. (2016). Achieving Kaiser Permanente quality. *Health Care Management Review*, *41*(3), 178–188. https://doi.org/10.1097/hmr.0000000000000070

McKenna, H., & Dunn, P. (2015). *Devolution: What it means for health and social care in England*. King's Fund. https://www.kingsfund.org.uk/publications/devolution?

Moisan, L., Fournier, P. -L., Lagacé, D., & Landry, S. (2021). The Integrated Performance Management System: a key to service trajectory integration. *International Journal of Integrated Care*, *21*(4), 25. https://doi.org/10.5334/ijic.5701

National Voices. (2013). *A narrative for person-centred coordinated care*. https://www.nationalvoices.org.uk/sites/default/files/public/publications/narrative-for-person-centred-coordinated-care.pdf

Mitchell, C., Tazzyman, A., Howard, S. J., & Hodgson, D. (2020). More that unites us than divides us? A qualitative study of integration of community health and social care services. *BMC Family Practice*, *21*(1), 1–10. https://doi.org/10.1186/s12875-020-01168-z

Office of National Statistics. (2020). *Impact of coronavirus in care homes in England: 26 May to 19 June 2020*. https://www.ons.gov.uk/peoplepopulationandcommunity/healthandsocialcare/conditionsanddiseases/articles/impactofcoronavirusincarehomesinenglandvivaldi/26mayto19june2020

RAND Europe, Ernst & Young LLP. (2012). *National evaluation of the Department of Health's integrated care pilot*. London: Ernst & Young LLP.

Shaw, S., Rosen, R., & Rumbold, B. (2011). *National evaluation of the Department of Health's integrated care pilot*. London: Nuffield Trust.

Suter, E., Oelke, N. D., Adair, C. E., & Armitage, G. D. (2009). Ten key principles for successful health systems integration. *Healthcare Quarterly (Toronto, Ont.)*, *13*, 16–23. https://doi.org/10.12927/hcq.2009.21092

Thorstensen-Woll, C., Wellings, D., Crump, H., & Graham, C. (2021). *Understanding integration: How to listen to and learn from people and communities*. King's Fund. https://www.kingsfund.org.uk/sites/default/files/2021-07/Understanding_integration_2021_guide_2.pdf

Valentijn, P. P., Schepman, S. M., Opheij, W., & Bruijnzeels, M. A. (2013). Understanding integrated care: a comprehensive conceptual framework based on the integrative functions of primary care. *International Journal of Integrated Care*, *13*, e010. https://doi.org/10.5334/ijic.886

Walshe, K., Lorne, C., McDonald, R., Coleman, A., & Turner, A. (2018). *Devolving health and social care: Learning from Greater Manchester*. Manchester: University of Manchester.

World Health Organization. (2016). *Integrated care models: an overview*. https://www.euro.who.int/__data/assets/pdf_file/0005/322475/Integrated-care-models-overview.pdf

WHO Regional Office for Europe. (2016). *Strengthening people-centred health systems in the WHO European Region: framework for action on integrated health services delivery*. Copenhagen: WHO Regional Office for Europe.

Further Reading

Thorstensen-Woll, C., Wellings, D., Crump, H., & Graham, C. (2021). *Understanding integration: How to listen to and learn from people and communities*. King's Fund. https://www.kingsfund.org.uk/sites/default/files/2021-07/Understanding_integration_2021_guide_2.pdf

6

The Background and Development of Integrated Care: International and UK Perspectives

Dr Kirsty Marshall

KEY CONCEPTS

- Perceptions of integrated care
- Drivers for integrated care
- International perspectives

INTRODUCTION

The following chapter introduces the political drivers and the vast range of integrated care implementation across the world. The chapter aims to contextualise the topic of integrated care and the different approaches, demonstrating that there is not a 'one size fits all' approach and that context, politics, and cultural expectation all play a role in the principles outlined in Chapter 5.

The chapter commences by introducing international perspectives before exploring a range of approaches adopted in different contexts. The UK perspective will be explored last, reflecting on how the Health and Care Act (2022) and the UK approach to integrated care draws influence from wider international implementation.

INTERNATIONAL PERSPECTIVE

It has long been known that there is a need to improve provision and access to quality health and social care across the world, and it is recognised that healthcare systems are straining under the cumulative effects of sociodemographic, economic, and environmental changes. In a response to these challenges. the World Health Organization (WHO) released The Astana Declaration of 2018 (WHO, 2018). This Declaration committed WHO member nations to the development of primary healthcare and health services. What is interesting about the commitment is that while it emphasises the need for services that are high-quality, safe, comprehensive, integrated, and accessible, it also commits the member states to creating and developing health-enabling environments. These environments should support individuals and communities to be empowered and engaged in maintaining and enhancing their health and wellbeing. Here we see the principles of integrated care (outlined in Chapter 5) underpinning international policy as there is a recognition that health is a product of not only the services provided but also the environment in which we are born, live, work, and die (Marmot et al., 2020). The following sections will explore several notable international examples of the development of integrated care, such as the population-based models of Kaiser Permanente (WHO, 2016), the commissioner/provider models of the Geisinger Health System (Curry & Ham, 2010), and the person-need-led models of Buurtzorg (De Blok, 2011). While these are key macro and meso examples, there are many more examples that have influenced integrated care across the world. Each of these policies and system-level approaches are interpreted at a local level, which all lead to difficulties in pinning down what we mean by 'integrated care'. The chapter concludes with a reflection on the Health and Care Act (2022) in the UK. In the UK, we see the influence of several different international models, providing an example of the evolutionary nature of integrated care.

European Perspective

Since the 1990s there has been recognition across several European countries that the treatment of illness through high-tech, hospital-based services is insufficient in the management of emergent demographic and epidemiological conditions which require multiorganisational, integrated, and system-wide approaches. In short, pathogenic hospital-centric healthcare is not an effective management strategy to manage populations with high levels of chronic and long-term health conditions (Antunes & Morerira, 2011).

Denmark—Skaevinge Municipality Home Care Service

One of the early examples of an integrated care model is the Danish system of applied integrated home care based on a self-care theory. This model was developed in Skaevinge Municipality in 1984 (Robertson, 2011; Wagner, 2001). This model predates many of the other examples and current literature, but the foundations of integrated care are clearly visible within the model, which centred on availability of support, especially within a person's own home. This model was multifaceted and included both a structural and cultural change. These changes included co-location, a municipality wide 24-hour Home Care Service, prioritisation prevention, and joint decision-making (Wagner, 2001). There was a shift in service delivery to enable responsibility and decisions to be taken by the person for the management of their care, what we would now call 'person-centred care'. In a 10-year review, Wagner (2001) found that more older people in 1997 (40.8%) assessed their own health as better in comparison with those of the same age in 1985 (28.9%). This was coupled with a reduction in the cost of service despite the increase in older people within the municipality.

Netherlands—Buurtzorg Model

Probably one of the most well-known models of integration of care can be observed in the Buurtzorg model from the Netherlands. The Buurtzorg model centres on prevention, self-management, and out-of-hospital care (De Blok, 2011) and has been a significant influence on a wide range of integrated care developments across the world. The Buurtzorg model started in 2007 (English translation, 'neighbourhood') and as De Blok (2011) explains, it was a reaction to a system that was highly bureaucratic and highly regulated. The model grew from a grassroots movement in nursing, providing an example of how systems can be transformed by those who deliver them as well as in policy chambers and head offices. Buurtzorg turned health delivery on its head as it removed much of the bureaucracy and developed a person-centred and personalised care approach providing greater freedom in planning and delivery of care (Monsen & De Blok, 2013). The model included the formation of self-directed teams that supported patients in maintaining their independence and self-care. Work by Drennan et al., (2018) in London and Maybin (2019) in West Suffolk demonstrate how the model has influenced neighbourhood development in the UK.

Teams work across professional boundaries and in geographical neighbourhoods, focusing on self-managing clients and self-managing teams. Shared human values underpin the ethos of the teams, including:

- People want control over their lives
- People want to maintain or improve the quality of their life
- Social interaction is important to people
- Relationships are important to people

In practice, this means that professionals proactively involve the client in decision-making and, where possible, a person's formal and informal networks are also included. Professionals seek to build trusting therapeutic relationships that foster self-care rather than dependency.

An area which garnered international attention was how the teams are formulated and work together. Buurtzorg teams have moved away from traditional hierarchy into self-governing teams where power is distributed, and professionals are provided freedom with responsibility to plan the care of people needing support.

Teams take active steps to embed themselves within the local community, building networks and relationships with local services and then utilising these networks to provide support to those that need it. Teams work on a grounding of share responsibilities and working with people to support independence and self-care (De Blok, 2011).

North American Perspective

The United States and Canada have both produced a wide range of innovative approaches to integration of care (Curry & Ham, 2010). It is difficult to compare between systems in Europe and the United States due to the complexity of health and social care systems and contexts. There are common challenges and drivers within both regions; however, there are significant differences in sociopolitical situations and cultural expectations (Rosen et al., 2011).

Rosen et al. (2011) highlighted that UK payment mechanisms did not support integrated care or provide high quality and efficiency, often disincentivising partnerships. Rosen et al. (2011) turned to the United States' accountable care organisations (ACOs) as an example of a mechanism for developing financial incentives for integration.

The basic premise for ACOs is that different organisations from the healthcare system are required to work together to improve the health of a population (Charles, 2022). Importantly, ACOs do not provide a single blueprint: rather, there are various types of delivery organisations, including multispecialty groups, physician-hospital organisations, and virtual physician organisations. Shortell et al. (2014) further explain that these organisations remain in the early years of development, and it will be some time before their effectiveness can be fully understood. It has been argued that due to the differences in historical context between the United States insurance-based healthcare systems and the NHS in terms of universal coverage, there is uncertainty about the cultural transferability of ACOs (Pollock & Roderick, 2018).

United States—Kaiser Permanente

For over a decade, Kaiser Permanente has been viewed as a healthcare system that has developed a successful vision and application of integrated health care (Curry & Ham, 2010). Kaiser was an early adopter of population health and chronic care approaches, focusing on empowering the population through prevention, self-management, and case management. Advocates of Kaiser's model highlight its focus on removing the artificial constructs of primary and secondary care, which remain a significant challenge for many health services. The model developed both vertical and horizontal integration approaches across all levels of the organisation which acted to incentivise partnerships and integration (Goodwin et al., 2014; McHugh et al., 2016). Kaiser is the largest integrated care system in the United States and is considered an exemplar in the delivery of quality services that support patients in maintaining health and wellbeing (McHugh et al., 2016).

Canada—PRISMA

The PRISMA programme established in Quebec is again frequently cited as another early example of best practice in integrated care (MacAdam, 2015). The aim was to implement a consistent integrated service that would improve the health, wellbeing, empowerment, and satisfaction of the frail elderly population. The programme included care coordination and self-care with a single point of entry. The programme's unique approach to governance and leadership garnered international attention because it did not advocate vertical or horizontal mergers, instead opting to adopt a coordination approach (Hébert et al., 2010; Leutz, 1999). Hébert et al. (2003) explain that coordination is required to be present at all levels: strategically, through a joint governing board which is inclusive of all relevant health, social care and wider organisations; managerially, with a service coordination committee; and operationally (clinically), with a multidisciplinary case management approach. This project showed a decreased incidence of functional decline among frail elderly people within the area (Hébert et al., 2003).

UK PERSPECTIVE

It is important to recognise that there is no unified UK perspective and healthcare in the UK is managed by each of the devolved nations. While English regions remain part of NHS England, regional devolution in areas like Greater Manchester has led to significant powers moving to a decentralised potion. This is further impacted by the formation of integrated care systems as mandated in the Health and Care Act (2022). Each nation and region have adopted different approaches to integration and are at different stages in their integration journey.

The Devolved Nations

The 1998 devolution agreements enabled each nation of the UK (Scotland, Wales, Northern Ireland [NI], and England) to define its own health and social care strategies (Bevan et al., 2014; Ham et al., 2013). The following examples demonstrate the differing approaches adopted across the nations of the UK.

Northern Ireland [NI]

NI has probably the most integrated of the UK's health systems, having had an administratively integrated health and social care service since 1973. The NI system has been described as 'one of the most structurally integrated and comprehensive models of health and personal social services in Europe' (Heenan & Birrell, 2006).

Heenan and Birrell (2009) explain that the NI model is based on closer managerial, organisational, and working arrangements between staff across disciplines, providing the opportunity for patients to move more effectively from acute to community settings. This is often seen in joint managerial positions across disciplines. The NI element also has a 'purchaser–provider split' which is viewed as enabling greater cooperation between services supported by commissioners (Donnelly & O'Neil, 2018). A 2011 review into NI health and social care indicated that, to improve the health outcomes of the NI population, there needed to be further reform of the system to strengthen the integrated care approach and place people at the centre of all healthcare decisions.

Scotland

Post-devolution Scotland has committed to the development of an integrated health and social care system and stronger partnerships (Pearson & Watson, 2018). The NHS Reform (Scotland) Act 2004 compelled NHS boards in Scotland to develop Community Health Partnerships (CHPs). These partnerships aimed to transform the relationships between primary and secondary healthcare and between health and social care, reducing gaps and increasing collaboration (Audit Scotland, 2012). CHPs took on the role of coordinating, planning, and providing primary and community health services. Two main types of approach are health-only and integrated health and social care CHPs. The 2011 audit of CHPs stated that while CHPs represented a significant step forward, there were several limitations, including a need for a more systematic approach to planning and resourcing, a system-wide approach to resourcing preventative services, and strengthening of governance and accountability. The Public Bodies (Joint Working) (Scotland) Act (2014) provided the legislation for the delegation of health and social care to joint integrated boards (Ham et al., 2013), providing the system-wide structural shift required to develop integration on an organisational, local, and community level (Pearson & Watson, 2018). Since 2016, integration of health and social care services in line with the requirements of the Public Bodies (Joint Working) (Scotland) Act 2014 have rapidly increased. Research by Person and Watson (2018) found that Scotland remains in the early stages of structural change to facilitate integrated practice. A 2021 study by the Nuffield Trust highlighted that while there have been real increases in health spending over the last decade, spending in social care has remained stagnant. As a result, health and care services have found it difficult to keep pace with population demand. Changing demographics and increasing morbidity continue to provide a significant challenge to services. In 2022, the Scottish government introduced a bill to develop a national care service. If implemented, Scottish Ministers would be responsible for the National Care Service and would have the power to make regulations, transferring health and social care functions to the institutions of the National Care Service with the aim of further integrating services (National Care Service (Scotland) Bill, 2022).

Wales

The structural drivers in Scotland have been highlighted, demonstrating how government policy guides legislation in the direction of integrated care. In Wales, their adopted approach included incentivising innovation through the introduction of an integrated care fund to act as a financial incentive for innovation in health and social care. This fund aimed to support the implementation of the Social Services and Well-being (Wales) Act (2014) and Well-being of Future Generations (Wales) Act (2015). The fund had a broad-spectrum mandate including funding through capital investment, the Community Care Information System, and the Dementia Action Plan. The fund was extended until mid-2022 to further 'pump prime' new models of care that encourage collaborative working. While it needs to be acknowledged that the Integrated Care Fund is still in the foothills of transformation, the 2022 evaluation found that the fund had:

- Supported the Welsh government's ambitions to transform health and social care
- Funded preventative actions to help sustain core services
- Improved working partnerships between organisations and across regions

England

Integrated care and integration have been embedded in English health policy for most of the past 30 years. Since the publication of the Five Year Forward View (NHS England, 2014) and Long Term Plan (NHS England, 2019), there has been an increasing drive towards a form of integrated care, which has cumulated in the Health and Care Act (2022); (Charles, 2022; NHS England, 2014, 2019).

The NHS Confederation 2020 report into the future of integrated care in England highlighted that for decades the legislative framework governing health has centred around the principle of competition to improve the quality of services. However, there is now a recognition that collaboration and integration are required to improve population health, deliver better-quality care, and make more efficient use of resources (Das-Thompson et al, 2020). The Health and Care Act (2022) was a significant restructuring of the health and care services in England which dismantled clinical commissioning groups and established integrated care systems (for example, Greater Manchester). Each system is led by an integrated care board (ICB) and integrated care partnerships, which take on the planning functions for that geographical location. Within each system, there are several localities with place-based partnership boards: these boards are multi-agency partnerships involving the NHS, local authorities, the voluntary sector, and local communities, and will provide leadership for their specific location. These geographical locations each contain neighbourhood areas (Charles, 2022). While the changes brought about by the Health and Care Act (2022) may support development of structures that support integration, the act is not without its flaws. As Alderwick (2022) explains, there are still gaping holes in the approach and it does little to acknowledge some of the existential threats to the health and care system, such as the backlog of unmet need, chronic workforce shortages, and increasing pressures on services. Others go further, pointing to the disconnect between the call for localisation and transferring of significant power to the secretary of state and therefore centralising decision-making (Moberly, 2022).

Greater Manchester—an example of regional devolution. One of the most interesting developments in health and social care in England was the widening of devolution to regional areas. Greater Manchester became a devolved region in 2016, and a 6-billion-pound budget was transferred from the central government. This was significant as it placed decisions on how to tackle health and wellbeing at a local rather than national level. The deal was decades in the making and required local leaders from health, local authorities, and communities to come together under the

Greater Manchester Combined Authority (GMCA) (GMCA, 2015). The Localism Act (2011) established the legal framework for devolution with the GMCA becoming the first devolved region.

From the start, Manchester aimed to move faster and further than the wider national agenda, understanding that the potential of the region was being hampered by health inequalities and poor health outcomes (Walshe et al., 2018). The GMCA is not one area but rather 10 local authorities, each with its own individual identity, history, and health and social care needs. For devolution to be successful, there needed to be a clear direction of travel with agreement but also flexibility for areas to develop programmes of work that met their population needs (some of these projects have been covered within this book). The pace of change was dramatic, as the system focused on a wholesale rather than incremental approach. This approach aimed to transform the culturally accepted norms of health and social care: community rather than hospital, increased prevention and self-care, and development of services based in 'place' and integrated to support individuals and communities to live healthier lives. As Manchester's devolution encompassed not just health and social but also wider public services, industry, communities, and a wide range of other stakeholders, the development of a cohesive vision was vital as these organisations were not tied together through contractual or organisational bonds. Lorne et al. (2019) explains that the complexity of the Manchester model comes from the double dynamics of solidity and fragility, where efforts are required to manage the contradictions and challenges of cross-organisational working.

This vision was set out in Stronger Together (GMCA, 2013) and has been a core communication theme throughout the devolution process. The vision included achieving sustainable economic growth, reform of public services, and integration of health and social care, with the ultimate aim of improving the prosperity of the population. This vision has been a key part of the Manchester approach as it allows all stakeholders to come together under a common goal.

IMPACT ON PEOPLE

Long-term and chronic conditions continue to replace communicable disease as the greatest challenge to the health, wellbeing, and prosperity of populations across the world. The COVID-19 pandemic laid bare the cracks within systems across the world and further demonstrated the need to address the fragmentation of services. However, there is an increasing understanding that integrated care should not just address structural challenges within existing services but also form part of a cultural shift and change in the relationship between services and the populations they service.

CONCLUSION

Outlined in this chapter are several approaches adapted to the implementation of integrated care. The international, national, and regional policy contexts for integrated care are complex, with several complicating factors. Political ideologies, culture, historical context, and geographical location alongside the demographics and epidemiologic characteristics of a population all influence how policies are developed, framed, and implemented. What is clear is that, increasingly, policy-makers are looking to integrated care to provide answers for the changes in society. However, a singular definition of integrated care remains elusive, and this provides challenges for policy-makers and those tasked with turning policy into action. The cases outlined are a small demonstration of how the concept of integrated care can be applied in different contexts.

References

Alderwick, H. (2022, April 29). *Health and Care Act passes but leaves unfinished business for the NHS and social care.* Health Foundation. https://www.health.org.uk/news-and-comment/news/health-and-care-act-passes-but-leaves-unfinished-business-for-the-nhs-and-social-care

Antunes, V., & Moreira, J. P. (2011). Approaches to developing integrated care in Europe: a systematic literature review. *Journal of Management & Marketing in Healthcare,* 4(2), 129–135. https://doi.org/10.1179/1753303 11X13016677137743

Audit Scotland, (2012). *Health inequalities in Scotland.* Edinburgh: Audit Scotland.

Bevan, G., Karanikolos, M., Exley, J., Nolte, E., Connolly, S., & Mays, N. (2014). *The four health systems of the United Kingdom: how do they compare?* London: Health Foundation, Nuffield Trust.

Charles, A. (2022). *Integrated care systems explained: making sense of systems, places and neighbourhoods.* King's Fund. https://www.kingsfund.org.uk/publications/integrated-care-systems-explained

Curry, N., & Ham, C. (2010). *Clinical and service integration: the route to improved outcomes.* London: King's Fund.

Das-Thompson, J., McQuade, K., Pett, W., & Ville, N. (2020). *The future of integrated care in England: Health leaders' views on how to make system working a success.* London: NHS Confederation.

De Blok, J. (2011). Buurtzorg Nederland: a new perspective on elder care in the Netherlands. *AARP The Journal,* 82–86.

Drennan, V. M., Calestani, M., Ross, F., Saunders, M., & West, P. (2018). Tackling the workforce crisis in district nursing: can the Dutch Buurtzorg model offer a solution and a better patient experience? A mixed methods case study.

BMJ Open, *8*(6), e021931. https://doi.org/10.1136/bmjopen-2018-021931

Donnelly, M., & O'Neill, C. (2018). Integration–reflections from Northern Ireland. *Journal of Health Services Research & Policy*, *23*(1), 1–3. https://doi.org/10.1177/1355819617741514

Goodwin, N., Dixon, A., Anderson, G., & Wodchis, W. (2014). *Providing integrated care for older people with complex needs: lessons from seven international case studies*. London: King's Fund.

Greater Manchester Combined Authority. (2013). *Stronger together*. https://www.greatermanchester-ca.gov.uk/media/1683/gm_strategy_stronger_together.pdf

Greater Manchester Combined Authority. (2015). *Greater Manchester Health and Social Care Devolution-Memorandum of Understanding*. http://web.archive.org/web/20150404034051/http:/www.agma.gov.uk/cms_media/files/mou.pdf

Ham, C., Heenan, D., Longley, M., & Steel, D. R. (2013). *Integrated care in Northern Ireland, Scotland and Wales: Lessons for England*. London: King's Fund.

Health and Care Act. (2022). London: Stationery Office.

Hébert, R., Durand, P. J., Dubuc, N., Tourigny, A., & PRISMA Group. (2003). PRISMA: a new model of integrated service delivery for the frail older people in Canada. *International Journal of Integrated Care*, *3*, e08. https://doi.org/10.5334/ijic.73

Hébert, R., Raîche, M., Dubois, M. F., Gueye, N. D. R., Dubuc, N., Tousignant, M., & PRISMA Group. (2010). Impact of PRISMA, a coordination-type integrated service delivery system for frail older people in Quebec (Canada): a quasi-experimental study. *Journals of Gerontology Series B: Psychological Sciences and Social Sciences*, *65*(1), 107–118. https://doi.org/10.1093/geronb/gbp027

Heenan, D., & Birrell, D. (2006). The integration of health and social care: the lessons from Northern Ireland. *Social Policy & Administration*, *40*(1), 47–66. https://doi.org/10.1111/j.1467-9515.2006.00476.x

Heenan, D., & Birrell, D. (2009). Organisational integration in health and social care: some reflections on the Northern Ireland experience. *Journal of Integrated Care*, *17*(5), 3–12. https://doi.org/10.1108/14769018200900032

MacAdam, M. (2015). PRISMA: Program of research to integrate the services for the maintenance of autonomy. A system-level integration model in Quebec. *International Journal of Integrated Care*, *15*, e018. https://doi.org/10.5334/ijic.2246

Leutz, W. N. (1999). Five laws for integrating medical and social services: lessons from the United States and the United Kingdom. *Milbank Quarterly*, *77*(1), 77–110. https://doi.org/10.1111/1468-0009.00125

Lorne, C., McDonald, R., Walshe, K., & Coleman, A. (2019). Regional assemblage and the spatial reorganisation of health and care: the case of devolution in Greater Manchester, England. *Sociology of Health & Illness*, *41*(7), 1236–1250. https://doi.org/10.1111/1467-9566.12867

Localism Act. (2011). London: Stationery Office.

Marmot, M., Allen, J., Boyce, T., Goldblatt, P., & Morrison, J. (2020). *Health equity in England: The Marmot review 10 years on*. London: Institute of Health Equity.

Maybin, J. (2019, September 26). *Going Dutch in West Suffolk: learning from the Buurtzorg model of care*. King's Fund. https://www.kingsfund.org.uk/blog/2019/09/buurtzorg-model-of-care

McHugh, M. D., Aiken, L. H., Eckenhoff, M. E., & Burns, L. R. (2016). Achieving Kaiser Permanente quality. *Health Care Management Review*, *41*(3), 178. https://doi.org/10.1097/HMR.0000000000000070

Moberly, T. (2022). Ten things you need to know about the Health and Care Bill. *BMJ (Online)*, *376*, o361–o361. https://doi.org/10.1136/bmj.o361

Monsen, K., & De Blok, J. (2013). Buurtzorg Nederland. *The American Journal of Nursing*, *113*(8), 55–59. https://doi.org/10.1097/01.NAJ.0000432966.26257.97

National Care Service (Scotland) Bill. (2022). Edinburgh: Scottish Parliament.

NHS England. (2014). *Five year forward view*. London: Stationery Office.

NHS England. (2019). *The long term plan*. London: Stationery Office.

NHS Reform (Scotland) Act. (2004). London: Stationery Office.

Pearson, C., & Watson, N. (2018). Implementing health and social care integration in Scotland: Renegotiating new partnerships in changing cultures of care. *Health & Social Care in the Community*, *26*(3), e396–e403. https://doi.org/10.1111/hsc.12537

Pollock, A. M., & Roderick, P. (2018). Why we should be concerned about accountable care organisations in England's NHS. *BMJ*, *360*, k343. https://doi.org/10.1136/bmj.k343

Robertson, H. (2011). *Integration of health and social care. A review of literature and models. Implications for Scotland*. Edinburgh: Royal College of Nursing Scotland.

Rosen, R., Mountford, J., Lewis, G., Lewis, R., Shand, J., & Shaw, S. (2011). *Integration in action: four international case studies*. London: Nuffield Trust.

Shortell, S., Addicott, R., Walsh, N., & Ham, C. (2014). *Accountable care organisations in the United States and England*. London: King's Fund.

Social Services and Well-Being (Wales) Act. (2014). London: Stationery Office.

The Public Bodies (Joint Working) (Scotland) Act. (2014). London: Stationery Office.

Wagner, L. (2001). Integrated health care for older people in Denmark-evaluation of The Skaevinge Project "ten years on". *Journal of Oita Nursing and Health Sciences*, *2*(2), 32–39. https://doi.org/10.20705/jonhs.2.2_32

Walshe, K., Lorne, C., McDonald, R., Coleman, A., & Turner, A. (2018). *Devolving health and social care: Learning from Greater Manchester*. Manchester: University of Manchester.

Well-being of Future Generations (Wales) Act. (2015). London: Stationery Office.

World Health Organization. (2016, April 15). *Framework on integrated, people-centred health services*. https://apps.who.int/gb/ebwha/pdf_files/WHA69/A69_39-en.pdf

World Health Organization. (2018). *Declaration on Primary Health Care*. https://www.who.int/primary-health/conference-phc/declaration

Further Reading

Book

Cottam, H. (2018). *Radical help: How we can remake the relationships between us and revolutionise the welfare state.* London: Hachette UK.

Provides a wide set of examples of different approaches to supporting people.

Article

Lewis, R. Q., Checkland, K., Durand, M. A., Ling, T., Mays, N., Roland, M., & Smith, J. A. (2021). Integrated care in England – what can we learn from a decade of national pilot programmes? *International Journal of Integrated Care, 21*(S2), 5. https://doi.org/10.5334/ijic.5631

This article examines integrated care implementation in the UK and provides some interesting insights on how to implement it.

7

Co-production in the Formation of Integrated Services

Dr Hayley Bamber, Dr Tracey Williamson, and Dr Elaine Ball

KEY CONCEPTS

- The author's experiences of co-production in practice
- What good co-production looks like
- The definition of co-production
- Rationale for the implementation
- The core characteristics of co-production

INTRODUCTION

Previous chapters have defined the term 'integrated care' and conceptualised multiple contexts which have led to increased interest in the topic. This chapter aims to build on this knowledge through consideration of how co-production can be utilised as a vehicle to support the implementation of integrated services. It will seek to define what co-production is and will outline the six core characteristics which are integral for effective co-production and thus the success of integrated care.

The case study used to support this chapter explores the implementation of co-production within a supported living environment. This case study was selected as a model example of how co-production can be successful when all key characteristics are utilised.

CASE STUDY **An Integrated Response to the Management of Vulnerable Adults in a Supported Living Service**

The chosen case study is that of KeyRing Living Support, which has been accessed via NESTA's co-production catalogue (NESTA, 2012). They are a supported living service for vulnerable adults who developed local networks which utilised individuals' skills and talents to ensure that mutual support was offered to increase individuals' independent living skills through linking people in the local community. As of 2013, there were 899 members in over 105 locations nationally. Each locality is composed of nine adult members (service users) and one volunteer, who developed their own support network. The ethos of the project was centred on people living independently but sharing their skills with one another and the wider community to maintain this independence (assets). The study accessed the community through a development philosophy that highlighted the need for social networks to promote good living (mutuality/reciprocity). Volunteers performed like good neighbours offering support to individuals when they experienced challenges, which then nurtured network development within the community (capacity).

Over time, mutual support networks (networks) were strengthened and solidified with all community members' contributions being valued. To support the empowerment of the project members, they themselves recruited staff and took up roles as trustees on the Board, which supported the blurring of the boundaries between recipients and service providers. Essentially, the developed networks were not only for vulnerable adults, but they also included a wide range of community residents, where individual assets were nurtured and maximised (equality/role blurring). The key finding highlighted that peer support networks improved outcomes for targeted individuals but also increased the scope for effectiveness of services (catalysts) (NESTA, 2012). All six core characteristics for co-production were present within the study.

INTRODUCING CO-PRODUCTION

The following section aims to provide an outline of the history of co-production and its progression into today's NHS healthcare system. There is a focus on mental health services to illustrate this sector's journey.

A Community Historical Timeline

A long-standing goal of the NHS has been the progression to community-based approaches to treatment, as opposed to hospital admissions (Edwards, 2014), albeit with limited success. It has been recognised that tapping into community resources can provide more effective care for individuals (Marshall & Bamber, 2022) whilst also being cost-effective for services; however, challenges have existed in progressing this approach. Over a period of 30 years, transformation ensued in three distinct stages: rapid de-institutionalisation, introduction and expansion of community systems, and diversification of services to address local needs (National Institute for Health and Care Excellence [NICE], 2015).

Changes to community-led care ascended from a growing evidence base (Tallack et al., 2020), with discussions peaking in the 1950s and 60s. In the 1970s, several scandals identified the ill-treatment of service users, which stressed the requirement for further change (NICE, 2015). Services were received in the home environment, with access to specialist hospitals available to support meeting longer-term needs (Naylor et al., 2015). Whilst institutional closures were deemed successful, community services' functions continuously revolutionised (Gilburt et al., 2014) in an endeavour to meet demand; however, this remained a struggle and focus shifted to person-centred care (Gilburt et al., 2014).

The Western World View of Co-production

Over the last 12 years, the NHS has been subjected to unprecedented pressure because of budget cuts, reduced resources (Farmer, 2011), coordinating a response to the COVID-19 pandemic (Hussain et al., 2020), and the subsequent backlog of ordinary hospital work (Maringe et al., 2020). The impacts of the pandemic on access to treatment, societal wellbeing, and staff mental health has strengthened the call for a reconsideration of service delivery from a deficit approach to one of asset utilisation (Holmes, 2019), thereby addressing the challenges of resource issues by facilitating care (Turner et al., 2015). Service provision can be delivered through various means, including third sector and local communities, ensuring that needs are met and resources retained. Co-production is a critical approach to public policy (Needham, 2009; Department of Health, 2010) but remains a Western construct and not a global construct.

In Fuchs, 1968 asserted that a new service economy approach including banking and healthcare differed greatly from the old industrial economy, which incorporated agriculture and manufacturing, within the United States. A changed relationship between producer and consumer was needed. In subsequent decades, political scientists and sociologists considered the use of co-production in educational and law enforcement services. Communities co-produced via neighbourhood-watch schemes and parent–teacher associations. In the 1970s, Ostrom utilised co-production to rationalise the increase in crime rates when officers were not actively patrolling the streets of Chicago (Ostrom, 1996), highlighting the imperative nature of community input (Stephens & Ryan-Collins, 2008). Ostrom (1996) contended that all citizens were motivated to co-produce; however, at that time economics was not considered. In 1980, Toffler decided to couple co-production with economics to exemplify links between previously separated functions of production and consumption. He noted that by using co-production, organisations could maximise opportunities whilst minimising cost (Toffler, 1980). Early co-production development revealed several positive organisational impacts via the development of a community of practice with a shared endeavour to achieve mutual benefit (Bamber, 2020).

Co-production within the UK progressed during the 1980s, when services were criticised for poor asset utilisation (Think Local Act Personal, 2018) and there was a renewed focus was on the doctor/service user relationship being reciprocal in nature to improve outcomes (Coote, 2002). However, within 10 years, co-production became superseded by the prioritisation of market-driven public service improvements (Centre for Market and Public Organisation, 2011). The provision of health and social care services was considered similarly to other goods, where service users were considered to need things done 'for' them. The mid-2000s saw a resurgence of co-production being applied across public and voluntary sectors due to the disability movement and the mental health user movement (Merseycare, 2013). The disability movement implied that society enforced environmental barriers that disabled individuals and advocated that individuals should independently determine how to live their lives (Pfeiffer, 1993). Similarly, the mental health user movement endorsed recovery and empowerment through equal relationships with professionals. Both movements advocated for a co-production approach to guarantee the active involvement of service users in their care.

Conceptualising Co-production and the Complexity in Definition

As outlined, co-production originated within the United States and in the 1980s journeyed to UK healthcare systems when the value of service user experience to service delivery was recognised (Clark, 2015). In response, the King's Fund emphasised that doctors required service users' input and proclaimed that there would be no benefit for anyone without the nurturing of the doctor/service user relationship (Coote, 2002).

Co-production is now more prominent within the NHS and, over recent years, discussions about how to implement the approach have continued to increase. However, debate remains around what co-production means and its subsequent application in practice (Social Care Institute for Excellence, 2015). Therefore, challenges exist in relation to implementing co-production in practice, determining if it has been effectively implemented, or even if it has been effectively interpreted. These challenges arise due to numerous existing definitions within the literature. Osborne et al. (2016) asserted that co-production is poorly defined, stressing that surrounding definitions are poorly formulated, with Clark (2015) noting that there is a requirement for a specific definition in mental health. Although academic evidence is disparate, Osborne et al.'s (2016) view was echoed by the New Economics Foundation (2010), who assert that no singular, agreed-upon definition exists (Boyle & Harris, 2009). This lack of clear definition presents problems in practice as the pace of change determined by policymakers risks distorting the meaning further (Stephens & Ryan-Collins, 2008). It is possible that the people implementing co-production could respond to these external pressure and implement the process too quickly (Department of Health, 2010), which increases the probability of all core characteristics not being effectively considered (Bamber, 2020). There have been occasions in practice where practitioners have interpreted the meaning differently, resulting in differences in function (Bhalla et al., 2011). Therefore, co-production requires defining to ensure effective communication, thereby enabling a shared understanding and producing better outcomes. Using a concept analysis, a clearer definition for co-production was developed.

Bamber (2020) defined co-production as:

'… the collaboration and equal distribution of power to maximise asset utilisation among stakeholders, to work towards an agreed, shared outcome. It requires the employment of reciprocal relationships to facilitate capacity development.'

Core Characteristics of Co-production

There are six core characteristics of co-production which have been identified (Bamber, 2020) and are supported by the Coalition for Personalised Care, whose co-production model focuses on the values required for successful co-production (NHS England & Coalition for Personalised Care, 2020). The model outlines the importance of ownership and acceptance of co-production by all, a culture of openness and honesty, a commitment to sharing power, clear communication, and a culture of valuing and respecting people to maximise the model's potential (Fig. 7.1).

Additionally, they consider a seven-stage 'how to do it' plan (Fig. 7.2) through attaining senior management support, using open and fair methods to recruit a variety of individuals, implementing systems, identifying areas where co-production could have the greatest impact, training, and constant evaluation (NHS England & Coalition for Personalised Care, 2020).

Whilst the above presents a suggested co-production model, it is noteworthy that this principle is newly developed and has not undergone rigorous testing to support

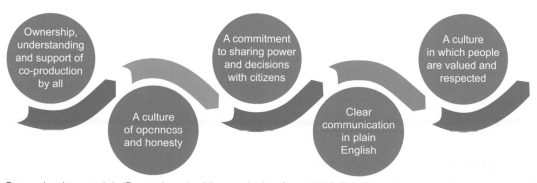

Fig. 7.1 Co-production model. (Reproduced with permission from NHS England & Coalition for Personalised Care.)

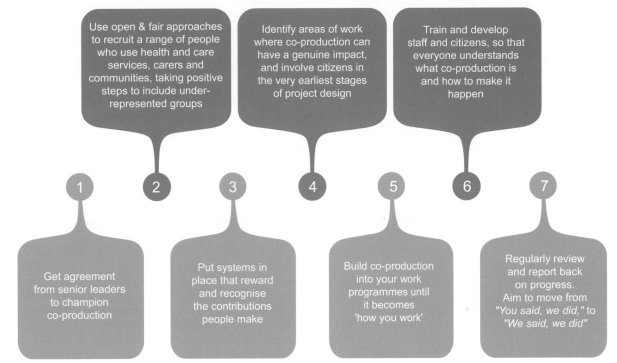

Fig. 7.2 The seven-stage plan. (Reproduced with permission from NHS England & Coalition for Personalised Care.)

its success or validity. While the Coalition for Personalised Care is developing a diagnostic tool to support organisations with identifying strengths and areas for improvement (NHS England & Coalition for Personalised Care, 2020), no current robust measurement guide can be utilised, leaving this model flawed. As a result, no agreed-upon model for co-production currently exists. However, there are six agreed characteristics and principles (confirmed in previous chapters): (1) assets, (2) equality/blurring roles, (3) capacity, (4) networks, (5) catalysts, and (6) reciprocity/mutuality, which many authors agree upon. Each of these are explored below.

(1) Assets. Asset utilisation is the acknowledgement that all individuals have unique skills and attributes which they can contribute to the development of a project (Bamber, 2020). McGeechan et al. (2016) have suggested that asset utilisation is a key component of co-production. Assets are qualities possessed by individuals such as abilities, time, and skills (Scottish Community Development Centre, 2011). This suggests that all parties engaged in co-production (including organisations, professionals, service users, and the community) must transform from passive recipients of care to active participants, where they become equal partners in service delivery (National Empowerment for Science, Technology and Arts, 2012). Through asset-based approaches, people are empowered to independently make decisions, which increases the likelihood of achieving the preferred outcomes (McLean et al., 2017). The acknowledgement of individuals' skills could revolutionise the professional/service user relationship, thus urging individuals to assume responsibility for their own wellbeing and foster their autonomy (Mental Health Foundation, 2013). Encouraging independent thinking about wellbeing can also support the current NHS movement towards preventative healthcare, reducing service demand and therefore saving money (Curry, 2006).

In relation to the previously discussed case study, part of KeyRing Living Support's success stemmed from the recognition that all individuals were able to contribute something to the scheme (NESTA, 2012). This resulted in individuals' increased confidence in their own abilities and subsequently meant that people were able to remain in their own homes and share their abilities to ensure that all individuals' needs were being met. Through asset utilisation, they were able to develop a community of purpose whereby all participants were valued and empowered (NESTA, 2012). Therefore, it is reasonable to assert that asset utilisation is integral to co-production's success as it is through the empowerment of individuals to take positions that professional boundaries are blurred.

(2) Equality or blurring roles. Equality is a critical part of co-production and encourages the development of effective and equal relationships (Pestoff et al., 2012). However, it is important to recognise that power imbalances that already exist between service users and professionals can inhibit the success of co-production in practice. Equality in this chapter refers to the acknowledgement that all individuals' views and opinions are equally important—no one is more privileged (Horton & Patapan, 2004). There is a need for continued concerted efforts to be made to change the existing power dynamics and reach an equilibrium where power is evenly distributed amongst all individuals involved (Fugini et al., 2016), thereby blurring roles to eliminate the defined boundaries (NESTA, 2012). Balance is therefore essential to make sure that greater expertise does not equate to greater power (Bamber, 2020). Therefore, central to the maintenance of balanced approach should be the recognition that individuals have assets and skills (Loeffler et al., 2013).

For KeyRing Living Support, their elevation of members to positions of recruitment and board members placed them ideally to blur the boundaries and become active participants in the distribution of power. Through these actions, individuals were empowered to utilise their assets to blur boundaries (NESTA, 2012). Therefore, this case study highlights the need to ensure that diversity and inclusion are considered. For example, within the mental health population, there is a significant under-representation of service users who engage with service development (Sclater, 2009). Various issues, including diagnosis, are critical for consideration as people with severe depression are more likely to struggle to actively engage in co-production in comparison to people with Parkinson's disease, which can impact on capacity development (Bamber, 2020).

(3) Capacity. Co-production aims to enrich strengths such as motivation, social capital, and networks (Scottish Community Development Centre, 2011). Filipe et al. (2017) assert that co-production requires changing the delivery model from the current deficit approach to one which promotes and focuses on asset utilisation (NESTA, 2012). However, there needs to be a recognition that both models are needed to ensure effective co-production. Whilst an asset-based approach focuses on the use of strengths to effect change, there remains a need to identify what needs to change and therefore it is important to consider deficits. KeyRing Living Support built capacity within their project through the development of a neighbourhood system whereby all individuals shared skills and talents. This meant that when challenges

arose, individuals' strengths and skills were called upon to resolve the issues, thereby increasing capacity (NESTA, 2012). It is therefore reasonable to assume that adopting an asset-based approach to healthcare provision with capacity building at its heart would encourage the engagement of all parties, promoting a cohesive, resilient community (Bamber, 2020).

(4) Networks. Networks are the foundation upon which activities are based (Bamber, 2020). If the right networks are not in place, then there is an increased likelihood that community-led programmes will not succeed and health improvement strategies will likely waver (Scottish Community Development Centre, 2011). In essence, networking requires effective collaboration between all stakeholders with the most advantageous method of knowledge transfer being through the engagement of professionals alongside both personal and peer networks (NESTA, 2012). In the case study, the actions of building capacity, asset utilisation, and role blurring led to the development of a community of practice. Over time, this community became an essential mutual support network which was essential for all participants to remain functioning independently (NESTA, 2012). Therefore, solid network development coupled with power distribution (among service providers and their users) is critical and has the potential to lead to reciprocal relationships, meaning there is a greater chance of success (Bamber, 2020). To enable these, development leaders must become facilitators, not directors.

(5) Catalysts. Being a catalyst involves engaging public service agencies to become facilitators (Sanderson & Lewis, 2012). To support facilitation, the issue of accessibility should be addressed to ensure changes to power imbalances. For example, when service development forums are held, these are often within NHS buildings as they are arranged by the organisation, which strengthens power imbalances and could affect the level of engagement due to stigma. Therefore, thinking about where meetings are held is critical, with community-based locations being recommended (Bamber, 2020). There is also a need to determine an agreement about what information can and will be shared. There should be transparency wherever possible; however, there can be issues in relation to confidentiality which could restrict access. Being open and honest about this and agreeing what information can be shared as a group helps to maintain the power balance (Bamber, 2020). Additionally, any co-production group needs to consider the groups' discourse. Professional discourse undoubtedly will have an impact on accessibility, as many service users and community members will not understand the different 'languages' being utilised. Thus, it is necessary to reiterate the point

that a shared language must be developed to ensure that all members feel involved, again supporting power distribution and reciprocal relationship development (Bamber, 2020). The case study noted that one of their key findings was that the peer support networks increased the scope of effectiveness of services as well as producing positive outcomes for the individuals within the project (NESTA, 2012). Therefore, it is evident that the development of equal, empowering, and solid networks with asset utilisation as a focus results in the potential expansion of service provision, meaning that there are more chances of needs being met as opposed to being highlighted as unmet and never being addressed (Bamber, 2020). To ensure there is this scope, there is a need for effective and reciprocal relationships to be developed.

(6) Mutuality or reciprocity. Reciprocity equates to an individual getting something in return for the effort and skills they have invested (Silverstein et al., 2002) and is a critical component of co-production. Mutuality provides a plethora of incentives to enhance and promote individuals' engagement with co-production. Therefore, mutuality can support people to develop and function/work in reciprocal relationships with professionals with shared expectations. When deciding to begin a co-produced activity, it is important that mutuality is considered as highlighting rewards and benefits can enhance developing positive relationships. KeyRing Living Support highlighted the benefits of community support and therefore developed a philosophy that stressed that social networks are essential to promote good living (NESTA, 2012).

CONCLUSION

When considering implementing co-production in practice, it is essential to consider how the term is defined, what its core components are, and how these can be applied to the chosen setting. Evidence has demonstrated that, for co-production to be successful, there is a need for all six core characteristics to be operating in conjunction with one another. The use of the KeyRing Living Support case study illustrates the positive, life-changing effects of utilising co-production to maintain independent living in the community though the application of the core characteristics.

References

Bamber, H. (2020). *Managers' and clinical leads' perspectives of a co-production model for community mental health service improvement in the NHS: a case study* [Professional Doctorate thesis, University of Salford].

Bhalla, V., Caye, J., Dyre, A., Dymond, L., Morieux, Y., & Orlander, P. (2011). *High-performance organizations: the secrets of their success*. Boston: The Boston Consulting Group.

Boyle, D., & Harris, M. (2009). *The challenge of co-production: how equal partnerships between professionals and the public are crucial to improving public services*. London: National Endowment for Science, Technology and the Arts.

Centre for Market and Public Organisation. (2011). *Research in public policy*. Bristol: Bristol University.

Clark, M. (2015). Co-production in mental health. *Mental Health Review Journal, 20*(4), 213–219.

Coote, A. (2002). *Claiming the health dividend: unlocking the benefits of NHS spending*. London: King's Fund.

Curry, N. (2006). *Preventive social care. Is it cost effective?* London: King's Fund.

Department of Health. (2010). *Practical approaches to co-production: Building effective partnerships with people using services, carers, families and citizens*. London: Department of Health.

Edwards, N. (2014). *Community services: how they can transform care*. London: King's Fund.

Farmer, M. (2011). *Cold tea and tears: it did happen to a dietician* (1st ed.). Beauchamp: Matador.

Filipe, A., Renedo, A., & Marston, C. (2017). The co-production of what? Knowledge, values and social relations in health care. *PLoS Biology, 15*(5), e2001403. https://doi.org/10.1371/journal.pbio.2001403.

Fugini, M., Bracci, E., & Sicillia, M. (2016). *Co-production in the public sector* (1st ed.). London: Springer International Publishing.

Fuchs, V.R. (1968). *The service economy*. Cambridge, USA: National Bureau of Economic Research. https://www.nber.org/system/files/chapters/c1154/c1154.pdf.

Gilburt, H., Peck, E., Ashton, B., Edwards, N., & Naylor, C. (2014). *Service transformation: lessons from mental health*. London: King's Fund.

Horton, K., & Patapan, H. (2004). *Globalisation and equality* (1st ed.). London: Routledge Taylor Francis Group.

Hussain, A., Balmforth, D., Yates, M., Lopez-Marco, A., Rathwell, C., Lambourne, J., Roberts, N., Lall, K., Edmundson, S., & BSC Group. (2020). The Pan London Emergency Cardiac Surgery service: coordinating a response to the COVID-19 pandemic. *Journal of Cardiac Surgery, 35*(7), 1563–1569. https://doi.org/10.1111/jocs.14747.

Holmes, J. (2019). *Brexit and the end of the transition period: what does it mean for the health and care system?* King's Fund. https://www.kingsfund.org.uk/publications/articles/brexit-implications-health-social-care.

Loeffler, E., Power, G., Boviard, T., & Hine-Hughes, F. (2013). *Co-production of health and wellbeing in Scotland*. Edinburgh: Governance International.

Maringe, C., Spicer, J., Morris, M., Purushotham, A., Notle, E., Sullivan, R., Rachet, B., & Aggarwal, A. (2020). The impact of the COVID-19 pandemic on cancer deaths due to delays in diagnosis in England, UK: a national, population-based, modelling study. *Lancet Oncology, 21*(8), 1023–1034. https://doi.org/10.1016/s1470-2045(20)30388-0.

Marshall, K., & Bamber, H. (2022). Using co-production in the implementation of community integrated care. *Primary Health Care*, *32*(6). https://doi.org/10.7748/phc.2022.e1753.

McGeechan, G. J., Woodall, D., Anderson, L., Wilson, L., O'Neill, G., & Newbury-Birch, D. (2016). A co-production community-based approach to reducing smoking prevalence in local community settings. *Journal of Environmental and Public Health*, *2016*, 5386534. https://doi.org/10.1155/2016/5386534.

McLean, J., McNeice, V., & Mitchell, C. (2017). *Asset-based approaches in service settings: striking a balance. An illustration of asset-based approaches in services, and an exploration of their potential for the future*. Glasgow: Glasgow Centre for Population Health.

Mental Health Foundation. (2013). *Starting today. The future of mental health services*. London: Mental Health Foundation.

Merseycare. (2013). *A disability history timeline. The struggle for equal rights through the ages*. Liverpool: Merseycare.

National Empowerment for Science, Technology & Arts. (2012). *UK innovation index: measuring the contribution of innovation to economic growth, and how this varies across sectors*. London: NESTA.

National Institute for Health and Social Care Excellence. (2015). *Transition between inpatient hospital settings and community or care home settings for adults with social care needs*. London: NICE.

Naylor, C., Alderwick, H., & Honeyman, M. (2015). *Acute hospitals and integrated care: from hospitals to health systems*. London: King's Fund.

Needham, C. (2009). *SCIE research briefing 31: Co-production: an emerging evidence base for adult social care transformation*. https://www.scie.org.uk/publications/briefings/briefing31/

NESTA. (2012). *People powered health co-production catalogue*. London: NESTA.

New Economics Foundation. (2010). *Right here, right now. Taking co-production into the mainstream*. London: NESTA.

NHS England and Coalition for Personalised Care (formerly Coalition for Collaborative Care). (2020, October 11). *A Co-production Model*. NHS, Umbrella partnership, C4PC. https://www.coalitionforpersonalisedcare.org.uk/resources/a-co-production-model/

Osborne, S. P., Radnor, Z., & Strokosch, K. (2016). Co-production and the co-creation of value in public services: a suitable case for treatment? *Public Management Review*, *18*(5), 639–653. https://doi.org/10.1080/14719037.2015.1111927.

Ostrom, E. (1996). Crossing the great divide: coproduction, synergy, and development. *World Development*, *24*(6), 1073–1087. https://doi.org/10.1016/0305-750X(96)00023-X.

Pestoff, V., Brandsen, T., & Verschuere, B. (2012). *New public governance, the third-sector and co-production* (1st ed.). New York: Taylor Francis Group.

Pfeiffer, D. (1993). Overview of the disability movement: history, legislative record, and political implications. *Policy Studies Journal*, *21*(4), 724–734. https://doi.org/10.1111/j.1541-0072.1993.tb02169.x.

Sanderson, H., & Lewis, J. (2012). *A practical guide to delivering personalisation: person-centred practice in health and social care*. London: Jessica Kingsley Publishing.

Sclater, E. (2009). *Practitioner's views on the most effective specific equality duties*. London: Equality and Human Rights Committee.

Scottish Community Development Centre. (2011). *Community development and co-production*. Glasgow: Scottish Community Development Centre.

Silverstein, M., Conroy, S. J., Wang, H., Giarrusso, R., & Bengtson, V. L. (2002). Reciprocity in parent-child relations over the adult life course. *The Journal of Gerontology*, *57*(1), 3–13. https://doi.org/10.1093/geronb/57.1.s3.

Social Care Institute for Excellence. (2015). *Co-production in social care: what it is and how to do it*. London: SCIE.

Social Care Institute for Excellence. (2018). *IMCA involvement in accommodation decisions and care reviews*. London: SCIE.

Stephens, L., & Ryan-Collins, J. (2008). *Co-production: a manifesto for growing the core economy*. London: New Economics Foundation.

Tallack, C. Charlesworth, A., Kelly, R., McConkey, R., Rocks, S. (2020). *The bigger picture: Learning from two decades of change*. NHS care in England. Retrieved from https://www.health.org.uk/publications/reports/the-bigger-picture.

Think Local Act Personal. (2018). *Where did co-production come from?* London: Think Local Act Personal. https://www.thinklocalactpersonal.org.uk/co-production-in-commissioning-tool/co-production/In-more-detail/where-did-co-production-come-from/

Toffler, A. (1980). *The third wave* (1st ed.). New York: Bantam Books.

Turner, A., Realpe, A. X., Wallace, L. M., & Koamala-Anderson, J. (2015). A co-produced self-management programme improves psychosocial outcomes for people living with depression. *Mental Health Review Journal*, *20*(4), 242–255. https://doi.org/10.1108/MHRJ-05-2014-0017.

PART II

System Level Integrated Care

8

Barriers and Challenges to Integrated Care

Dr Hayley Bamber and Dr Kirsty Marshall

KEY CONCEPTS

- Change management
- Professional and change
- Power in change
- Organisational change

INTRODUCTION

In part one, the theoretical basis for integrated care was presented. As we move from theory to practice, it is important to consider the following question: if the benefits of integrated care are obvious, why are we not all doing this in practice? The reality is that there are significant barriers and challenges which impact on the practicalities of implementing integrated care within individual services. This chapter seeks to consider some of these barriers and acts as a signpost to chapters which endeavour to address these issues.

THE POLITICAL MOTIVATION FOR INTEGRATED CARE

In Chapter 5, we grappled with what integrated care is and explored the challenges presented by integrated care, being a complex and diverse concept with multiple definitions and approaches. Chapter 5 advocates focusing integrated care activities on underpinning principles (World Health Organization [WHO], 2016), rather than ridged definitions as this will enable integrated care to be viewed through a wider lens. Zonneveld et al. (2018) similarly argue that a value-based approach could enable an increased understanding of integrated care and the behaviours embedded within its implementation. Furthering this, they state that a focus on values could support the development of guidance or governance. Focusing on principles may provide a tool to explore

motivations at all levels during the transition to integrated care.

However, before the 'what', we need to consider the 'why' of integrated care: what are the motivating factors at a macro, meso, and micro level and how do these motivators act as both drivers and challenges (Chapter 5)? As Raus et al. (2020) explain, a population's health and the healthcare provided to a population is profoundly political, and therefore the political context of any policy requires understanding to appreciate the drive and direction of the policy (Chapter 1). For example, while many policy papers talk in terms of improving population health and wellbeing, there is also a significant economic driver for integrated care. This economic driver can be viewed as the continual drive toward more efficient and cheaper healthcare, or, in its wider context, the neoliberal view that health is an economic asset; both are commodities governed by market principles (Viens, 2019). However, many European health systems have endured several years of austerity which have had an impact on the social determinants of health, health inequality, and ultimately health outcomes (Marmot et al., 2012). In the UK, Marmot et al. (2020) demonstrate that there has been a change in health outcomes during this time of austerity, especially deprived areas, including a reduction in life expectancy for women in the most deprived areas. However, it is not just at a macro level that motivation comes into play. As Kaehne (2018) explains, there remains a debate amongst integration researchers on how to conceptualise the politics of integration programmes. Kaehne (2018) further explains that viewing organisational interests through the wider political context can provide useful insights into the potential challenges of integration. These insights then have the potential to inform the development of policy and supporting research.

Complex Systems

Health and social care systems are extremely complex with multiple organisations, financial models, cultures, professional groups, and legal responsibilities. Often the journey to integrated care starts with an exploration on how to fit the pieces of the jigsaw together differently. This structural approach only tells half of the story of integrated care and could explain why it is difficult to truly answer the question of what if integrated care was perceived through the lens of people and communities rather than systems and services. As Hughes et al. (2020) explain, the structures of integrated care are only a small proportion of the multifaceted and multiorganisational networks people draw on to manage their lives. It is also important to recognise that people's lives are not defined within the context of health and social care: people in communities use a wide range of organisations and places, many of which will influence their health and wellbeing. Therefore, when considering integrated care, we need to consider the system and place where people live within their widest context, including but not limited to the environment (for example, safe green spaces), financial stability (employment), and housing. Hopkins and Rippon (2015) state that an asset-based approach is important in how services approach health and care in that there needs to be a focus on promoting and strengthening the factors that support good health and wellbeing and that foster communities and networks that sustain health. However, for this to be achieved there would need to be a systemic shift in the culture and structure of current systems. Chapter 9 provides an exploration of how systems leadership is needed to support integrated care transformation and Chapter 12 provides an example of how social prescribing is bringing about shifts in thinking across whole systems.

Restructure, Restructure, Restructure

One significant challenge which exists within health, social, and third sector care settings is the propensity for service development and change (Bamber, 2020). Whilst the notion of progression and improvement seems to be a clearly desirable ideal (WHO, 2018) there are significant practical issues with continually changing processes (Bamber, 2020). Change management theorists such as Kotter (1997) and Maurer (1996) highlight the need to engage staff in the change process and take the time to embed new practices. However, there seems to be a culture of 'restructure, restructure, restructure' (from our experience especially within the NHS) (Bamber, 2020). The implications on how this change occurs are significant. If organisations seek to placate staff to agree to predetermined changes, then they risk losing the respect and goodwill of tired and stretched frontline workers (Bamber,

2020). In Bamber's (2020) study exploring managerial perspectives of the implementation of a co-production model, it was evident that staff felt that their voices were not heard when discussing concerns about restructures and this therefore led to disengagement from the process, reduced job satisfaction, and increased the likelihood of significant retention issues. It was also noted, however, that senior managers have little control over the pace of change (Bamber, 2020). Therefore, it is reasonable to assume that, to minimise the impact of restructuring, it is imperative that organisations are honest and upfront about the drivers for the change and the level of flexibility that exists within that change, and then share the ownership with practitioners through an integrated approach with co-production at the core (Bamber, 2020; Marshall, 2020; Marshall & Bamber, 2022). Co-production is explored in Chapters 7, 19 and 24.

Power. For integration to successfully occur, issues of status, power, and resource distribution must be addressed and equally distributed (Kaehne, 2018). Whilst this sounds like a simple concept, it is laced with many significant challenges. One issue is the power struggle which inevitably occurs when collaborative processes are instigated and people in power positions attempt to retain their power (Bamber, 2020). Many authors have considered the challenges with endeavouring to distribute power in practice (Coen & Kearns, 2012; Dalgarno & Oates, 2017; Edgren, 1998; Mayer & McKenzie, 2017; Olsen & Carter, 2016). Edgren (1998) states that the possession of power influences an individual's role definition and a sense of achievement. Possession can then impact on the desire to relinquish this power (Coen & Kearns, 2012). This was noted within Bamber's (2020) study where participants highlighted power as a significant barrier to co-production's success. It was purported that some people with positions of power on the board of directors were uncomfortable being responsible for actions of others, which led to them actively working against a co-production model to retain this power (Bamber, 2020). However, Edgren (1998) argues that it is possible for power to be distributed equally and this can have a positive impact on service user care, suggesting that finding an equilibrium is possible.

A further consideration is the subtle hierarchies of power which exist and can be a challenge to undo, such as the power between professionals and service users. Coen and Kearns (2012) questioned if power can truly be shared equally between service users and professionals with preexisting hierarchies in action. Throughout services, binary opposites exist, including doctor/service user, professional/service user, or professional/carer which impact on the distribution of power. However, Dalgarno and Oates (2017) demonstrated that a consensus can be achieved through joint working, evidencing that co-production could be a useful vehicle to promote integration in practice. Chapter 7 provides an overview of the theory of co-production including its use in rebalancing power.

Therefore, for power to be distributed in practice to support an integration approach, it is essential that people re-evaluate their 'expert' roles (Dalgarno and Oates, 2017) and the development of reciprocal relationships with equity at the heart (Bamber, 2020). It is also essential that work continues to help redefine the identity of service users to empower them to actively engage in all aspects of their care and service progressions (Mayer and McKenzie, 2017). If individuals feel empowered, then greater equilibrium is achievable and better outcomes are attained.

Professional practice. When considering any joint endeavour, it is critical to be mindful of the power of professional identity (Trede et al., 2012). Change is challenging at most times but when people may view the change as seeking to dilute their specialist skills and knowledge, which are at the core of their identity, then resistance is likely to follow and achieving outcomes is less probable (Fullan, 2007). Maintaining professional identity is important for professionals and for the success of integration in practice. Professionals work hard to attain their qualification and become their chosen registered professional and then spend years specialising and developing their skills (Hoeve et al., 2014). Issues do arise when this identity is challenged and the suggestion of the addition of generic roles is made (Ling et al., 2012). For example, within mental health care, coordination is a generic role which led to some challenges where professionals experienced decreased job satisfaction and increased staffing issues, as staff left posts as they felt that they were not using the skills that they were training to use (Culverhouse & Bibby, 2008; Waller et al., 2013). Therefore, it is clear to see why integration could be challenging in practice and there is a need for a focus on individuals' strengths and skills as opposed to asserting a generic approach which may be perceived to devalue professionals (McGeechan et al., 2016). Chapter 16 provides an example of the challenges and opportunities during times of professional change.

Managing large-scale change is tough as there are lots of different people with lots of different experiences and values which may not always align, which is likely to cause conflict (NHS England, 2018). As explored in the previous subsection, power is something which people aim to retain; therefore, asking professionals to develop skills which historically were deemed to be those of a fellow professional is likely to cause friction and conflict amongst people (Bamber, 2020). It is essential that the human element is not lost in efforts to implement integration in practice as this would be a disservice to staff and to the aims

of integration NHS Institute for Innovation and Improvement, (2005). Working with teams to enhance reciprocal relationships where individuals' voices are heard is essential to supporting the progression of integration (Bamber, 2020; Marshall, 2020).

Dominance of the medical profession is another major challenge when seeking to implement integration. Historically, medical staff have been better represented within management structures with therapy staff being less so (Greengross et al., 1999). Where there is not equity of representation 'around the table,' a power imbalance is introduced along with an increased likelihood of disengagement from the minority or their voices being quietened by the group. This means that a truly co-produced approach will not be in place and there is a high chance that the endeavour will fail (Bamber, 2020). If we are unable to ensure fair, equitable representation for all professionals and stakeholders, then it seems unlikely that we will be able to effectively represent service users which is essential for successful integration of services (Marshall, 2020).

People's expectations and experience. Often, a significant challenge for organisations looking to implement any large-scale change is the communication of vision and expectations (Cummings & Angwin, 2015). If everyone is not working towards an agreed shared outcome, then people may be frustrated and unhappy and the chances are that that change will be unsuccessful (Bamber, 2020). It is therefore evident that communication is essential to communicating the agenda for integration. When communication is sporadic and disparate, the role out of the process can be hindered (Bamber, 2020), impacting on overall success. There are a few key points which are likely to support managing people's expectations, including an effective communication strategy, modelling desired behaviour, affording individuals ownership over how they meet the overall agreed outcome, and inclusion of all relevant parties from the development stage.

Significant implications exist in practice when unclear communication is present, which has been highlighted through most serious incident reviews; hence, communication needs to be consistent, accurate, and disseminated via a strategy. Therefore, the start of the communication process needs to be with all individuals at the head of an organisation subscribing to integration and a willingness for a co-production approach (Bamber, 2020). Without this unity, there will be confusion and a diluted message being illustrated to frontline workers (Phillips et al., 2022). When all agree, there is also a requirement for a clear and equitable communication strategy to ensure that all parties are clear of what is expected of them and what the requirements of them are (Bamber, 2020). When clarity is absent, people disengage quickly from the process and do not fulfil their roles, impacting on the success of the change (Bamber, 2020).

Another approach to trying to manage the challenges of people's expectations is to model the behaviours which you are wanting others to follow (Bellomo et al., 2016). Through doing so, people can see that the change is clearly adopted by senior managers, they can see the value, and they are more inclined to amend their behaviour to be more in line with the change process (Bellomo et al., 2016). Staff want to see that a change is for a purpose, as they experience so many in practice that never seem to be sustained or long-term which impacts on morale, wellbeing, and job satisfaction (Bamber, 2020)

As part of the change process, ownership needs to be given to individuals to ensure that people remain engaged and enthused about the change process. When people do not have control or input into how change occurs, they feel 'done to' and 'unheard' which can lead to them becoming passive recipients of direction (Bamber, 2020). This results in poor morale, poor mental health, and poor opportunities for innovation, which directly affect the success of the intended change (Bamber, 2020). Therefore, it is reasonable to assert that giving individuals ownership over how integration is achieved within their localities is going to result in positive outcomes (Pierce et al., 2003).

It is also critical to consider who needs to be included in the provision of information surrounding the vision and expectations. It is essential that organisations think outside of the norm and consider how they can include service users and the community in their discussions and communication strategy. As will be established throughout this book, integration is about more than an organisation but about the co-production between organisations, communities, and service users to work towards an agreed shared outcome (Bamber, 2020). If service users are not included and communicated with, then they are not empowered to 'blur the boundaries' and become empowered to be equal partners in change which will impact on the success of integrations (Bamber, 2020).

CONCLUSION

This chapter introduced some of the challenging aspects of why integrated care is not a simple approach to adopt, from conceptualising the political and social influences through to the interpersonal relationships that are key to making integrated care happen in practice. As you interact with other chapters in the book, you will read a wide range of practical examples where organisations from across systems have overcome these challenges (at least in part) and developed innovative solutions. These practical case

studies will be supported by theory and evidence to illustrate their wider implications.

References

Bamber, H. (2020). *Managers' and clinical leads' perspectives of a co-production model for community mental health service improvement in the NHS: a case study* [Professional Doctorate thesis, University of Salford].

Bellomo, N., Clarke, D., Gibelli, L., Townsend, P., & Vreugdenhil, B. J. (2016). Human behaviours in evacuation crowd dynamics: from modelling to "big data" toward crisis management. *Physics of Life Reviews, 18*, 1–21. https://doi.org/10.1016/j.plrev.2016.05.014

Coen, L., & Kearns, N. (2012). Co-producing innovation or innovating co-production? Responding to the contact needs of non-resident parents in the Republic of Ireland. *Child and Family Social Work, 18*(2), 207–216. https://doi.org/10.1111/j.1365-2206.2011.00823.x

Culverhouse, J., & Bibby, P. (2008). Occupational therapy and care coordination: the challenges faced by occupational therapists in community mental health settings. *British Journal of Occupational Therapy, 71*(11), 496–498. https://doi.org/10.1177/030802260807101108

Cummings, S., & Angwin, D. (2015). *Strategy builder: how to create and communicate more effective strategies*. London: John Wiley & Sons.

Dalgarno, M., & Oates, J. (2017). The meaning of co-production for clinicians: an exploratory case study of practitioner trainers in one Recovery College. *Journal of Psychiatric Mental Health Nursing, 25*(5-6), 349–357. https://doi.org/10.1111/jpm.12469

Edgren, L. (1998). Co-production – an approach to cardiac rehabilitation from a service management perspective. *Journal of Nursing Management, 6*(2), 77–85. https://doi.org/10.1046/j.1365-2834.1998.00054.x

Fullan, M. (2007). *Leading in a culture of change*. London: John Wiley & Sons.

Greengross, P., Grant, K., & Collini, E. (1999). *The history of development of the UK national health service 1948-1999*. London: DFID Health Systems Resource Centre.

Hoeve, Y. T., Jansen, G., & Roodbol, P. (2014). The nursing profession: public image, self-concept and professional identity. A discussion paper. *Journal of Advanced Nursing, 70*(2), 295–309.

Hopkins, T., & Rippon, S. (2015). *Head, hands and heart: asset-based approaches in health care*. London: Health Foundation.

Hughes, G., Shaw, S. E., & Greenhalgh, T. (2020). Rethinking integrated care: a systematic hermeneutic review of the literature on integrated care strategies and concepts. *The Milbank Quarterly (Toronto, Ont.), 98*(2), 446–492. https://doi.org/10.1111/1468-0009.12459

Kaehne, A. (2018). Values, interests and power: the politics of integrating services. *Journal of Integrated Care, 26*(2), 158–168. https://doi.org/10.1108/JICA-01-2018-0007

Kotter, J. P. (1997). *Leading change*. Cambridge, MA: Harvard Business School Press.

Ling, T., Brereton, L., Conklin, A., Newbould, J., & Roland, M. (2012). Barriers and facilitators to integrating care: experiences from English Integrated Care Pilots. *International Journal of Integrated Care*, *12*, e129. https://doi.org/10.5334/ijic.982

Marmot, M., Allen, J., Bell, R., Bloomer, E., Goldblatt, P., & Consortium for the European Review of Social Determinants of Health and the Health Divide. (2012). WHO European review of social determinants of health and the health divide. *The Lancet*, *380*(9846), 1011–1029. https://doi.org/10.1016/s0140-6736(12)61228-8

Marmot, M., Allen, J., Boyce, T., Goldblatt, P., & Morrison, J. (2020). *Health equity in England: The Marmot review 10 years on*. London: Health Foundation.

Marshall, K. (2020). *An exploration of neighbourhood team members experiences of the transition from traditional health and social care teams to integrated care systems, within a defined health and social care economy* (Publication No. 595618) [Professional Doctorate thesis, University of Salford].

Marshall, K., & Bamber, H. (2022). Using co-production in the implementation of community integrated care: a scoping review. *Primary Health Care*, *32*(6). https://doi.org/10.7748/phc.2022.e1753

Maurer, R. (1996). Using resistance to build support for change. *The Journal for Quality and Participation*, *19*(3), 56.

Mayer, C., & McKenzie, K. (2017). '…it shows that there's no limits': the psychological impact of co-production for experts by experience working in youth mental health. *Health and Social Care in the Community*, *25*(3), 1181–1189. https://doi.org/10.1111/hsc.12418

McGeechan, G. J., Woodall, D., Anderson, L., Wilson, L., O'Neill, G., & Newbury-Birch, D. (2016). A coproduction community-based approach to reducing smoking prevalence in local community settings. *Journal of Environmental and Public Health*, *2016*, 5386534. https://doi.org/10.1155/2016/5386534

NHS institute for innovation and improvement. (2015). *Managing the human dimensions of change*. Personal and organisational development. Retrieved from: https://www.england.nhs.uk/improvement-hub/wp-content/uploads/sites/44/2017/11/ILG-3.4-Managing-the-Human-Dimensions-of-Change.pdf

NHS England. (2018). *Leading large scale change: a practical guide*. London: NHS England.

Olsen, A. M., & Carter, C. (2016). Responding to the needs of people who have learning disabilities and have been raped: co-production in action. *Tizard Learning Disability Review*, *21*(1), 30–38. https://doi.org/10.1108/TLDR-04-2015-0017

Phillips, G., Kendino, M., Brolan, C. E., Mitchell, R., Herron, L. M., Korver, S., Sharma, D., O'Rielly, G., Poloniati, P., Kafoa, B., & Cox, M. (2022). Lessons from the frontline: leadership and governance experiences in the COVID-19 pandemic response across the Pacific region. *The Lancet Regional: Western Pacific*, *25*, 100518. https://doi.org/10.1016/j.lanwpc.2022.100518

Pierce, J. L., Kostova, T., & Dirks, K. T. (2003). The state of psychological ownership: integrating and extending a century of research. *Review of General Psychology*, *7*(1), 84–107. https://doi.org/10.1037/1089-2680.7.1.84

Raus, K., Mortier, E., & Eeckloo, K. (2020). Challenges in turning a great idea into great health policy: the case of integrated care. *BMC Health Services Research*, *20*(1), 130. https://doi.org/10.1186/s12913-020-4950-z

Trede, F., Macklin, R., & Bridges, D. (2012). Professional identity development: a review of higher education literature. *Studies in Higher Education*, *37*(3), 365–384. https://doi.org/10.1080/03075079.2010.521237

Viens, A. M. (2019). Neo-liberalism, austerity and the political determinants of health. *Health Care Analysis*, *27*(3), 147–152. https://doi.org/10.1007/s10728-019-00377-7

Waller, H., Garety, P., Jolley, S., Fornells-Ambrojo, M., Kuipers, E., Onwumere, J., Woodall, A., & Craig, T. (2013). Training front-line mental health staff to deliver "low intensity" psychological therapy for psychosis. A qualitative analysis of therapists and service user views on the therapy and its future implementation. *Behavioural and Cognitive Psychotherapy*, *43*(3), 298–313. https://doi.org/10.1017/s1352465813000908

World Health Organization [WHO]. (2016). *Framework on integrated, people-centred health services*. Retrieved from: http://apps.who.int/gb/ebwha/pdf_files/WHA69/A69_39-en.pdf?ua=1&ua=1

World Health Organization, Organisation for Economic Co-operation and Development, & The World Bank. (2018). *Delivering quality health services: a global imperative for universal health coverage*. Geneva: World Health Organization.

Zonneveld, N., Driessen, N., Stüssgen, R. A., & Minkman, M. M. (2018). Values of integrated care: a systematic review. *International Journal of Integrated Care*, *18*(4), 9. https://doi.org/10.5334/ijic.4172

Further Reading

Article

Hughes, G., Shaw, S. E., & Greenhalgh, T. (2022). Why doesn't integrated care work? Using Strong Structuration Theory to explain the limitations of an English case. *Sociology of Health & Illness*, *44*(1), 113–129. https://doi.org/10.1111/1467-9566.13398

A research paper which takes a case of a group of NHS organisations and councils and used ethnographic methods to explore the links between individual patients and professionals and organisational strategy and decision-making.

Report

Hopkins, T., & Rippon, S. (2015). *Head, hands and heart: asset-based approaches in health care*. London: Health Foundation.

9

System Leadership

Helen Kilgannon

KEY CONCEPTS

- The NHS expectation of leaders
- Why integration requires a different approach to leadership
- System leadership at a strategic and team level
- The emerging characteristics of system leaders

INTRODUCTION

Leadership can be defined as 'the action of leading a group of people or an organization' (Oxford English Dictionary, 2021).

The complex world of health and social care is comprised of multiple different roles and professions, where care for an individual is delivered across many different settings, teams, and organisations from traditional hospital-based services to people's homes and less traditional settings such as barber shops and supermarkets. Traditional management and leadership approaches characterised by the above definition were developed during the industrial revolution based on a mechanistic approach to supporting people. They relied on proximity of the workforce and employment through a single organisation and are therefore unlikely to be effective in the complex world of health and social care. In a more integrated health and social care system, effective leadership which sees the whole system is key. In some circumstances, leadership is practiced by those in managerial positions; however, more recently, the concept of distributed and system leadership which is not related to position or power is of increasing importance.

The NHS describes the expectations of its leaders in the Healthcare Leadership framework through the description of behaviours across nine interconnected dimensions. The dimensions cover strategic leadership behaviours such as sharing the vision, connecting our services, and more operational behaviours such as leading with care and holding to account.

In the UK, the NHS People Plan (NHS England, 2020) describes the expectation of leaders and the NHS workforce to support the delivery of safe and effective care. The People Plan highlights the need for leaders to be compassionate, inclusive, and representative of the people the NHS supports, and refers to certain styles of leadership: for example, clinical, distributed, and collaborative. It is anticipated that a new leadership compact describing the expected behaviours will be co-designed with leaders in the NHS and published in 2022/23. With so many different narratives, descriptors, and expectations for leaders in health and social care, this chapter seeks to explore some of the key considerations for leaders in integrated care. A study by Harris et al. (2022) funded by The National Institute for Healthcare Research Leadership for Integrated Health and Social Care provides a helpful starting point for the evidence base for leadership in integrated care. The study identified seven areas of consideration for leaders in integration:

1. Inspiring intent to work together
2. Creating the conditions to work together
3. Balancing multiple perspectives
4. Working with power
5. Taking a wider view
6. Commitment to learning and development
7. Clarifying complexity

We will use a case study to explore these aspects in relation to team-level leadership.

CASE STUDY

The Advancing Quality Alliance (Aqua) is an NHS improvement organisation in northwest England. Aqua has a long history of supporting the development of models of integrated care and supporting leaders to develop their expertise to support this, as described by Fillingham and Wier (2014). They identified that the behaviours and qualities required to lead integrated care would need to be different from traditional leadership and management approaches.

In 2016, Aqua launched the leading integrated teams programme. The programme supports the leaders of integrated teams to develop systems expertise, share their learning about integrated models of care and support, and improve their team's performance in delivering high-quality services. The programme also incorporates the Affina Team Journey tools (Affina Organisational Development, 2022), which have been developed based on research and evidence from across health and social care including the national NHS staff opinion survey on effective team working.

This case study reflects the experience of a participant and their leadership journey during and after the programme, showing their personal commitment to learning and development. The practice examples demonstrated leadership requirements at a team level, leading an integrated multidisciplinary team of people (nursing, social workers, community assessment officers, mental health practitioners, pharmacists, and pharmacy technicians) employed by several different organisations (an NHS mental health trust, an NHS acute and community trust, a clinical commissioning group, and the local authority).

Leadership consideration (Harris et al., 2022)	Practice Example—Leader's Experience
Inspiring intent to work together	The leader described how the team were established as a pilot initially with no manager or leader in position and how this was quickly rectified. To bring focus to work, the leader described the importance of defining the cohort of people they would support, creating a mission statement which put the people at the centre of care, and using stories from each other's experience to focus on how the service could make a difference. The leader also described how they ensured that they were personally visible, committed, and sought to empower and motivate the team.
Creating the conditions to work together	As all members of the team were employed by different organisations, a key role of the leader was to bridge between different employment arrangements, policies, procedures, and support systems (e.g., budgets, information technology support). These differences could well be a source of tension or ultimately lead to conflict. The Affina Team Journey provided a structure to support the leader to hold discussions and reach consensus on how the team would work together including ground rules The leader referenced the importance of the culture across the team and how their role was to create a safe environment for all.
Balancing multiple perspectives and taking a wider view	The leader described how they introduced a key worker model, where key workers were able to work with an individual and access support from across the team to address health, care, and social needs. This was not without challenges, as there was such a breadth of support available across the different professionals and services. However, the leader believed this was a key source of learning for the team to really understand the opportunities that each other's skills, experiences, and professions would bring to an individual and family. The team then wrote several case studies to demonstrate the impact of the key worker role and ensured that this was shared with each organisational governance framework and board. The case studies show the breadth of interventions the team could support which require both health and care support and how this can be achieved within a single team without need for complicated referrals. In one of the case studies, the team was also able to mobilise support for a carer whose health was deteriorating.

Leadership consideration (Harris et al., 2022)	Practice Example—Leader's Experience
Working with power	The leader clearly referenced power in discussion and particularly how some members of the team had come from a culture where they had freedom to solve problems. The leader described how they set up a process for teams to discuss complex cases; however, the team did not come forward with cases. On closer discussion, the team stated that they collectively 'get on with it' and will bring anything they cannot resolve to the team leader's attention. This is a clear example of how this leader has created the right conditions for the team but is also able to put their positional power to one side.
Clarifying complexity	Complexity was a key feature of the leading integrated teams programme, with participants exploring theories and methodologies with them to support solutions to challenges. The leader saw a key part of their role as sense-making across the different policies and procedures, enabling the team to effectively function. They also described taking responsibility for raising through governance systems where the different policies and approaches were impacting the team and seeking to resolve the issue, in both the systems that support care and employment practices.

WHY DOES INTEGRATION NEED A DIFFERENT LEADERSHIP APPROACH?

The case study demonstrates that leadership in integrated systems has specific challenges. The delivery of health and care is led and managed by a range of organisations including the provider organisation, local government, commissioners, and third-sector organisations. Each organisation will be underpinned by its own governance, assurance, and regulation frameworks. The board or organisational leaders will determine the culture and leadership approach for each organisation and these leadership and governance differences can make it difficult to align approaches to a common goal and work in collaboration to move towards integrated care. Within the NHS, there has been an added dimension of the creation of an internal market in 1990 where the NHS organisations competed against each other for business (Department of Health, 1997). The very nature of competition encourages leadership behaviours based on power, performance, short-term goals and success, which the King's Fund (2012) has defined as a pace-setting style. If there is a predominance of this style within the NHS, how has the NHS started to move to alternative styles which will support integration?

The UK government's Health and Care Act (2022) outlines a new legal framework for integration and includes a clear duty to collaborate across providers of health and care and with public involvement from individuals, carers, and representatives of people receiving or likely to receive care. The act also removes the requirement for competition

within the system, looking to a new integrated care system (ICS) to have oversight of planning and delivery of care. The act gave the legal framework to enable better movement to the World Health Organization's (WHO) Core Principles of Integrated Care (WHO, 2016), detailed in Chapter 5. These are a great starting point to understand why delivery of integrated care requires a different approach to leadership. The principles of care, which are comprehensive, continuous, holistic, empowered, and co-produced, not only move care to require multidisciplinary working but also a shift in the relationship between caregivers/arrangers and individuals, calling for a change in approach at the team level which we have explored in the case study. The described principles around the organisation and management of care, such as coordination, collaboration, and governance through shared accountability, signify the need to work across organisational and sector boundaries and call for a change at a system level. These new arrangements require a different approach at the system level (i.e., across organisations), defined as systems leadership.

"The collaborative leadership of a network of people in different places and at different levels in the system creating a shared endeavor and cooperating to make a significant change"

Ghate et al., 2013

The UK system is making similar changes to other healthcare systems across the world, as governments attempt to find solutions to ageing populations and changing demographics. The core purpose and shared endeavour of the ICSs is to improve outcomes for the population, tackling inequalities, enhance productivity, and help the NHS to support social and economic development. The purpose of ICSs cannot be realised by organisations working in isolation or competition as in previous legislation. It requires new governance and leadership. The ICS board guidance (NHS England, 2021) describes the constitution for the boards to include the following representatives: independent executives, executive representatives from the ICS, NHS trusts, primary care NHS services, and local authorities. Collectively, they will be accountable for ensuring an effective partnership, aligning ambitions, purpose, and strategies across partner organisations. For the ICS to create this alignment will require their leadership to focus on opportunities for collaboration and co-operation as described in the above definition. Furthermore, it will not only be the role of the representatives of the board to make changes but for all leaders at all levels in the multiple organisations, particularly team leaders as described in the case study.

Senge et al. (2015) further describe systems leadership as having three core capabilities:

- The ability to see the larger system
- Fostering reflective and generative conversations
- Collective focus on reactive problem solving to co-creating the future

In practice, this can be seen as:

1. **The ability to see the larger system**—Recognising the contribution of all aspects of the health and care system, not just a single team or organisation. Coupled with the need to view multiple organisations is the requirement to consider the wider social determinants of health and wellbeing, such as education, housing, and employment. The Health and Care Act (2022) legally establishes the functions of ICSs which were described in NHS England's (2021) guidance. ICSs are intended to be a partnership between organisations that deliver health and care for a defined population. They are governed via an integrated care board which brings together all NHS resources and an integrated care partnership which brings all health and care partners together including organisations who represent those receiving care (e.g., Healthwatch, a UK organisation aimed at making sure decision-makers hear the voice of and use the feedback from people and communities to improve care) to agree upon the strategy and approach for care locally. This change in health and care structure is specifically designed to support leaders to see the larger system and how each part impacts the population's health and wellbeing. The case study shows multiple examples of seeing the wider system, like the key worker role and the leader's responsibility for making sense of the various policies and governance.

2. **Fostering reflective and generative conversations**—Focusing on thinking, questioning, and listening to avoid making assumptions based on previous experience. The Health and Care Act (2022) describes how competition will be removed from the health system allowing organisations to concentrate on meeting health needs. However, the removal of this alone may not change behaviours or conversations between senior leaders. System leaders at all levels must move from being experts in their own area and the pace-selling style to asking questions to support new and innovative solutions. The *Designing Integrated Care Systems* paper (NHS England, 2019) describes a maturity framework for ICSs, which clearly describes how to move from an emerging system to a thriving system the system leaders are to have different conversations. The maturing ICS is seen as one that has 'a culture of learning and sharing with system leaders solving problems together and drawing in the experiences of others' (NHS England, 2019).

3. **Collective focus on reactive problem-solving to co-creating the future**—The traditional management approach leads us to fix individual issues; however, systems leadership and systems thinking are becoming equally as important. Systems thinking encourages us to see the world through its connections and understand how change impacts each part of the system, and through this understanding we can build sustainable change. Most importantly, the WHO (2016) Principles of Care describe the need for a change in relationship between caregiver and receiver, often referred to as co-production. Co-production is an equal partnership between those who use health and care services, communities, and those who deliver and lead services (Coalition for Personalised Care, 2021). It requires system leaders to meaningfully engage communities in every stage of health and care design. This should ensure that rather than fixing issues from the professional perspective, they engage with communities to understand their perspective and how to truly improve services and co-create. The NHS England (2019) guidance makes clear that for an ICS to move through the maturity framework, they must start by actively engaging voluntary services and communities in the decision-making process, be able to show how this is happening at all levels of the system, and ultimately produce a narrative for the ICS that will deliver the ambition of communities and impact wellbeing. Secondly, they must move from a position of organisational leadership to strong collaborative and inclusive leadership across health, local government, and voluntary sectors. These approaches are not

new: local authorities such as Wigan have been working in these ways since 2011. Naylor and Wellings (2019) detail the local authorities' approach with citizens to tackle a financial deficit and create a new approach to public services which was based on working with the assets of people, services, and communities.

Senge et al. (2015) show how systems leadership is about creating new relationships between the different health and care organisations and the community they support. In the UK, this has now been formalised via the Health and Care Act (2022). For many who advocate for systems leadership and system thinking, this change of emphasis to ICSs and integrated team leadership is very welcome. However, the history of the health and care system being led, managed, and governed through separate organisations and their own hierarchical management systems may take some time to change.

CONCLUSION

The studies by Harris et al. (2022) and Senge et al. (2015) are both helpful frameworks for leaders regardless of whether they work at the system or team level. The evidence base for system leadership is continuing to increase, and at the heart of the change is each leader consciously changing their leadership behaviours and relationships between different professionals and across organisations. With the needs of the health and social care system and individuals becoming more complex, real change will come when the system is truly co-produced with individuals, families, and communities. The introduction of representation on the integrated care boards from organisations such as Healthwatch is very welcome and will further support the move to different leadership approaches for integration.

References

Affina Organisation Development. (2022). *The Affina Team Journey.* https://www.affinaod.com/team-tools/affina-team-journey/

Coalition for Personalised Care. (2021). *A Co-production Model: Five values and seven steps to make this happen in reality.* https://coalitionforpersonalisedcare.org.uk/wp-content/uploads/2021/07/C4PCCo-production-model.pdf

Department of Health. (1997). *The new NHS: modern. dependable.* London: Stationery Office.

Fillingham, D., & Weir, B. (2014). System leadership: Lessons and learning from: *Aqua's Integrated Care Discovery Communities.* London: King's Fund.

Ghate, D., Lewis, J., & Welbourne, D. (2013). *Systems Leadership: Exceptional leadership for exceptional times: Synthesis paper.* Nottingham: Virtual Staff College.

Harris, R., Fletcher, S., Sims, S., Ross, F., Brearley, S., & Manthorpe, J. (2022). Developing programme theories of leadership for integrated health and social care teams and systems: a realist synthesis. *Health and Social Care Delivery Research, 10*(7). https://doi.org/10.3310/WPNG1013

Health and Care Act. (2022). London: Stationery Office.

King's Fund. (2012). *Leadership and engagement for improvement in the NHS.* London: King's Fund.

Naylor, C., & Wellings, D. (2019, June 26). *A citizen-led approach to health and care: Lessons from the Wigan Deal.* https://www.kingsfund.org.uk/publications/wigan-deal

NHS England. (2019, June). *Designing integrated care systems (ICSs) in England.* https://www.england.nhs.uk/wp-content/uploads/2019/06/designing-integrated-care-systems-in-england.pdf

NHS England. (2020). *NHS People Plan.* https://www.england.nhs.uk/ournhspeople/

NHS England. (2021). *Integrated care systems: guidance.* https://www.england.nhs.uk/publication/integrated-care-systems-guidance

Oxford English Dictionary. (2021). Oxford: Oxford University Press.

Senge, P., Hamilton, H., & Kania, J. (2015). The dawn of system leadership. *Stanford Social Innovation Review, 13*(1), 27–33. https://doi.org/10.48558/YTE7-XT62

World Health Organization. (2016). *Open mindsets: participatory leadership for health.* https://apps.who.int/iris/handle/10665/251458

Further Reading

Websites

For System Leadership across public services, see the Leadership Centre and the King's Fund. https://www.leadershipcentre.org.uk/publications/

To explore leadership in integrated health and social care services. https://www.kingsfund.org.uk/topics/system-leadership

To explore a citizen-led approach to health and care design, https://www.kingsfund.org.uk/projects/lessons-wigan-deal

https://www.leadershipacademy.nhs.uk/resources/healthcare-leadership-model/

Study

Harris, R., Fletcher, S., Sims, S., Ross, F., Brearley, S., & Manthorpe, J. (2022). Developing programme theories of leadership for integrated health and social care teams and systems: a realist synthesis. *Health and Social Care Delivery Research, 10*(7). https://doi.org/10.3310/WPNG1013

At the heart of the systems leadership model is relationships and seeing each other and those who receive care as humans. To further understand the compassionate leadership approach, explore:

West, M. (2021). Compassionate leadership: Sustaining wisdom, *humanity and presence in health and social care.* London: The Swirling Leaf Press.

10

Improving Outcomes for Children and Young People with Special Educational Needs—Outcomes-Based Accountability

Dr Kirsty Marshall, Steve Kay, and Charlotte Michell

KEY CONCEPTS

- Children and young people
- Special educational needs and disabilities
- Outcomes-based accountability
- Narratives
- Change

INTRODUCTION

This chapter focuses on how outcome-focused approaches can support and guide the implementation of policy and the setting of strategic direction. A case study from Rochdale in Greater Manchester will be used to illustrate how an outcomes-based accountability framework was used to guide a multiorganisation systems approach to an integrated special educational needs and disabilities (SEND) system in Rochdale. Drawing on the case study, this chapter will explore the challenges and opportunities of implementing multiple policy agendas within complex systems and the interconnection between strategy, policy, and evaluation, including the role of narrative and outcomes in supporting system-wide person-centred change. The chapter explores how placing the needs and outcomes for children and families at the heart of the change process enabled a more positive, sustainable, and impactful result.

LEARNING DISABILITIES AND HEALTH OUTCOMES

In the UK in 2022, the percentage of pupils across all state-funded nursery, primary, secondary, and special schools, non-maintained special schools, pupil referral units, and independent schools with special educational need support was 12.6% (1,129,843 pupils) and 4% (355,566) of pupils had education, health, and care plans (i.e., a formal assessment has been made and a plan is in place). Both figures had shown an increase on previous years (Department of Education [DE], 2022). The types of need which presented most often were autistic spectrum disorder and speech, language, and communication needs for those with special educational needs (SEN). While autistic spectrum disorder was the largest presented need, it is important to recognise that pupils present with a large variety of needs, including social, emotional, and mental health; specific learning difficulties; moderate learning difficulties; physical disability; and visual, hearing, and multisensory impairment. Despite the existence of many national, regional, and local structures to support people and legal frameworks to prevent discrimination, people with learning disabilities in the UK still experience significant health inequalities and worse physical and mental outcomes (White et al., 2022).

On average, men and women with a learning disability die 22 and 26 years younger than the general population, respectively (White et al., 2022). Inequalities were magnified during the COVID-19 pandemic as the Local Government Association (2022) found people with learning disabilities reported a traumatic loss of routine, activities, and contact with family and carers which was isolating and difficult to cope with. This loss of routine was coupled with the increased risk of dying from the disease compared to the general population. In the UK, the NHS reported that children and young people with SEN were more likely to experience mental health disorders (NHS Digital, 2022). Alongside the impact on mortality and morbidity, young people with learning disabilities face significant challenges as they transition to adulthood with significant structural limitations to their entry to the workforce which can have a significant impact on their ability to reach their potential and live fulfilling and healthy lives. A European report by Antwerp Management School found that there were significant difficulties for people with learning disabilities in finding long-term, sustainable jobs. The study states that despite people's desire to work and ability to work, prejudices exist that result in a lack of opportunities and unemployment or long-term sick leave (Van Hoofstadt et al., 2020). In the UK, *The SEND Review: Right support, right place, right time* government consultation on SEND and the alternative provision system in England (DE, 2022) reported that, by the age of 27, children with SEN are less likely to be in sustained employment and are at greater risk, including becoming a victim of crime and other societal harms.

It is from this backdrop that the project within the case study developed. The project commenced with the principle that the needs and outcomes of the children and their families would be privileged and that this would be the main driver for change. This was important because the long-term ambitions for children with learning disabilities are the same as for those children without learning disabilities: children and young people should be able to obtain optimal health and wellbeing, to able to meet their daily needs, engage in education, obtain long-term employment, partake in meaningful activity, and ultimately be able to participate in their community at the level they desire and have agency in their lives (National Academies of Sciences, Engineering, and Medicine, 2018).

UK Provision

It has long been recognised that fragmentation within services for children and young people with SEND can have a detrimental impact on the long-term outcomes and their health and wellbeing (DE, 2022). Therefore, in the UK, the Children and Families Act (2014) was introduced, containing new legal duties in relation to children and young people with SEND. These duties were developed into guidance in the form of a code of practice for children and young people aged 0–25 years who have SEND (DE, 2022). The responsibilities for enacting the legal responsibilities sat with local partnerships. The partnerships were to include local authorities, health commissioners, providers, early-years settings, schools, and post-16 further education. The aim of these partnerships was to ensure compliance with legal duties but also to improve service provision, reduce fragmentation, and ultimately support children and young people, all of which have improved outcomes. Following the royal assent of the Health and Social Care Act in April 2022, integrated care systems were established across England to oversee delivery of joined-up health and care within local regions. In 2022, *The SEND Review: Right support, right place, right time* (DE, 2022) aimed to set the strategic direction in addressing three key challenges:

- Challenge 1: outcomes for children and young people with SEN or in alternative provision are poor
- Challenge 2: navigating the SEND system and alternative provision is not a positive experience for children, young people, and their families
- Challenge 3: despite unprecedented investment, the system is not delivering value for money for children, young people, and families
  (DE, 2022)

As with other areas of health and social care, children and young people's services are affected by the wider governmental and societal changes. Using the UK as an example, recent years have witnessed a significant influencing factor that have impacted on the strategic and organisational planning, implementation, and access of services. Fig. 10.1 outlines the societal drivers and key policy developments within the UK.

The case study outlined below explores how the Rochdale (UK) system came together to develop an approached to the integration agenda and how they used outcomes-based accountability (OBA) to support an ambitious agenda to improve the outcomes for children with SEN within their local area by developing an integrated SEND service that incorporated partners from across the local system.

To meet the outcomes, the strategy included (but not exclusively) the development of Family Hubs, co-located single access points for families; Connect the Classroom, high-speed broadband to be available in all schools; development of Multi-Academy Trusts, to increase and improve school provision; and Poverty Proofing Schools, to reduce stigma and remove barriers to learning. These interventions stretched across the whole system as it was recognised that, to effectively support children and young people, no single agency could deliver alone. Rather, the system placed the outcomes set by the children and families as the starting point and used these outcomes to develop programmes that would support the achievements of the outcomes. This is a distinctly different approach to setting outcomes based on the outputs of organisations.

The strategy drove the impetus for closer integration of services. It was important to all members of the partnership that the changes led to significant and meaningful transformation and real-world improved outcomes. Therefore, to ensure these outcomes, the Council for Disabled Children (CDC) was commissioned to support the strategic development and develop an OBA approach. The rationale for the adoption of an OBA approach was to bring together organisations and SEND services under overarching goals and a common set of measurable objectives.

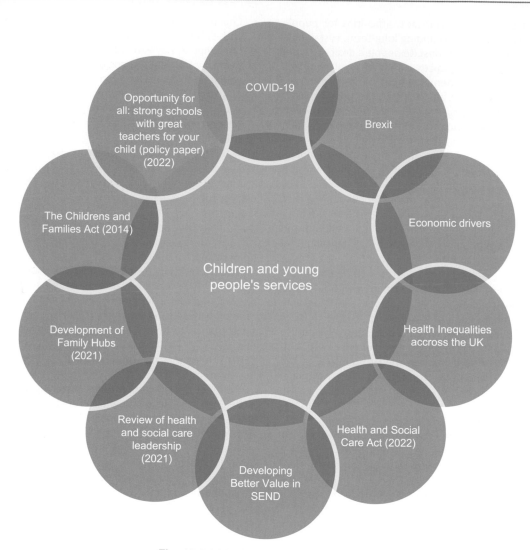

Fig. 10.1 UK influencing drivers.

There are many aspects of the change approach adopted in the case study that deserve greater analysis; however, three key areas will be focused on. The importance of a systems approach, stakeholder involvement, and introduction of OBA were core enablers of the programme.

Getting People Together—'Let's Talk'

At the start of the process, there was a commitment to bringing the system together to guide the strategic direction for SEND services. This included developing a common goal and vision. The stakeholder-led activities formed part of the OBA approach which underpinned the programme of work and was supported by the CDC. From the beginning, there was a commitment from senior leaders to support strong stakeholder engagement including supporting parents and families to be involved and have their voice heard. This approach was important to build trust across the system and parents who often find themselves the position of having to be *'warrior parents'* often having to fight the system and finding *'conflict in place of trust'* (Lamb, 2009; Ofsted, 2021).

The systems commitment was an important factor in the development of both the outcomes approach and as a counterbalance to challenges. This is because, as Evans et al. (2018) reported, when implementing large-scale change

CASE STUDY

The Rochdale system (including education, health, social care, and wider partners) set out an ambitious plan to transform services for children and young people with SEN. A core foundation of this plan was that there was to be focus on making a meaningful improvement to the outcomes of children with SEN and their families, privileging these needs over those of individual organisations and traditional ways of working. This approach included ensuring that all parts of the partnership placed the children and young people at the centre for the integration. At the commencement of the project, three workshops were delivered in the first half of 2021 which brought together key stakeholders from across education, health, social care, and voluntary and community sectors (VCS), and parent carer representatives.

Children and young people had engagement sessions alongside the wider multiagency events. The output of these events was to produce a clearer child-centred vision for the future of SEND services and ensure that the children's and young people's voices were heard and formed part of the planning process. The outcomes identified are presented in Table 10.1. It is important to recognise that as part of this process there were feedback opportunities, and these opportunities enabled the children and young people to remain central to the strategic planning. Feedback from the children directly altered the strategic outcomes, as they were able to comment on wording, emphasis, and meaning to ensure that the final outcomes matched their aspirations for the services that supported them.

TABLE 10.1   Strategic outcomes for an integrated SEND system in Rochdale

My opinions are valued	All children and young people are supported to share their views, taking into account their communication needs, and their thoughts are respected. Children and young people have choices, are allowed to take managed risks, and have a say in their own lives.
I am emotionally well	Children and young people are happy/content and are supported to recover from difficult times. They are mentally healthy and can access good mental health support.
I am as healthy as possible	Young people's health needs are met quickly, they are supported to be active, and pain is well managed.
I am safe and supported at home, at school, and in the community	Young people are well supported by a range of adults who understand what matters to them and how to meet their needs. They have stable and safe home and educational environments, and have access to adequate food, clothing, and living conditions. Safeguarding and mental health support helps young people to be safe.
I am active and involved	I have opportunities in my community. I can choose from a range of groups that meet my interests and needs and I am supported to participate. I can make friends, learn skills, help others, and have fun. I belong to wider networks, and my sensory and social needs are met.
I am hopeful and prepared for the future	I have goals and aspirations for my future. I am supported to take steps towards being independent and am developing life skills and confidence. I have information about jobs and adulthood. I have options and can make my own choices.
Those that care for me are supported	Parent carers, siblings and family, and those who care for me are well supported to do so. They can easily access support for themselves and for me, and do not need to repeat their story to get support.

(Council For Disabled Children, 2022)

which requires the engagement of multiple stakeholders it is to be expected that divergent views amongst stakeholders are likely to occur and these may have a negative impact on any co-ordinated action required for change. This study is supported by several integrated care studies that highlight the need for attention to be given to how stakeholder groups work together. CLAHRC Greater Manchester (2016) highlighted that the hierarchies between different professions may exacerbate difficulties in interdisciplinary work, with professions such as nurses, occupational therapists, and physiotherapists feeling inhibited in expressing their opinions in the presence of professionals they perceive as holding greater power. Mitchell et al. (2020) further highlighted 'social care vs. health service issues', identifying a perception among social care staff that they were dominated by the much larger NHS (health) sector, and this impacted how they felt about their role in integration. These were important considerations when bringing together the system to transform SEND. However, of equal importance was ensuring that the children, families, community, and wider partners also felt they had equity of voice within the meetings. Beacon (2015) cautions that for a shared purpose to be established, core professionals need to develop trusted relationships and work together; they must, however, also recognise the roles of people, the community, and the volunteer sector as these have often been undervalued. Shaw et al. (2011), RAND Europe and Ernst and Young LLP (2012), and Rosen et al. (2011) further this, emphasising that there is a need for any shared vision to include views of those using the service as this will help build staff commitment and a strong sense that integration is doing the right thing. This was achieved within this project through ensuring the following steps were in place: engaged and committed leadership from across the system, facilitated opportunities for sharing opinions and ideas, equity in engagement in the stakeholder events, and keeping focus on supporting successful outcomes for the children and young people and their families.

One practical example of how equity and opportunity for involvement was created was stakeholder engagement for children and young people. These events provided children and young people with their own opportunity to develop the outcomes which the services would be assessed on. The children and young people had additional facilitated meetings in which they could explore what was important to them and provide insight into their experiences. Engaging stakeholders from the early stages of the process enabled a commencement of a discussion on the very relationships that were dominant within how children with SEN were supported. Denis et al. (2011) state that for successful delivery of integrated provision, it is not just the relationship between professionals and organisations that need to change but the wider perceptions that stakeholders have of their roles and relationships must also evolve. This view links with current thinking on asset-based approaches which argue that greater emphasis needs to be given to recognising people assets and strengths (Foot & Hopkins, 2010).

Implementation of an OBA Approach

For the approach adopted by the Rochdale system to be successful, it was important for the team to understand each other and come together under a common set of goals that could inspire change and drive improvement. As discussed earlier, system events were a vital part of this; however, they were only part of the story. The development of the outcomes under the OBA framework enabled the teams to pivot away from output (what is being delivered/how the systems are working) to being outcomes-focused (what difference is being made).

The teams were facilitated using OBA. This model was developed by Mark Friedman (2005) and outlined in his book *Trying Hard Is Not Good Enough*. An OBA framework is a method of enabling organisations and systems to plan, implement, and evaluate a strategic approach. Within the approach, there are two distinct areas of accountability: population accountability and performance accountability.

Birrell and Gray (2018) explain that OBA is driven by data and is action-orientated, taking communities and systems from 'problem-talking' to taking the required actions to solve the problems. However, they caution that it is important to understand that the term 'outcome' is used differently in the OBA framework than in other frameworks. While the framework is data-driven, the outcomes are normative rather than empirical statements.

In this case study, including all stakeholders in the outcome development was key and the team placed a strong emphasis on wide involvement. One example of placing the children and young people at the heart of the process was the returning of the outcomes to the group so they could ensure the outcomes were meaningful; at this stage, changes were made to reflect comments. There were several benefits to this, including developing a strong basis for change, gaining buy-in, developing a common set of goals, and building trust with the children and young people. Once the outcomes were defined, teams worked backwards to identify the means to achieve the outcomes (a process referred to as 'turning the curve').

Birrell and Gray (2018) state that it is also important to consider that, by their very nature, OBA outcomes can be very vague, general, and often unmeasurable. Within the programme of work, this was managed through the development of a logic model to manage the process and link the required outputs to outcomes. Logic modelling is a very useful strategy that breaks down a program to its components, outputs, and outcomes. The logic model correspondingly assists in placing the programme within its context and supports identification of factors affecting program operations and outcomes.

The team identified key learning points in developing outcomes as follows:

- Listen closely to those involved in and impacted by the outcomes
- Work with a wide range of partners
- Ensure the focus remained on children and young people with SEND living a good life
- The system needs to be led by what is needed to deliver and to enable children to reach these positive life outcomes
- Making the important measurable, not the measurable important
- There is importance in developing strong evidence to underpin actions

CONCLUSION

In conclusion, the development of an integrated SEND service to support children and young people was an ambitious and innovative approach to bringing about large-scale change, and an important feature that underpinned the approach was the adoption of the OBA framework. This framework was facilitated by the CDC and placed a strong emphasis on ensuring that the outcomes were meaningful and important to the children, young people, and their families.

References

Beacon, A. (2015). Practice-integrated care teams–learning for a better future. *Journal of Integrated Care, 23*(2), 74–87. https://doi.org/10.1108/JICA-01-2015-0005

Birrell, D., & Gray, A. M. (2018). Outcomes-based approaches and the devolved administrations. In C. Needham, E. Heins, & J. Rees. (Eds.), *Social policy review 30: Analysis and debate in social policy, 2018* (pp. 67–86). Bristol: Policy Press.

Council for Disabled Children. (2022). *Case Study: Developing a strategic outcomes framework and an integrated SEND system in Rochdale*. Rochdale Council: Unpublished internal company document.

CLAHRC Greater Manchester. (2019). *Understanding and supporting the integration of health and social care at a neighbourhood level in the city of Manchester. Report part A: Rapid scoping review*. Manchester: CLAHRC.

Denis, J. L., Davies, H. T. O., Ferlie, E., & Fitzgerald, L. (2011). *Assessing initiatives to transform health care systems: lessons for the Canadian health care system*. Ottawa: Canadian Health Services Research Foundation.

Department of Education. (2022, September 19). *Academic Year 2021/22: Special educational needs in England*. https://explore-education-statistics.service.gov.uk/find-statistics/special-educational-needs-in-england/2021-22#contact-us

Evans, J. M., Grudniewicz, A., & Tsasis, P. (2018). Trial and error, together: divergent thinking and collective learning in the implementation of integrated care networks. *International Review of Administrative Sciences, 84*(3), 452–468. https://doi.org/10.1177/0020852318783063

Foot, J. & Hopkins, T. (2010) *A glass half-full: how an asset approach can improve community health and well-being*. https://www.local.gov.uk/sites/default/files/documents/glass-half-full-how-asset-3db.pdf

Friedman, M. (2015). *Trying Hard Is Not Good Enough*. Bloomington: Trafford Publishing.

Lamb, B. (2009). *Lamb Inquiry: Special Educational Needs and Parental Confidence*. London: DCSF Publications.

Local Government Association. (2022). *Health inequalities:learning disabilities and covid-19*. https://www.local.gov.uk/our-support/safer-and-more-sustainable-communities/health-inequalities-hub/health-inequalities-1

Mitchell, C., Tazzyman, A., Howard, S. J., & Hodgson, D. (2020). More that unites us than divides us? A qualitative study of integration of community health and social care services. *BMC Family Practice, 21*(1), 1–10. https://doi.org/10.1186/s12875-020-01168-z

National Academies of Sciences, Engineering, and Medicine. (2018). *Opportunities for improving programs and services for children with disabilities*. Washington, DC: The National Academies Press.

NHS Digital. (2022). *Rate of Mental disorders among 17-19 year olds increased in 2022*. https://digital.nhs.uk/news/2022/rate-of-mental-disorders-among-17-to-19-year-olds-increased-in-2022-new-report-shows#:~:text=The%20Mental%20Health%20of%20Children,2021%20to%2025.7%25%20in%202022.

Ofsted. (2021, June 16). *Research and analysis: SEND: old issues, new issues, next steps*. https://www.gov.uk/government/publications/send-old-issues-new-issues-next-steps/send-old-issues-new-issues-next-steps

RAND Europe, Ernst & Young LLP. (2012). *National evaluation of the department of health's integrated care pilot*. London: Ernst & Young LLP. https://www.rand.org/content/dam/rand/pubs/technical_reports/2012/RAND_TR1164.pdf.

Rosen, R., Mountford, J., Lewis, G., Lewis, R., Shand, J., & Shaw, S. (2011). *Integration in action: four international case studies*. London: Nuffield Trust.

Shaw, S., Rosen, R., & Rumbold, B. (2011). *What is integrated care*? London: Nuffield Trust.

The Children and Families Act. (2014). London: Stationery Office.

Van Hoofstadt, A., Bastien, T., Maenhout, L., & Cambré, B. (2020). *My Talents. For Diversity: The European research and the lessons learnt*. Antwerp Management School, Antwerp.

White, A., Sheehan, R., Ding, J., Roberts, C., Magill, N., Keagan-Bull, R., Carter, B., Ruane, M., Xiang, X., Chauhan, U., Tuffrey-Wijne, I., & Strydom, A. (2022). *Learning from Lives and Deaths - People with a learning disability and autistic people (LeDeR) report for 2021 (LeDeR 2021)*. London: King's College.

11

Governance and Accountability in Integrated Care

Dr Kirsty Marshall, Jason Gravestock, Dave Wilson,
Paula Bell, and Joanne Finnerty

KEY CONCEPTS

- Governance during change processes
- Accountability across organisations
- Collaboration in health and social care

INTRODUCTION

Ensuring robust governance within any integrated care endeavours is vital, as clear lines of accountability are key to maintaining safety, quality, and effective use of public monies (Kershaw, 2018). This chapter introduces the concepts of governance and accountability and commences by outlining the concepts and context within the sectors engaged in integrated care and then explores challenges and opportunities at different levels (macro, meso, micro). To contextualise the issues, a case study of a project in Greater Manchester which introduced blended roles has been used and the project leads have supported the development of the chapter by providing their insights into their journey.

GOVERNANCE OF INTEGRATED CARE

By its very nature, integrated care requires interorganisational collaboration, which presents a challenge for governance. Integrated care is often delivered on a geographical footprint and has multiple organisations working together (Local Government Association [LGA], 2021). These organisations often come with different levels of governance and accountability as well

as difficult differing legal frameworks (Minkman, 2017). For example, local authorities in the UK have statutory responsibilities, such as licencing, environment protection, care of children, and wider safeguarding responsibility (Ministry of Housing, Communities & Local Government, 2011). There will also be contractual and financial differences across organisations; for example, general practice contracting. There will also be compliance and monitoring requirements within each organisation, such as the Care Quality Commission in the NHS. If these were not complex enough, integrated care aims to bring in wider partners from across a geographical place, including the community, voluntary, and faith sectors and the private sector who may be unfamiliar with the complex governance arrangements found in health, social care, and other statutory bodies. As D'Amour et al. (2008) explain, interprofessional and interorganisational collaboration are impacted by multiple interactional, organisational, and sociopolitical factors. Minkman (2017) also argues that if we are to deliver local (place-based) governance that supports integration around people's needs, there is an imperative to free us from terms such as 'primary care', 'secondary care', and 'tertiary care' or other professional and organisational terms that place divisions into the system, as these build barriers rather than enable integration. Integrated governance is an important factor in overcoming the current fragmented and complex health and social care arrangements which often lead to the people using the services struggling to navigate impersonal and bureaucratic systems.

CASE STUDY

The case study is taken from a project within Tameside, Greater Manchester. The Tameside and Glossop Integrated Care NHS Foundation Trust and the Tameside local authority have been implementing transformation to integrated care since 2016 and this project is one initiative aimed at supporting this transformation. The drivers for the project were the experiences of people living at home and requiring support from multiple agencies. Service users often found care was delivered in a disjointed way and there was a focus on tasks rather than an asset/strength-based approach, and communication between health and social care teams was often poor.

The project aimed to re-design district nurse (NHS) and care worker (private sector commissioned through the local authority) roles and saw some support roles transferred from district nurses to care workers. The transference of roles aimed to improve the quality of home care

delivery, enhance patient/service user experiences, foster better working conditions, and enhance clinical effectiveness. The project also supports a wider re-design of the care worker role, which had seen job roles, pay, and training re-designed to support recruitment, retention, and employee satisfaction in all roles.

The pilot included:
- Introduction of safety huddles for home care providers and district nurse teams
- Introduction of joint care planning and care bundles
- Training and competency framework for care workers
- Greater co-location, spending more time within neighbourhood offices

The initial project focused on pressure-area care with plans to expand to a wider range of other roles. The district nurses provided training and support to care workers who then took on a wider range of activities.

GOVERNANCE AND ACCOUNTABILITY

Governance, put simply, is the act of governing something (Cambridge English Dictionary, 2022). However, when applied to health and social care, governance is a complex and dynamic process across systems, organisations, and professionals. Gordon et al. (2020) explain that governance can be regarded as the interface between governmental policy (system-wide rules) and the strategic decisions of organisational leaders. This interface results in a set of organisational policies and practices that set the acceptable organisational activity.

Within the UK health service, governance is a system through which:

'NHS organisations are accountable for continuously improving the quality of their services and safeguarding high standards of care by creating an environment in which excellence in clinical care will flourish.'

Scally and Donaldson 1998, p.61

Fundamentally, governance in health care involves the process of monitoring systems and delivery to assure patient safety and quality of care across an organisation. These processes include audits and monitoring, risk management, quality and safety performance, and patient safety alongside internal and external monitoring.

The Council of Europe developed 12 principles for good governance (Table 11.1).

The 12 principles demonstrate that alignment can be seen between governance priorities for health and local authorities; however, different lenses, working practices, and political agendas may act as barriers to joint governance arrangements. Minkman (2017) explains that traditional governance *within* organisations does not necessarily transfer to governance *between* organisations, furthering this by stating that when network governance is required it needs to be more horizontal, nonhierarchic, and focus on trust as a basic value.

The requirement for networks based on trust are important in integrated care as there is often a power imbalance between organisations (Ansell & Gash, 2008). An example of this is the 'social care vs. health service issue' described by Mitchell et al. (2020), whose research identified that there is a perception among social care staff that they were dominated by the much larger NHS (health) sector and had the potential to impact their role in integration. This power divide is further magnified when considering the role of the community and voluntary sector within integration. Many integrated care developments, such as integrated care systems (ICSs) in the UK place a strong emphasis on community and voluntary sector involvement; however, there have been countless studies that have highlighted that voluntary sector services do not always get an effective seat at the table during integrated care development (Beacon,

TABLE 11.1   The Council of Europe (2008) 12 Principles

Principle	
1. Fair Conduct of Elections, Representation, and Participation	This principle covers fair elections, including placing citizens at the centre of public activity. The principle highlights the need to ensure all men and women have a voice in decision-making and that attention is given to the inclusion of the voices of the less privileged in society.
2. Responsiveness	Citizen needs are considered when planning objectives, rules and procedures. Complaints are responded to.
3. Efficiency and Effectiveness	Best possible use of resources; performance is monitored (audits).
4. Openness and Transparency	Access to information; public are aware of how decisions are made.
5. Rule of Law	Abiding with the law and judicial decisions.
6. Ethical Conduct	Measures against corruption; public good is placed before individual interest; conflicts of interest are addressed.
7. Competence and Capacity	The skills of those who deliver governance are continually developed.
8. Innovation and Openness to Change	Effective solutions to problems are sought and there is a readiness to be involved in wider projects.
9. Sustainability and Long-term Orientation	Sustainability of community; active plans solve rather than transfer problems to future generations (environmental, structural, financial, economic, or social).
10. Sound Financial Management	Risks are managed; fair sharing of burdens, benefits, and reduction of risks.
11. Human Rights, Cultural Diversity and Social Cohesion	Human rights are respected, protected and implemented; discrimination on any grounds is combated; cultural diversity is an asset.
12. Accountability	Responsibility for decisions whether they be collective or individual.

2015). There are a several reasons for this, including the size of organisations, capability and understanding of complex governance, and structural arrangements of large statutory organisations. Therefore, when considering voluntary and community organisations within ICSs, it is very important that power imbalances are considered in the governance development, ensuring that practical elements such as attendance at meetings is addressed in the early stages to enable full engagement. An area to consider in particular is the impact of the coronavirus pandemic. During the pandemic, many voluntary and community sector organisations were unable to fundraise and this will have an ongoing impact on the funding and capacity going forward. Therefore, when considering inclusion within ICSs, larger statutory organisations need to consider how they use their governance arrangements to support smaller voluntary sector services to engage and contribute (King's Fund, 2022).

Governance arrangements were particularly important within the case study as the project works across different organisations, the NHS, and the local authority. The care staff who would be adopting new roles worked for private sector organisations (commissioned by the local authority). Governance arrangements were further complicated as the project required the movement of roles traditionally done by nursing staff to care staff. This is important as nurses in the UK are governed by their Nursing and Midwifery Council (NMC) professional code of conduct (NMC, 2018) and therefore continue to have accountabilities for all duties or tasks which are delegated onto others. The project managed this through a co-production approach, enabling teams to be active members in the development of the project and raise and discuss accountability and governance questions. They utilised training and a competency framework to ensure safety and audited the process regularly. While the initial project drivers came from capacity and resource management, the project leads ensured that the project centred around the people receiving services, their safety, and service quality. This approach enabled individual members in each team to tap into the shared values that underpin their work and created a positive narrative. Marshall (2020) similarly found that a narrative aligned with the shared values is important in integration as it enables the breaking down of organisational and professional barriers.

Approaches to System Risk

Risk management has been defined as the systematic identification, assessment, and evaluation of risk (Cottee & Harding, 2008). When considering governance in integrated care, risk is particularly important. This can be seen in the case study which demonstrates that, when adopting a place/neighbourhood approach, there will be a process of transforming traditional professional and organisational roles, which introduces risk. In the case study, this was the movement of roles from NHS teams to home care teams. Kerzner (2018) explains that risks arise in projects due to the temporariness and instability brought about by the nature of the project work. These include aspects such as loss of secure relations, sense of reputation, achievement, and professional boundaries. Within integrated care transformations, these risks are carried across multiple organisations, making shared management of these risks and benefits an important aspect of governance arrangements (LGA, 2021). Beacon (2015) explains that there is a need for the development of a shared vision and establishment of a common need amongst partners that enable shared risk, with a recognition of shared benefits across the system. A challenge to the development of shared risk lies in traditional cultural behaviours. Goodwin et al. (2012) highlight that NHS culture demonstrates a fundamentally risk-averse managerial approach and this has the potential to reduce innovation. Therefore, the planning of integration needs to have a risk management plan that enables innovation and positive risk to enable change.

Within the case study, regular discussion of risks started even before the project started and continued throughout. The first example of this was how the project was framed. Initially, there was caution on the movement of activities away from the nurses to home care staff (as discussed previously), and the risk here was being viewed from the service and professional perspective. However, as Stoop et al. (2020) explain in their European case research, older people living within their own home may experience limitations in multiple domains of their life that pose risks to their ability to live safely. Therefore, it is important to view risk from person- and family-centred

perspectives. In taking a person-centred approach to risk, the team were able to frame and discuss the changes from a different perspective. One example was exploring the pathogeneses of everyday tasks. Many of the suggested changes were to enable home care staff to support people with activities they would have previously completed themselves. Traditionally, once a person could not complete a task themselves, nurses were brought in to complete the tasks, therefore medicalising the process. Taking a person-centred view on risk, the team were able to adopt a comprehensive, interdisciplinary, salutogenetic, and proactive approach which reduced the medicalisation of a person's life while also addressing problems and risks of safety at home.

Leadership and Governance

Denis and Gestel (2015) state that for reform to be significant, there needs to be the capacity to bring about changes not only in structures but also in perceptions of roles, practices, and activities. The case study demonstrated that effective leadership in integrated care transformation is vital as it enables actors within the change process the space and permission to challenge and innovate to develop new ways of working. The project benefited from leaders who followed a systems leadership approach. The social care and health leads adopted a shared, participatory, adaptive, and solution-focused leadership approach. Importantly, this scanned across the system and not just within their traditional organisations. One way they demonstrated this approach was through the application of governance. In early meetings, the leaders took the decision to plan and implement relatively quickly, resolving issues as the process developed rather than spending long periods at the start ensuring all processes were planned in advance. For this approach to be successful, those leaders developed a sense of shared accountability, strong communication, and an effective feedback process; any issues could be resolved quickly to maintain safety and quality of care. The process adopted in the case study is reflective of an action-learning set approach, where small groups explore and reflect on actual actions and changes to learn and influence future actions (Walia & Marks-Maran, 2014). In this case study, the project leadership and team met regularly to reflect on processes; manage any challenges, risks, and issues; and plan for next stages. This was particularly useful as it enabled the project to be nimble and adaptive while maintaining governance oversight.

Governance as an enabler rather than a barrier. Permission to challenge past ways of working and the transference of power was cited by the team as an important enabler. The team reported that key to positive risk management and governance was leaders providing permission to change. The approach adopted in the case study was collaborative, flexible, and mixed formal and informal activities. The approach taken followed the three key elements highlighted by Minkman (2017) in that it was horizontal (having the right people from across the organisations, including stakeholders who would be making the changes), nonhierarchic, took a co-production approach, and provided equity of voice in meetings through positive leadership. Finally, trust as a basic value was important as it enabled the building of strong relationships between services and the dismantling of stereotypes and barriers that can derail cross-sector collaborations (Cairns & Harris, 2011).

Governance and population health across an integrated system. As previously discussed in Chapter 1, population health is at the core of integrated care development. However, the adoption of a population health approach requires a significant shifting of focus within systems (Buck et al., 2018). Farmanova et al. (2019) state that for successful integrated care implementation, there needs to be a set of strategies aimed at preventing disease, addressing social determinants of health, and improving health. They suggest that these interventions need to include:

- Focusing on health and wellness
- Embracing intersectoral action and partnerships
- Targeted initiatives to affect health in vulnerable groups
- Re-designed interventions, including creative and innovative ways of addressing clinical and nonclinical issues

The role of the system is important in the development of population health as organisations hold cultural and historical bias that may not align with population health. Tension between organisations may be a barrier to the development of shared governance and accountability (Gordon et al., 2020). Adebowale (2022) explains that the voluntary community and social enterprise sector need to be key and equal partners in the delivery of health and care to enable them to build on the work they undertake in supporting populations. In their analysis of collaborative governance, Ansell and Gash (2008) warn that collaborative governance processes are prone to manipulation by stronger actors within systems if stakeholders do not have the capacity, status, or resources to participate on an equal footing. Furthering this, Gordon et al. (2020) explain that starting conditions need to be addressed for a truly collaborative approach to governance of integrated care to be achieved. Within the case study, the use of informal meetings was seen as key to addressing concerns and building a basis from which to build collaboration. The team stated that, before the project started, there was a process of getting to know each other and each other's

organisation; in doing this, they were able to have cultural conversations that focused the project on the reality of its context.

Meta-Level Governance and Accountability

The World Health Organization (2022) states that leadership and governance require effective oversight, accountability, regulation, coalition-building, and attention to system design. Importantly, they also state that policy frameworks must exist with these requirements to determine both the governance and the health system. Debie et al. (2022) highlight that the pandemic has demonstrated the importance and need for a systems-governance approach.

At a system level, the integration agenda must be underpinned by effective governance arrangements that reflect the responsibility, the stakeholders, and the scale of delivery (Nicholson et al., 2013). Nicholson et al. (2013) emphasise the importance of gaining consensus about integration targets which must be put into a strategic framework and agreed upon by partners to fulfil common integration goals. An example of this can be seen in the Greater Manchester (GM) Health and Social Care Partnership, which was established with 37 NHS organisations and councils and has the mandate to oversee devolution, when GM received a £6-billion health and social care budget from the central government in 2016 (GMCA, 2015a, 2015b). As part of the Memorandum of Understanding between organisations, there was a clear commitment to a joint governance and financial pathways which built on existing partnership arrangements and would strengthen them. The GM model is significant as it starts with system-level engagement and the building of a framework that enabled the multiple organisations to align within the system.

Alongside ensuring there is an effective framework for change, the system 'meta' level needs to set and guide the strategic vision and goals, as these are important enablers in the development of integrated care and its underpinning governance. To be effective, strategic alignment needs to inspire and speak to the shared values of multiple stakeholders to enable people to challenge and test traditional boundaries. Marshall (2020) found that in the development of neighbourhoods, team members would deconstruct and use visions to support the change processes, creating lived visions that were meaningful for them and their service users (discussed further in Chapter 16).

Within the case study, strategic alignment was important as it enabled the project to be embedded within a larger framework and, importantly, gain system-level support for implementation. One way the project team achieved strategic alignment was positioning the project within the GM Adult Social Care Transformation programme priorities 'Living well at home' and being a trailblazer project. This approach anchored the project but also enabled effective reporting, spread, and adoption. Another advantage of placing the project with the wider 'meta' or system level was the ability to draw down knowledge and resources. An example of this was that the project was able to link with the system-level quality improvement (QI) teams who could advise on QI methodology and provide project structure, thus enabling wider dissemination of results and lessons.

Meso-Level—Organisational Governance and Accountability

When organisations move towards integrated care developments, there is an acknowledgment that individual organisations cannot tackle 'wicked' societal problems alone, and that collaboration, shared risk, and accountability are needed to begin to build more effective solutions (Emerson et al., 2012). Organisations need to be in a place where they understand their interdependence (Bryson et al., 2015). However, there are significant challenges in collaborative approaches even when all partners are engaged and supportive of partnerships (Coxon, 2005). The very complex nature of these partnerships makes them challenging and often leads those within the system to have a reduced understanding of the ambition of the integration or partnership (Smith & Barnes, 2013).

At a system level, it is important not to make assumptions regarding organisational commitment towards the networks and integration as these may not automatically present. This will impact on the development of shared risk and governance (Minkman, 2017). Gordon et al. (2020) state that attention needs to be given to bringing together partners as institutional design is vital, as it sets the basic ground rules for collaboration and can act as an enabler or barrier to the development of shared governance. The framework for collaborative governance Emerson et al. (2012) identifies several important drivers, including leadership, resources, setting a tone of collaboration, and distribution of power.

Within the case study, each organisation had motivating factors for engaging in the programme of work and development of shared governance. The district nurses needed to release capacity and the social home care model needed to evolve to provide greater job satisfaction and career progression; together, they held the shared motivator of improving care for people within their own homes and preventing unnecessary hospitalisation. These motivators became the drivers and enablers to support teams to challenge their traditional models and adopt new working practices, which was supported by positive leadership.

A wide range of previous research has discussed the inherent and multiple complexities, conflicts, and inconsistencies within cross-sector alliances and partnerships (Cairns & Harris, 2011; Cramm et al., 2013; Radermacher et al., 2011). It is important to note that, when considering the development of governance structures, that there is a cultural organisational shift required to enable partnerships to flourish and enable what Emerson et al. (2012) call principled engagement. Principled engagement enables people with differing contexts and organisations to develop relational and identity goals that work across their respective institutional, sectoral, or jurisdictional boundaries. This enables them to solve problems, resolve conflicts, and create value. Importantly, this approach requires organisational leadership at all levels and a leadership approach that is comfortable working across systems (leadership is covered in Chapter 9). In the case study, principled engagement was present through the involvement of key leaders in health and social care but also in engaging those who would affect and were affected by the change; for example, district nurses who would be delegating responsibilities and home care teams who would be adopting new working practices and responsibilities. A key leader within the project was the district nurse team leader, as she needed to create an environment that was enabling of change and ensure that governance arrangements would be robust but also enable positive risk within professional boundaries.

Meso-Professional-Level Governance and Accountability

The meso level moves from organisational governance to how actors within the field of health and social care work within governance arrangements. Taking a system-wide approach provides challenges and opportunities and how shared governance and accountability is a key enabler (Chapter 13). Chapter 19 explores in greater detail the importance of professional practice within an integrated framework and learning from, with, and about each other in interprofessional education and interprofessional development.

The case study presented in this chapter highlights several real-life governance and accountability challenges faced when moving to more integrated practice, and these challenges can be transposed to several situations faced in integration. One key issue is that of professional boundaries and cultures. Professional groups within health and social care have strong professional identities developed during their education and work life (Cairns & Harris, 2011). As explained in the seminal work of Tajfel

(1974) and Tajfel (2010), people hold multiple social identities which are formed through dynamic, contextual, and responsive processes. Importantly, people hold an emotional significance to this social classification and these social identities become part of our self-concept. A consequence of this social grouping is that individuals engage in assessments and comparisons which reinforce group membership and the othering of those from other groups. This is important when considering the dynamics of governance at a professional level as consideration needs to be given to how group identity may act as a barrier to the adoption of new working arrangements. An example can be seen in the CLAHRC Greater Manchester (2019) report that found that medical culture could present a difficulty in integration as professions such as nurses, occupational therapists, and physiotherapists may feel inhibited in expressing their opinions and reducing challenges.

Professional identity is often reinforced through professional standards and regulations which underpin each professional group and act to provide an ethical framework for practice. These standards are important as they guide professional practice and, importantly, their scope is to protect the public, but they are often risk-adverse, and do not sit comfortably in a changing professional environment (Stahlke Wall, 2018). If we consider the change in the case study, the nurse's underpinning framework is the NMC code of conduct and they will have considered this during the implementation. For example, the code states that nurses are accountable for their decisions to delegate tasks and duties to other people and should only delegate duties that are within the other person's scope of competence (NMC, 2018). To ensure engagement of the nurses within our case study, these professional standards were brought into the change processes and underpinned the design, including named delegation, a competency framework, training, shared documentation, and audits. The adopted approach turned governance into an enabler for change and integration by ensuring safe and compassionate care which built confidence and trust between teams.

Impact on People's Accountability to Local People and Patients

The principles behind the practice of integrated care teams are that patients should be empowered to self-manage their conditions, understand their needs, and manage their own health and health care (Beacon, 2015). However, Minkman (2017) found that clients are not always considered and, if clients are involved, this is often via the professionals rather than through co-produced health. Integrated governance needs to be developed in a way that enables people to have more control of their

care and decisions regarding their health and wellbeing. This will require the system to redress its relationship with each other and with the communities and individuals they service. Morton and Paice (2016) describe a strategic co-production approach adopted in northwest London. The initiative saw lay partners included in the strategic design process where they were encouraged to provide challenges, encourage innovation, improve communication, and hold partners to account to ensure people remained central to the development and pushing the agendas further. They adopted the principle that everyone comes to the table as an equal partner: lay people were viewed as bringing experiences and skills and an understanding of the communities that they lived in, and this approach enabled a cultural shift in professional perspectives and enhanced the programme development. This approach can be seen during the development and implementation of the case study and continues to be the approach taken for new projects.

CONCLUSION

To conclude, during the development of the 'blended roles' project, there was a consistent approach of system leadership to bring together a range of stakeholders to develop new and equitable models of care delivery. The team focused on meaningful and significant reform to bring about changes that were not only in structures but also supported the cultural, role, and practice changes. The case study demonstrated that effective leadership in integrated care transformation is vital as it enables actors within the change process the space and permission to challenge and innovate to develop new ways of working.

References

Adebowale, V. (2022). *The voluntary sector: a game-changer in integrated care systems*. https://www.nhsconfed.org/articles/voluntary-sector-game-changer-integrated-care-systems

Ansell, C., & Gash, A. (2008). Collaborative governance in theory and practice. *Journal of Public Administration Research and Theory*, *18*(4), 543–571. https://doi.org/10.1093/jopart/mum032

Beacon, A. (2015). Practice-integrated care teams–learning for a better future. *Journal of Integrated Care*, *23*(2), 74–87. https://doi.org/10.1108/JICA-01-2015-0005

Bryson, J. M., Crosby, B. C., & Stone, M. M. (2015). Designing and implementing cross-sector collaborations: needed and challenging. *Public Administration Review*, *75*(5), 647–663. https://doi.org/10.1111/puar.12432

Buck, D., Baylis, A., Dougall, D., & Robertson, R. (2018). *A vision for population health: towards a healthier future*. London: King's Fund.

Cairns, B., & Harris, M. (2011). Local cross-sector partnerships: tackling the challenges collaboratively. *Nonprofit Management & Leadership, 21*(3), 311–324. https://doi.org/10.1002/nml.20027

Cambridge English Dictionary. (2022). Cambridge: Cambridge University Press.

Cottee, C., & Harding, K. (2008). Risk management in obstetrics. *Obstetrics, Gynaecology & Reproductive Medicine, 18*(6), 155–162. https://doi.org/10.1016/j.ogrm.2008.04.003

CLAHRC Greater Manchester. (2019). *Understanding and supporting the integration of health and social care at a neighbourhood level in the city of Manchester: Report part A: Rapid scoping review*. Manchester: CLAHRC.

Council of Europe. (2008). *12 Principles of Good Governance*. https://www.coe.int/en/web/good-governance/12-principles#{%2225565951%22:[11]}

Coxon, K. (2005). Common experiences of staff working in integrated health and social care organisations: a European perspective. *Journal of Integrated Care, 13*(2), 13–21. https://doi.org/10.1108/14769018200500012

Cramm, J. M., Phaff, S., & Nieboer, A. P. (2013). The role of partnership functioning and synergy in achieving sustainability of innovative programmes in community care. *Health & Social Care in the Community, 21*(2), 209–215. https://doi.org/10.1111/hsc.12008

D'amour, D., Goulet, L., Labadie, J. -F., Martin-Rodriguez, L. S., & Pineault, R. (2008). A model and typology of collaboration between professionals in healthcare organizations. *BMC Health Services Research, 8*(1), 1–14. https://doi.org/10.1186/1472-6963-8-188

Debie, A., Khatri, R. B., & Assefa, Y. (2022). Successes and challenges of health systems governance towards universal health coverage and global health security: a narrative review and synthesis of the literature. *Health Research Policy and Systems, 20*(1), 1–17. https://doi.org/10.1186/s12961-022-00858-7

Denis, J. L., & Gestel, N. V. (2015). Leadership and innovation in healthcare governance. In E. Kuhlmann, R. H. Blank, I. L. Bourgeault, & C. Wendt (Eds.), *The Palgrave international handbook of healthcare policy and governance* (pp. 425–440). London: Palgrave Macmillan.

Emerson, K., Nabatchi, T., & Balogh, S. (2012). An integrative framework for collaborative governance. *Journal of Public Administration Research and Theory, 22*(1), 1–29. https://doi.org/10.1093/jopart/mur011

Farmanova, E., Baker, G. R., & Cohen, D. (2019). Combining integration of care and a population health approach: a scoping review of redesign strategies and interventions, and their impact. *International Journal of Integrated Care, 19*(2), 5. https://doi.org/10.5334/ijic.4197

Greater Manchester Combined Authority (GMCA). (2015a). *Taking charge of our health and social care in Greater Manchester*. http://greatermanchester-ca.gov.uk/download/downloads/id/125/taking_charge_of_our_health_and_social_car e_in_greater_manchester.pdf

Greater Manchester Combined Authority (GMCA). (2015b). *Greater Manchester Health and Social Care Devolution-Memorandum of Understanding*. http://web.archive.org/web/20150404034051/http:/www.agma.gov.uk/cms_media/files/mou.pdf

Goodwin, N., Smith, J., Davies, A., Perry, C., Rosen, R., Dixon, A., Dixon, J., & Ham, C. (2012). *Integrated care for patients and populations: improving outcomes by working together*. London: King's Fund.

Gordon, D., McKay, S., Marchildon, G., Bhatia, R. S., & Shaw, J. (2020). Collaborative governance for integrated care: insights from a policy stakeholder dialogue. *International Journal of Integrated Care, 20*(1), 3. https://doi.org/10.5334/ijic.4684

Kershaw, M. (2018). *Developing governance to support integrated care: a bumpy ride?* https://www.kingsfund.org.uk/blog/2018/10/developing-governance-support-integrated-care-bumpy-ride

Kerzner, H. (2018). *Project management best practices: Achieving global excellence*. London: John Wiley & Sons.

Kings Fund. (2022). *Integrated care systems explained: making sense of systems, places and neighbourhoods*. https://www.kingsfund.org.uk/publications/integrated-care-systems-explained

Local Government Association. (2021). Must know: Integrated health and care - How do you know your council is doing all it can to promote integration to improve health and social care outcomes at a time of change? https://www.local.gov.uk/publications/must-know-integrated-health-and-care-how-do-you-know-your-council-doing-all-it-can

Marshall, K. (2020). *An exploration of neighbourhood team members experiences of the transition from traditional health and social care teams to integrated care systems, within a defined health and social care economy* (Publication number – 595618) [Professional Doctorate thesis, University of Salford].

Minkman, M. M. (2017). Longing for integrated care: the importance of effective governance. *International Journal of Integrated Care, 17*(4), 10. https://doi.org/10.5334/ijic.3510

Ministry of Housing, Communities & Local Government. (2011). *Review of local government statutory duties: summary of responses*. https://www.gov.uk/government/publications/review-of-local-government-statutory-duties-summary-of-responses--2

Mitchell, C., Tazzyman, A., Howard, S. J., & Hodgson, D. (2020). More that unites us than divides us? A qualitative study of integration of community health and social care services. *BMC Family Practice, 21*(1), 1–10. https://doi.org/10.1186/s12875-020-01168-z

Morton, M., & Paice, E. (2016). Co-production at the strategic level: co-designing an integrated care system with lay partners in North West London, England. *International Journal of Integrated Care, 16*(2), 2. https://doi.org/10.5334/ijic.2470

Nicholson, C., Jackson, C., & Marley, J.A. (2013). Governance model for integrated primary/secondary care for the health-reforming first world – results of a systematic review. *BMC Health Services Research, 13*, 528. https://doi.org/10.1186/1472-6963-13-528. Erratum in: *BMC Health Services Research, 17*(1), 569. https://doi.org/10.1186/s12913-017-2444-4

Nursing & Midwifery Council. (2018). *The code: Professional standards of practice and behaviour for nurses, midwives and nursing associates.* http://www.nmc.org.uk/globalassets/sitedocuments/nmc-publications/revised-new-nmc-code.pdf

Radermacher, H., Karunarathna, Y., Grace, N., & Feldman, S. (2011). Partner or perish? Exploring inter-organisational partnerships in the multicultural community aged care sector. *Health & Social Care in the Community, 19*(5), 550–560. https://doi.org/10.1111/j.1365-2524.2011.01007.x

Scally, G., & Donaldson, L. J. (1998). Clinical governance and the drive for quality improvement in the new NHS in England. *BMI, 317*(7150), 61–65. https://doi.org/10.1136/bmj.317.7150.61

Smith, N., & Barnes, M. (2013). New jobs old roles – working for prevention in a whole system model of health and social care for older people. *Health & Social Care in the Community, 21*(1), 79–87. https://doi.org/10.1111/j.1365-2524.2012.01089.x

Stahlke Wall, S. (2018). The impact of regulatory perspectives and practices on professional innovation in nursing. *Nursing Inquiry, 25*(1). https://doi.org/10.1111/nin.12212

Stoop, A., Lette, M., Ambugo, E. A., Gadsby, E. W., Goodwin, N., MacInnes, J., Minkman, M., Wistow, G., Zonneveld, N., Nijpels, G., Baan, C. A., de Bruin, S. R., & SUSTAIN Consortium. (2020). Improving person-centredness in integrated care for older people: experiences from thirteen integrated care sites in Europe. *International Journal of Integrated Care, 20*(2), 16. https://doi.org/10.5334/ijic.5427

Tajfel, H. (1974). Social identity and intergroup behaviour. *Information, International Social Science Council, 13*(2), 65–93. https://doi.org/10.1177/053901847401300204

Tajfel, H. (Ed.). (2010). *Social identity and intergroup relations* (vol. 7). Cambridge: Cambridge University Press.

Walia, S., & Marks-Maran, D. (2014). Leadership development through action learning sets: an evaluation study. *Nurse Education in Practice, 14*(6), 612–619. https://doi.org/10.1016/j.nepr.2014.06.004

World Health Organization. (2022). *Effective Health System Governance for Universal Health Coverage UHC.* https://www.who.int/health-topics/health-systems-governance

Further Reading

Report

Nesta. (2013). *Co-production catalogue.* http://www.nesta.org.uk/publications/co-production-catalogue

Articles

Ansell, C., & Gash, A. (2008). Collaborative governance in theory and practice. *Journal of Public Administration Research and Theory, 18*(4), 543–571. https://doi.org/10.1093/jopart/mum032

Gordon, D., McKay, S., Marchildon, G., Bhatia, R. S., & Shaw, J. (2020). Collaborative governance for integrated care: insights from a policy stakeholder dialogue. *International Journal of Integrated Care, 20*(1), 3. https://doi.org/10.5334/ijic.4684

12

Social Prescribing Within an Integrated System

Dr Michelle Howarth, Dr Michaela Rogers, and Lynne Bowers

KEY CONCEPTS

- Social prescribing
- Asset-based community development
- Health disparities
- Personalised care

INTRODUCTION

In this chapter, we will explore the concept of social prescribing and how this approach to wellbeing has enabled communities and individuals to take more control of their wellbeing. The chapter will explicate the social prescribing movement within the context of the NHSE Personalised Care movement. A focus on the operationalisation of social prescribing through asset-based community approaches will be used to explore how health disparities can be addressed through an integrated agenda.

Traditional medical responses based on a pathogenic paradigm do little to stem or support the growing numbers of long-term conditions both in the UK and globally. Alternative nonmedical approaches based on asset-based community methods have been used as part of a 'social prescription' to promote wellbeing for a range of populations (Howarth et al., 2020). Social prescribing provides a holistic model predicated on the need for integrated working thats empower communities and individuals. This chapter will discuss how social prescribing schemes use integrated methods of working to support personalised approaches to care for individuals and communities. The evidence-based case study about Alice will help the reader to explore how social prescribing has supported an individual's wellbeing through a range of nonmedical services. The chapter will explicate how integrated working is used within social prescribing to help reduce health disparities and support collaborative communities.

WHAT IS SOCIAL PRESCRIBING?

In 2007, the Government Policy review highlighted the import of a personalised approach in supporting the individual in decision-making – they stated, *'the overall vision is that the state should empower citizens to shape their own lives and the services they receive'* (HM Government, 2007). Since this time, social prescribing has gained momentum as an asset-based movement (described below) that utilises personalised approaches to support those most in need. There are a range of definitions of social prescribing. However, the National Academy of Social Prescribing (NASP) has defined social prescribing as a process that supports people *'via social prescribing link workers, to make community connections and discover new opportunities, building on individual strengths and preferences, to improve health and wellbeing'* (NASP, 2020). Social prescribing is a process used to refer people with nonclinical needs to a community link worker to facilitate a wellbeing conversation with the aim of determining 'what matters' to the person, rather than determining 'what is the matter with a person' (National Health Service England [NHSE], 2019). This approach is underpinned by a salutogenic paradigm that underpins the question 'what makes people healthy' rather than 'how do we treat disease'. Salutogenic approaches are predicated on a person's strengths rather than their deficits (Henry & Howarth, 2018) and offer a promising means of supporting the wellbeing of people and communities. Howarth et al. (2020) argue that the approach mirrors that supported through social prescribing because of the precedent placed on the person, as opposed to the illness.

Increasing numbers of people with long-term conditions has led to a call to prioritise how we can keep people well through lifestyle choices and improved resilience. This call to action, initiated in the original Marmot report (2010) and further highlighted in the NHS Five Year Forward View (Department of Health, 2014), has helped secure asset-based approaches as one of the key strategies in promoting wellbeing (Howarth & Donovan, 2019). Additionally, the recently formed Office for Health Improvement and Disparities (n.d.) is working with integrated services to help improve health and *on levelling up health disparities to break the link between background and prospects for a healthy life*.

'Asset-based' community approaches that utilise community groups to support resilience can be prescribed through a social prescription. Arguably, engaging fully in community life and groups can promote good physical and mental health by focusing on the things that matter most (NHSE, 2019). Community assets are typically delivered through the third sector ecosystem, such as the voluntary, community & social enterprise (VCSE) sector, housing, welfare, and private industries, which help to reduce health and social inequalities. Social prescribing is gaining momentum and is frequently being used by health professionals (Husk et al., 2017). Whilst the concept of social prescribing is considered to be a contemporary revolution, its origins can be located within asset-based community approaches, familiar to many community-based nurses (Hopkins & Rippon, 2015). The use of community assets to support the wellbeing of individuals has arguably been a staple of the VCSE, who have provided support and guidance for communities over the last 20 years. It is reported that these asset-based approaches have gained popularity because of their ability to help tackle health disparities through utilisation of community resources (Cassetti et al., 2020). Social prescribing has emerged as a movement that uses asset-based, nonmedical approaches to support wellbeing (Howarth & Lister, 2019). Social prescription schemes are largely funded through primary care networks (PCNs) or well-established community voluntary sectors (CVSs). However, the range of services that they can refer to often fall out of the PCN offer and predominantly involve the VCSE. There is a myriad of services which provide nonmedical opportunities that support wellbeing. This can include gardening clubs, yoga groups, and walking associations, through to more developed social prescribing schemes operated within the PCNs and integrated care systems (ICSs). Whilst the VCSE sector provides the majority of social prescription provision, private organisations can also provide socially prescribed services. However, the evidence-base reporting on the impact of social prescribing is mixed, largely due to the diverse interventions and models used that have unpredictable outcomes and are a challenge to measure (Cassetti et al., 2020). Other challenges predicated on a lack of sustainable funding have also been reported which has resulted in a lack of investment for VCSE and local authority provision. Limitations caused through funding disparities have caused some resentment towards a centralised NHS-led approach that has seemingly funded link workers without also funding the referral destination.

Salutogenesis

Furthering the introduction to salutogenesis in Chapter 3, we explore the subject here within the context of social prescribing. In advocating the wider determinants of health, there is increasing recognition for nonmedical approaches that support wellbeing, as opposed to just supporting health, prompting an emerging critique questioning the effectiveness of the pathogenic model (Howarth & Lister, 2019). Global interest in salutogenic approaches that prioritise the wider determinants of health as part of the life continuum has been stimulated by these critiques. Antonovsky's (1967) salutogenic model is most frequently cited as an established public health concept because it advocates the individual's capacity and ability to utilise resources that create health and wellbeing and help develop a 'sense of coherence' (Lindström & Eriksson, 2005). This is reflected through a paradigm shift within global health policy, which has influenced the development of service models predicated on an asset-based rather than deficit-based approach.

As a salutogenic approach, social prescribing involves focusing on personalised approaches that prioritise the individual in decision-making based on their needs and not just their pathogenic state (NHSE, 2019). These nonmedical approaches have been embedded within public health policies as key strategies to promote wellbeing (Cook et al., 2019). Subsequently, there is now an emphasis on health systems to move away from medical-based, curative, pathogenic models towards person-centred, integrated care that meets a person's individualized needs (World Health Organization [WHO], 2015).

These shifts represent worldwide changes as contemporary public health strategies that promote wellbeing through global health initiatives (Cook et al., 2019) and social prescribing are increasingly recognised as effective solutions to help ameliorate the preconditions of chronic diseases. Arguably, these dichotomous paradigms of pathogenesis and salutogenesis are reflected in the WHO's 1948 original definition of health, which highlights wellbeing *and* health as key aspects of health and *not merely the absence of disease or infirmity*'. Thus, salutogenic principles may have historically performed an intrinsic role, albeit they have gotten lost in the dominance of pathogenic approaches. Importantly, salutogenic principles resonate with the individual's functional ability which incorporates both the person's inherent capacity and the physical and social environments they interact with (WHO, 2017). Moreover, salutogenic approaches are ideal in the support of people living in poverty or deprivation because the focus on the person and the wider determinants of health and wellbeing can facilitate an empowering approach that is able to support the social capital of a community through asset-based practices.

How Social Prescribing Promotes Integrated Working

According to McManus et al. (2016), long-term conditions (LTCs) often manifest in increased general practitioner (GP) attendance for social rather than clinical issues. People with LTCs present with comorbidities that require complex, multidisciplinary, and multiagency integrated working (Howarth et al., 2020). Many people with LTCs represent populations from some of the most deprived communities (Marmot, 2010). Marmot et al.'s (2010) Fair Society report highlighted the symbiotic relationship between social and health inequalities. In 2020, Polley argued that Marmot's seminal report was influential in changing mindsets within the health sector and lent credibility to the asset-based approaches used within social prescription. Personal support offered to individuals with complex needs can often involve working across agencies and disciplines such as housing, health, and social welfare (Polley et al., 2020), often requiring a level of integration that enables a more holistic response to that individual. However, there are recognised barriers to effective integrated working caused by data protection issues, lack of a single data entry for people, and limited understanding of the beneficiary journey. The lack of integrated systems, poor communication, competing or different demands or objectives can lead to practical difficulties in implementation.

ICSs have the potential to alleviate some of the challenges to integrated working. ICSs are NHS bodies that aim to produce the strategic direction of integrated care and bring together organisations that will help improve population health and tackle health disparities. This partnership will collaborate in bringing a wide range of system partners together that will work to address health, social, and public health needs. They are based on a collaborative paradigm and, in recognition that the VCSE sector is a key partner in the integration of services, the model is designed to embrace the VCSE sector as equal partners.

In doing so, nonmedical approaches, services, and social prescribing schemes that operate as part of the wider VCSE sector have an opportunity to work within an ICS to ensure that services are truly integrated. According to the ICS guidance on partnerships in the VCSE sector, 'VCSE is a key strategic partner in helping shape, improve and deliver services' (NHS England, n.d.). There is a strong emphasis on 'place-based' partnerships that work alongside the NHS, council, local authority, and VCSE organisations through *'close working with the sector as a strategic partner in shaping, improving and delivering services, as well as developing and delivering plans to tackle the wider determinants of health'* (NHS England, 2021). Since 2018, the VCSE sector has actively participated in a leadership system to enable VCSE organisations to facilitate partnership working. The programme was also designed to support the work of the VCSE sector and create impactful alliances within the ICSs. There is now a greater incentive for the VCSE sector to be integrated within ICSs so that they are able to provide sustainable support. According to Charles (2021), major questions exist pertaining to the operationalisation of the partnership and how care and health partnerships will work and relate to each other. For example, isolated voices from the VCSE sector or local authorities may face challenges in terms of representation amidst the predominance of the NHS. Integrated working and proactive mindsets are required at the start to ensure that non-healthcare organisational voices are not minimised.

Brymer et al. (2019) state that there are a range of activities that can be used to promote health and wellbeing for people who may be vulnerable or who are socially excluded. Subsequently, there has been a rise in the use of asset-based community approaches to integrate nature as a means of improving the wellbeing of the community (Burls, 2007) with an emerging evidence base to suggest that this is also beneficial in engaging vulnerable or socially excluded communities (Marmot, 2010). The appetite for nature-based interventions presents an opportunity to embed salutogenic principles as a social prescription that could benefit vulnerable or socially excluded people. For example, evidence suggests that socially prescribed nature-based activities can reduce social isolation and improve social connectedness (Howarth et al., 2016).

The following case study illustrates how multiple agencies and organisations collaborated through

---

CASE STUDY   Alice 'With the Trousers'

Alice, a 74-year-old woman, attends Newtown Women's Aid which is led by Mary (all people and organisations referred to in this case study are anonymised for confidentiality purposes). Newtown Women's Aid is a domestic violence and abuse (DVA) specialist service offering refuge accommodation and community-based support. When Alice

CASE STUDY   Alice 'With the Trousers'—cont'd

started attending a craft session run by Newtown Women's Aid, she confided that this was the first time in decades that she had been able to get out of the family home and engage in an activity without her husband, Arthur. Alice had been married to Arthur for 56 years and they had three adult children who lived in other parts of the country.

Over time, Alice let small details slip into the conversation with Mary about the ways in which Arthur had controlled Alice and her life, limiting her ability to forge friendships or develop interests outside of the family home. Eventually she disclosed that Arthur had been controlling, manipulative, and emotionally abusive throughout their marriage and that during the early years he had been physically violent. Alice had been terrorised within her own home, forced into adopting a regime where she was not allowed to work or to make her own decisions. Arthur decided what Alice would wear, who she could talk to, and where she could go.

Over the past 5 years, 76-year-old Arthur's mobility had deteriorated after a fall. He was more reliant on Alice than ever before. Alice too had declining mobility due to arthritis. With Arthur in tow (he did not allow Alice to attend appointments alone), Alice had visited her doctor to discuss the management of her arthritis. Her doctor felt that engaging in a weekly physical activity would help prevent further deterioration in her mobility (and the social isolation that he suspected Alice was experiencing). The doctor suggested that he made a referral to a social prescribing link worker, who could work with Alice to understand what matters to her and identify how her physical activity could be supported. Alice met with Daisy, the social prescribing link worker who referred Alice to the Newtown Gardening Group. Arthur (reluctantly) agreed as he needed Alice to be physically able to care for him and manage his needs. Alice thrived on the contact with other older people and on engaging with nature and nature-based activities.

Alice begun to work with Daisy, and, with regular support from Daisy, Alice decided that she wanted to leave Arthur and enjoy the rest of her life abuse-free. Daisy liaised with Newtown Women's Aid to prepare a package of support and with the local housing office to secure Alice a small flat in sheltered housing with a scheme manager living on-site to support residents. Alice flourished. She continued to attend Newtown Gardening Group and each week she also attended the craft session run by Newtown Women's Aid. One week she turned up to the craft session wearing a pair of trousers. Arthur had restricted Alice's autonomy, and controlled everyday aspects of her life, to the extent to which Alice had never been 'allowed' to wear trousers in her adult years; this was an empowering moment for Alice (who became known as 'Alice with the trousers').

The remit of Newtown Women's Aid was to deliver specialist services and they also did awareness-raising and training of other practitioner groups. The chief officer, Mary, realised that older people like Alice were a hidden group of victims/survivors and she organised a programme of work that included training religious leaders across the region on the complexities of DVA and barriers to help-seeking, as well as a number of events where she would go to community church groups to talk about DVA. Alice volunteered and worked with Mary to raise awareness of DVA amongst older communities. Alice gained a sense of reward at being able to contribute to conversations that might help someone like her recognise their experiences of abuse and seek help. Through working with Daisy and Newtown Women's Aid, Alice had found her voice.

The integrated approaches used within Alice's case study highlights the multiple agencies involved in a social prescription. The need to ensure that Alice's needs were identified and that what matters to Alice was prioritised meant that several agencies worked together to ensure the support and safety of Alice.

---

social prescribing to support an older lady regain her independence.

Impact on Older People

Alternative nonmedical approaches based on asset-based methods have been used as part of a 'social prescription' to promote wellbeing for a range of populations (Howarth & Lister, 2019). Hence, the impact of social prescribing has far-reaching consequences and influences an individual's mental, physical, and spiritual wellbeing (Polley et al., 2020). Social prescribing is increasingly recognised as an effective solution to

help ameliorate the preconditions of chronic diseases and social issues that characterise this age cohort as, across the globe, it is reported that the impact of reduced social contact and greater isolation can worsen associated poor health outcomes (Perissonotto et al., 2012). For example, this is indicated by increased mental health difficulties, which can subsequently lead to depression and social isolation and exacerbate the vulnerability of older people (WHO, 2017). However, traditional medical responses which integrate a pathogenic paradigm do little to stem or support the complexity of older people's health and wellbeing needs.

As highlighted in the case study of Alice, older people in particular are thought to benefit from nature; studies have reported that engagement with nature can increase longevity (Takano et al., 2002). Significantly, nature-based activity can help reduce and slow down decline in physical health and limit the effect of LTCs, such as reducing the incidence of diabetes (Dalton et al., 2016). Access to nature-based activities can influence wellbeing for a range of populations, but it is reported to have significant benefits for older adults (Brymer et al., 2019). It is understood that older people may not exercise as often as required because of the negative impact that the ageing process has on health and mobility (McPhee et al., 2016). Poor health and comorbid conditions represent major barriers that preclude older adults from getting outdoors and engaging with nature which can increase social isolation (McPhee et al., 2016). Hence, access to nature is important and, equally, the ability to access a green space that is close by can significantly improve social interaction (Cook et al., 2019).

CONCLUSION

This chapter has argued for social prescription as an alternative, nonmedical approach as effective in treating health needs for a range of populations. Social prescription and its underpinning asset-based community methods are rooted in salutogenesis, an established public health concept that moves away from a deficit-based approach and instead takes an individual's ability to utilise resources to enhance their health and wellbeing as the point of departure. The case study of Alice illuminates the ways in which social prescribing can be delivered across services through an integrated, collaborative approach and in ways which are holistic and person-centred. The case study also draws attention to the effects of social prescription and the ways in which it was experienced by Alice as empowering, enabled through her partnership with Mary and Daisy. By offering a case study centring on Alice, the chapter highlights the ways that social prescribing can be effective with a specific target population. The notion that social prescription can benefit older people is highlighted through an increasing evidence base which simultaneously demonstrates how both chronic disease and social conditions often associated with older age (such as isolation) can be addressed by personalised social prescription. Finally, whilst this evidence base illustrates the benefits of social prescription for older people, additional research also highlights the value of asset-based approaches for other populations and, as such, the great potential for improved physical, mental, and spiritual welbeing.

References

Antonovsky, A. (1967). *Unravelling the mystery of health. How people manage stress and stay well.* San Francisco: Jossey-Bass.

Brymer, E., Freeman, E., & Richardson, M. (2019). Editorial: one health: the well-being impacts of human-nature relationships. *Frontiers in Psychology, 10*, 1611. https://doi.org/10.3389/fpsyg.2019.01611

Burls, A. (2007). People and green spaces: promoting public health and mental well-being through ecotherapy. *Journal of Public Mental Health, 6*(3), 24–39. https://doi.org/10.1108/17465729200700018

Cassetti, V., Powell, K., Barnes, A., & Sanders, T. (2020). A systematic scoping review of asset-based approaches to promote health in communities: development of a framework. *Global Health Promotion, 27*(3), 15–23. https://doi.org/10.1177/1757975919848925

Charles, A. (2021, August 19). Integrated care systems explained: making sense of systems, places and neighbourhoods. https://www.kingsfund.org.uk/publications/integrated-care-systems-explained

Cook, P., Howarth, M., & Wheater, P. (2019). Biodiversity and health in the face of climate change: implications for public health. In M. R. Marselle, J. Stadler, H. Korn, K. N. Irvine, & A. Bonn. (Eds.), *Biodiversity and health in the face of climate change: Challenges, opportunities and evidence gaps.* New York: Springer International Publishing.

Dalton, P. S., Ghosal, S., & Mani, A. (2016). Poverty and aspirations failure. *The Economic Journal, 126*(590), 165–188. https://doi.org/10.1111/ecoj.12210

Department of Health. (2014). *Five year forward view.* London: Stationery Office.

Henry, H., & Howarth, M. L. (2018). An overview of using an asset-based approach to nursing. General Practice. *Nursing, 4*(4), 61–66.

HM Government. (2007). *Putting people first.* London: Stationery Office.

Hopkins, T., & Rippon, S. (2015). *Head, hands and heart: asset-based approaches in health care.* London: Health Foundations.

Howarth, M. L., Withnell, N., McQuarrie, C., & Smith, E. (2016). The influence of therapeutic horticulture on social integration. *Journal of Public Mental Health, 15*(3), 136–140. https://doi.org/10.1108/JPMH-12-2015-0050

Howarth, M., & Lister, C. (2019). Social prescribing in cardiology: rediscovering the nature within us. *British Journal of Cardiac Nursing, 14*(8), 1–9. https://doi.org/10.12968/bjca.2019.0036

Howarth, M. L., & Donovan, H. (2019). Social prescribing: the whys, wherefores and implications. *Journal of Prescribing Practice, 1*(2), 94–98. https://doi.org/10.12968/jprp.2019.1.2.94

Howarth, M. L., Brettle, A. J., Hardman, M., & Maden, M. (2020). What is the evidence for the impact of gardens and gardening on health and well-being: a scoping review and evidence-based logic model to guide healthcare strategy decision making on the use of gardening approaches as a social prescription. *BMJ Open, 10*(7), e036923. https://doi.org/10.1136/bmjopen-2020-036923

Husk, K., Lovell, B., & Garside, R. (2017). Prescribing gardening and conservation activities for health and wellbeing in older people. *Maturitas, 110,* A1–A2. https://doi.org/10.1016/j.maturitas.2017.12.013

Lindström, B., & Eriksson, M. (2005). Salutogenesis. *Journal of Epidemiology & Community Health, 59*(6), 440-442.

Marmot et al. (2010). *Fair society, healthy lives: the Marmot Review: strategic review of health inequalities in England post-2010.* London.

McManus, S., Bebbington, P., Jenkins, R., & Brugha, T. (Eds.). (2016). *Mental health and wellbeing in England: Adult Psychiatric Morbidity Survey 2014.* Leeds: NHS Digital.

McPhee, J. S., French, D. P., Jackson, D., Nazroo, J., Pendleton, N., & Degens, H. (2016). Physical activity in older age: perspectives for healthy ageing and frailty. *Biogerontology, 17*(3), 567–580. https://doi.org/10.1007/s10522-016-9641-0

National Academy for Social Prescribing. (2020). *A social revolution in wellbeing: Strategic Plan 2020-23.* London: National Academy for Social Prescribing.

NHS England. (2019). *The long term plan.* London: Stationery Office.

NHS England. (n.d.). *Voluntary, community and social enterprises (VCSE).* https://www.england.nhs.uk/ourwork/part-rel/voluntary-community-and-social-enterprises-vcse/.

NHS England. (2021). *Building strong integrated care systems everywhere ICS implementation guidance on partnerships with the voluntary, community and social enterprise sectorhttps.* https://www.england.nhs.uk/wp-content/uploads/2021/06/B0905-vcse-and-ics-partnerships.pd.

Office for Health Improvement and Disparities (n.d.). https://www.gov.uk/government/organisations/office-for-health-improvement-and-disparities

Perissinotto, C. M., Cenzer, I. S., & Covinsky, K. E. (2012). Loneliness in older persons: a predictor of functional decline and death. *Archives of Internal Medicine, 172*(14), 1078–1084. https://doi.org/10.1001%2Farchinternmed.2012.1993

Polley, M., Whiteside, J., Elnaschie, S., & Fixsen, A. (2020). What does successful social prescribing look like? *Mapping meaningful outcomes.* London: University of Westminster.

Takano, T., Nakamura, K., & Watanabe, M. (2002). Urban residential environments and senior citizens' longevity in megacity areas: the importance of walkable green spaces. *Journal of Epidemiology & Community Health, 56*(12), 913–918. https://doi.org/10.1136/jech.56.12.913

World Health Organization. (2015). *Summary: World report on ageing and health.* Luxembourg: WHO Press.

World Health Organization. (2017, December 12). Mental health of older adults. https://www.who.int/news-room/fact-sheets/detail/mental-health-of-older-adults

Further Reading

Bickerdike, L., Booth, A., Wilson, P. M., Farley, K., & Wright, K. (2017). Social prescribing: less rhetoric and more reality. A systematic review of the evidence. *BMJ Open, 7*(4), e013384. https://doi.org/10.1136/bmjopen-2016-013384

Chatterjee, H. J., Camic, P. M., Lockyer, B., & Thomson, L. J. M. (2017). Non-clinical community interventions: a systematised review of social prescribing schemes. *Arts & Health, 10*(2), 97–123. https://doi.org/10.1080/17533015.2017.1334002

Morris, D., Thomas, P., Ridley, J., & Webber, M. (2022). Community-enhanced social prescribing: integrating community in policy and practice. *International Journal of Community Well-Being, 5*(1), 179–195. https://doi.org/10.1007/s42413-020-00080-9

Younan, H.-C., Junghans, C., Harris, M., Majeed, A., & Gnani, S. (2020). Maximising the impact of social prescribing on population health in the era of COVID-19. *Journal of the Royal Society of Medicine, 113*(10), 377–382. https://doi.org/10.1177/0141076820947057

PART III

Organisational Influences and Application of Integrated Care

13

Management of Change in Integrated Services

Dr Naomi Sharples

KEY CONCEPTS

- Complex adaptive systems
- Kurt Lewin's components of change
- Deming's change tool
- Virginia Satir's change model

INTRODUCTION

The following chapter will provide an overview of three change management theories that can be used to support change within integrated services. This chapter will offer frameworks and a narrative that reflects the complex nature of systemic change. As such, it will exemplify the application of the change theories which can be applied by teams at conceptual and operational levels.

The change theories have been chosen to show the reader how change can be understood from the broad conceptual level in the case of complex adaptive systems, through to the change processes offered by Kurt Lewin, and finally as a 'tool' for change management as captured by the Deming wheel (Fig. 13.1).

CONCEPTUAL FRAMEWORK FOR CHANGE

We can confidently say in the 21st century that we are moving away from the belief that organisations, systems, structures, cultures, and the humans within them function in a Newtonian, mechanistic, linear manner. However, the common depiction of organisational culture, structure, and systems often portrays a simplistic view that can obfuscate the complex reality.

Understanding that we are part of and function within complex and ever-changing systems allows us to explore and understand the relationship between social behaviour and organisational transformation more fully (Miller, 2007).

Complex Adaptive Systems

To understand complexity theory, we work to leave behind simplistic 'single-loop', cause-and-effect, linear, simplistic approaches to understanding change. By moving away from a reductionist perspective, we instead engage with the patterns, connections, relationships, and interdependencies of organisations people, cultures, and systems (Obolensky, 2014).

Complex adaptive systems (CAS) theory is not new: it has roots in the natural world, with examples as diverse as ant colonies, where individual ants working together sustain the health of the colony, as in the case of the leaf-cutter ant. They also relate to, respond to, and sustain the life and health of the fungus that is also their symbiotic home (Fig. 13.2).

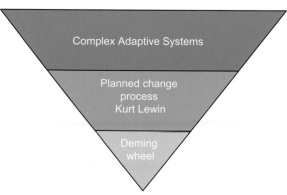

Fig. 13.1 Change management theories.

CASE STUDY

The focus of the chapter will be on the integration of integrated care systems (ICSs) within a mixed rural/urban area of the northwest of England. The area has a population of 2.5 million people and faces a wide variety of challenges, from delivering services to urban populations, to focused work with marginalised and socially deprived populations in rural and coastal areas.

Prior to the COVID-19 pandemic, there was extensive engagement with service deliverers, analysis of health outcomes, and community focus groups across the partnership to understand the key health and wellbeing issues for our people and communities.

This engagement reinforced the need to address several significant and well-documented challenges. These are not unique to this area and demography, and include locally specific challenges, such as stroke, suicide, alcohol-related harm, death from violent crime, and the need for improved services in the most deprived areas. These often interrelated areas of challenge were identified for whole-system action.

The four areas for development included establishing:

The Integrated Care Board (ICB)—responsible for planning and procuring services at a regional level.

The Integrated Care Partnership (ICP)—where the NHS, local authority, and stakeholder partners are responsible and accountable for generating an integrated care strategy to improve health and care outcomes and experiences for the population.

Place-Based Partnerships—accountable to the ICB, delivering place-based services across the boroughs.

Provider Collaboratives—incorporating one Acute and Specialist Trust and a mental health, community, and learning disability collaborative, agreeing upon objectives with the ICB, to contribute to the delivery of the strategic priorities. Focusing on collaborative working to deliver benefits of scale and support across multiple places or systems.

The ICP will work to prevent ill-health by channelling human and financial resources 'upstream' where there is more benefit to population health.

The provider collaboratives will join to become ICPs across the NHS, local authority, and third-sector services. One ICP will focus on ill-health prevention, supported self-care, and delivering personalised care closer to home. This will focus interventions on a public health and community services model—with dedicated focus on primary and preventative interventions in the medium to long-term, there will be less reliance on secondary/hospital services.

- Improve population-level interventions including:
  - Improve access to employment and workplace health and education
  - Develop services and support people and families by growing community resilience
  - Enable people to live well and self-care where appropriate
  - Improve end-of-life care, developing the concept of 'compassionate communities'
- Move resources, including staff and services, out of hospital and into the community
  - Deliver accessible GP and community services closer to where people live and reduce demand for hospital services
  - Marshal community assets, including buildings, social networks, and people to build and enhance population wellbeing
  - Partner with housing, community-based assets, and third-sector providers in supporting people to be well
  - Facilitate collaboration between organisations
- Integrate health and social care services for holistic joined-up care
  - Strengthen our multidisciplinary and multi-agency teams, ensure mental health support and provision is on par with physical health for people throughout their lives
  - Establish democratic oversight of integrated care provision through purposeful community engagement
- Exploit the use of digital health technology for the benefit of service users
  - Enhance service user independence, wellbeing, and service user experience, and improve services
  - Enhance health data reporting and analysis to progress the design and delivery of targetted interventions.

This refocusing and redesign of services requires a range of huge and systemically complex changes in an ICP, requiring dedicated and skilled resources to assess, plan, implement, and evaluate the complex structural and social changes.

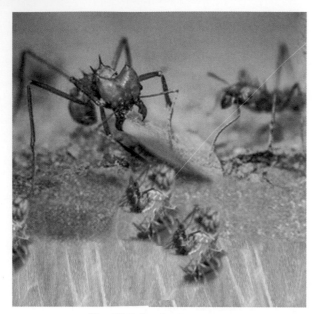

Fig. 13.2 Leafcutter ants.

We see complexity theory in viral mutations, where the behaviour of a myriad of dynamic complex agents relate, mutate, and create novel forms of infections, adapting to environmental challenges and becoming increasingly problematic until the environment responds to 'defend' itself.

We live within a wide variety of systems that are nested within each other, such as the virus within the human body, the human family system, the human within the community system, the health organisation, and the health and care national system, each with a myriad of systems nested within. To visualise this dynamic, we can explore a nested system to help understand (Fig. 13.3).

Managing the change required to implement an ICS, or even one component of the ICS, requires an awareness and appreciation of the complex, competing, and systemic components involved (Fig. 13.4).

Here, the agents are the individuals in the various voluntary, statutory, and health and care communities. They are influenced by the external and internal environment and receive and emit information across the systems as well as responding to feedback, which will continually reinforce new actions, decisions, behaviours, processes, and feedback that reduce certain actions, decisions, behaviours, and processes.

Through the constant feedback, self-organised networks emerge to deliver health and social care within care communities, resulting in complex adaptive systems that support the new health and social care paradigm.

The defining qualities of CAS include:

Nested systems—systems live within other systems.

Emergence—the system agents interact in random ways, patterns emerge from the interactions, the patterns inform the behaviour of the agents and, in turn, the behaviour of the system.

Co-evolution—a system is on its own and at the same time part of its environment; when the environment changes, the system must adapt (e.g., when the ICP is formed, the services and systems within must adapt—and they are, at the same time, the ICP environment).

Sub-optimal—a complex system does not need to be perfect to be healthy, it just needs to be 'good enough' to be effective.

Requisite variety—the more diverse the agents within the system, the more the system will thrive. Contradictions and uncertainty within the system creates novel ideas and greater creative potential. Diversity in the workplace offers new and creative opportunities, whereas an exclusionary culture offers very little to the health of the systems and environment.

Connectivity—as expressed in a gestalt configuration, the whole as a connected system is greater than the sum of the individual agents. The power comes from the relationships.

Simple rules—the system itself is not complex, nor are the rules that govern the system. However, the emerging patterns can be very complex because of the variety and connectivity.

Iterative—the feedback loop within the system creates an ever-increasing reaction, resulting in adjustment, action, and reaction. The COVID-19 variants are poignant examples of this iterative behaviour.

Self-organising—no controlling agent, no hierarchy of agents, no management. The system is in a state of constant self-organisation through the iterative feedback mechanism and adjusting to the environment. In organisations, we find this a challenge to believe due to our understanding of organisational structures. If we strip away the structures into their component parts, they become people/agents with different and sometimes competing agendas. As the agents network and relate, patterns of behaviour emerge that create the organisational environment. We all know agents with leadership titles who do not lead, or agents without officially ascribed power who do lead—it's all about the relationships.

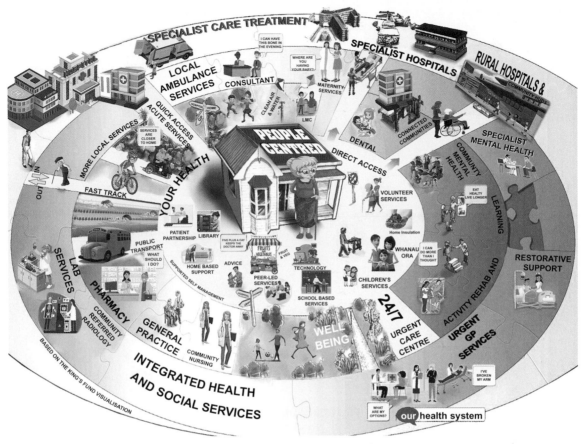

Fig. 13.3 Healthcare organisation.

We are already witnessing the variation in function and design of ICBs, ICPs, and place-based solutions as they emerge across ICSs. This variation is evident in that relationships driven through approaches to internal and external communication and networking will yield a variety of results, even when applying the same ICS frameworks.

Within each organisation and associated subgroups, there are multilevel dynamic challenges. Services must go through the process of analysing the current state of provision, developing a clear vision of the desired state, analysing the gap between current and desired, and then producing changes within the organisational systems, structure, and culture, all whilst continuing to provide complex health and care systems and services. These developments rely heavily on the establishment of a 'platform for change' where individuals across organisations can create an environment where dynamic complex change can emerge.

As we write in 2021/22, this work is also being completed against a backdrop of a global pandemic, which has created sustained pressure on already pressurised services.

Having outlined CAS theory, this will be used as the overarching backdrop through which we can consider the application and alignment of change models.

Change Management Models

All change management models aim to get us (i.e., an organisation or system) from a current to a desired state. In ICS implementation, we hope to be moving from an 'emerging' through to a 'thriving' ICS (NHS, 2019). Taking the case study as an example, the ICP would be moving some hospital-based services to community-based services, such as the people, buildings, and support systems. In turn, the Provider Collaboratives will be required to work together in new and novel ways to meet the health needs at a neighbourhood level.

Change management theories range from the apparently 'simple' to more complex theories and everything between. The important issue is applying the model to

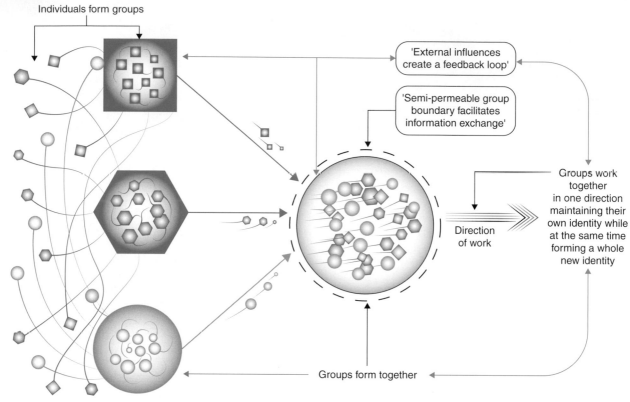

Individuals form groups

'External influences create a feedback loop'

'Semi-permeable group boundary facilitates information exchange'

Direction of work

Groups work together in one direction maintaining their own identity while at the same time forming a whole new identity

Groups form together

Fig. 13.4 Complex adaptive systems.

support the process of transformation, or, more specifically, applying the model to create the platform for change. To frame the chapter, we will firstly be looking at the most used, and possibly most misunderstood, change process theory developed by Kurt Lewin. As we will see, Lewin's work complements and aligns with CAS theory.

We will then go on to look at Dening's (2012) Plan Do Study Act (PDSA) as one of many tools to assist the process of transformation.

Kurt Lewin

Kurt Lewin (1890–1947) takes his place as 'Grandee' of change management theory with his reassuringly clear model. As a child psychologist, Lewin was initially focused on social psychology. It was here he developed his field theory, which was designed to facilitate change in situations of family/relational conflict. His three-step change approach developed from his field theory to later become the cornerstone of organisational change theory.

Lewin offers us a comprehensive range of theories to apply to situations where one needs to facilitate movement from a current to a desired situation (Burns, 2020). Using our case study example of moving some

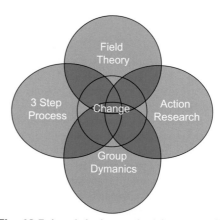

Fig. 13.5 Lewin's theoretical framework.

hospital-based services to community-based services, we can consider how Lewin's theoretical frameworks (Fig. 13.5) can assist the change process.

- **Field theory**—Where the forces that sustained a situation (e.g., current hospital-based services) and those that drive or restrain change (i.e., what is driving the move to community-based provision and what is restraining this move) are articulated as a life space, or the mapped representation of the environment with dynamic forces identified (CAS supports the concept that we all live within many life spaces at the same time, including home, relationships, work, leisure, community…).

- **Group dynamics**—The nature and composition of groups, how people within groups interact with those within and external to the group based on emotions and feeling, and how these create group-held beliefs and norms. In relation to the example—which groups are involved in the move from hospital to community services? How would the group norms, beliefs, and values need to develop? What are the emotions and feelings involved? Who has power? Who needs more power?

- **Action research**—Where what forces and dynamics understood from the field and the group are acted upon in a way to engage change towards the desired outcome. The actions are simultaneously researched for effectiveness through critical reflection. As the process of service change is acted out, action research can support the analysis of the process through the repeated cycle of planning, acting, observing, and reflecting.

- **Three-step change approach**—Focused on the unfreezing of the current forces and group dynamics (hospital-based services, systems, teams and culture) to implementing a new way of being (community-based services, systems, teams and culture), which is closer to the behaviour required for the desired outcome, and then finally embedding the changes to secure a new field and new group dynamics.

It should be noted at this point that whilst Lewin spoke and wrote about the process of change, moving from one situation to finally embedding change in a desired situation, he did not design the three-step model as we see it today—this was done after his death in 1947 by Crosby (2020).

Field theory and group dynamics give the practitioner the understanding of an individual's or group's behaviours, motivations, and relationships, and then action research and the three-step change process offer a framework and reflection or focus to be able to act on the field and the group dynamics to secure a desired transformation.

As a social psychologist, Lewin was heavily influenced and applied a gestalt framework in the development of his theories. Taken individually, any one of the four 'tools' would be lacking, and therefore open to critique. By using a gestalt position and understanding the role of each of the tools in the whole (i.e., the use of all the tools together is different to or greater than the sum of the individual tools), the application of Lewin's change theories becomes a meaningful option and a further lens through which to navigate CAS.

Having analysed the organisation life space and the group dynamics before any change takes place, we understand the 'current situation' in relation to a range of factors or component parts, which need to go through a transition process (altered states) to become the new and desired outcome. Lewin focuses on the creation of energy and of locomotion/movement to begin the fission needed to process through the change. In the unfreezing process, the current equilibrium requires unbalancing to achieve a fluidity in a once-balanced field (organisational paradigm). In considering the 'fission' required to change, we can then think of that fission creating the energy between the agents and triggering motion, interpersonal connections, and communications to begin the random process that will form the emerging order from the dynamic/nonlinear systems (Burns, 2004).

When we consider the reorganisation required to form the partnerships, we understand that we are dealing with organisations that have very different 'life spaces', as illustrated by New Local (Fig. 13.6), an independent think tank and network of local councils. They are epitomising CAS by working as an emergent adaptive system, transforming public services, releasing the power of communities (agents and networks), and influencing political stakeholders at the same time.

To move from one paradigm to the other takes effort, focus, understanding, and a desire not only to embrace change but to let go of your 'known' way of working. This may also mean letting go of power, position, and reconstructing relationships.

Applying Lewin's force field analysis at this stage helps to orientate the agents to a high-level outcome. By forming the desired outcome in the central semipermeable space—in this example we use a workforce transformation high-level aim—the drivers of change and the restraining factors can be added and analysed.

Drivers and restrainers are illustrated differently, sometimes with strengths indicated numerically, or as in Fig. 13.7, with the considered 'power' of the driver or restraint. However, this is a representation that is based on one individual's perspective and as such may differ from one person to the next according to their agenda.

Areas for action and implementation. With this example, there are four specific areas for action to take place. Turning the restraints into areas for action means that these are the four specific areas for analysis, planning, implementation of plans and subsequent behavioural change, and finally evaluation.

Applying Lewin's process, we are in the 'unfreeze stage' where the analysis and planning is taking place. At this point, we could apply the 'Deming wheel' (Deming, 2012). The Plan, Do, Study, Act (PDSA) cycle is an 'improvement learning cycle', as illustrated in the following, using the second restraint as an example.

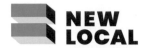

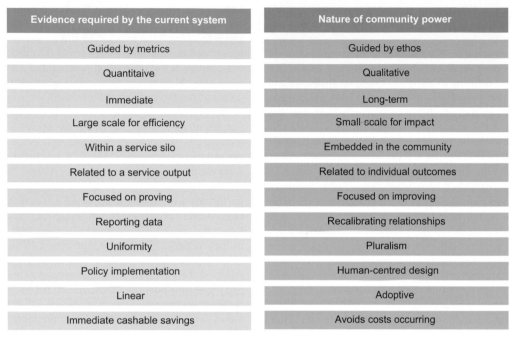

Evidence required by the current system	Nature of community power
Guided by metrics	Guided by ethos
Quantitaive	Qualitative
Immediate	Long-term
Large scale for efficiency	Small scale for impact
Within a service silo	Embedded in the community
Related to a service output	Related to individual outcomes
Focused on proving	Focused on improving
Reporting data	Recalibrating relationships
Uniformity	Pluralism
Policy implementation	Human-centred design
Linear	Adoptive
Immediate cashable savings	Avoids costs occurring

Fig. 13.6 Organisations with different 'life spaces'. (From https://www.newlocal.org.uk/research/community-power/)

Unclear Data on Primary Care, Voluntary, Social Care Staff Ethos, Skills, and Scope, Impacting on Service Design
1. **Plan**—we plan to / this will produce:
   a. To review and map human resources (HR) data sources and reporting functions to support workforce analysis.
   b. Using process mapping and patient journey experience—analyse the roles, responsibilities, and job descriptions of primary/community care staff with a focus on scope of practice, duplication of responsibilities, and gaps in provision.
   c. Analyse the differences in organisational culture and staff ethos through a range of cross-cutting forum discussions and narrative creation events.
   d. Steps to execute—implementation:
      i. Director X to speak to HR leads in the five lead health and care organisations to understand the HR data held and collect and collate the job descriptions of the healthcare staff. To understand the reporting functions available to the Workforce Development Team (WDT) implementation team.
      ii. Manager X to bring together the service managers or equivalent of the five health and care providers to undertake an externally facilitated process-mapping exercise, including a patient journey narrative. Identify areas of role cross-over/duplication, opportunity to extend scope, and gaps in provision.
      iii. Working party/task and finish group established with representatives from each organisation to facilitate monthly forums aimed at eliciting, understanding, and analysing organisational cultures and staff ethos, to reframe and develop an agreed-upon underpinning philosophy.
2. **Do**—what was observed—evaluation? Carry out the plan; note down observations, barriers to plan, systems/structures/cultures that facilitate the plan and those that create blockages.
3. **Study**—what was learned? Analyse the emerging structures and outcomes of the cross-organisation working groups. Was the plan active? Are there more areas to consider? Has something come up in the execution that requires further attention/work?
4. **Act**—what can be concluded from this first cycle? The conclusions then become the areas for further cycles until the team is satisfied with the outcome.

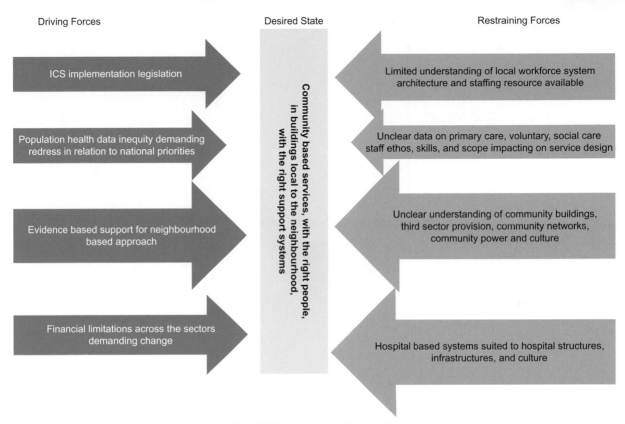

Fig. 13.7 Drivers and restrainers.

The PDSA cycle is used often within health and care organisations. Deming's work is accessible, with a strong sense of being a 'rational approach' which supports people to understand and apply this change management process. Whilst seemingly 'rational', the structure is broad enough to form a supportive structure within a CAS theory approach. Essentially, it is a tool to frame the changes whilst working within a CAS paradigm.

People and changing. Change is often considered as 'unusual' or 'uncomfortable', challenging or energising, even despite change being ever-present. Some change models help people to understand the emotional journey people take through change processes (e.g., Bridges model; Kubler-Ross's change curve (EKR Foundation, 2022), which helps articulate the emotional response to change; and Virginia Satir's model (Fig. 13.8), which focuses on the emotive process of accepting change (Satir, 1994)).

Lewin's process. Satir describes the emotional journey through change, helping people to reflect on and consider their stage in the change process, or the experience of others within the process. By adding Lewin's process to the model, we can illustrate the points at which people may excel or struggle. Whilst we need to guard against linear models, the arrow on the Y axis represents the unerring ability for people and organisations to move up and down the change process before the new status quo is fully experienced (see Fig. 13.8).

Supporting staff through transformation is vital in that it firstly reflects leadership awareness and understanding of compassion for people undergoing a change process. Secondly this compassion will support followership, communication, narration, and adoption of the changes. If leaders do not show compassion or understand the emotional component of change, people will still go through the range of emotions they attach to the paradigm shift, but these emotions will go unrecognised, unnoticed, and unheard.

Leading change and following the change agents. Leadership theory will be focused on in greater detail in a later chapter; however, you cannot think about change without considering people. Applying the 'Pareto rule',

Virginia Satir Change model

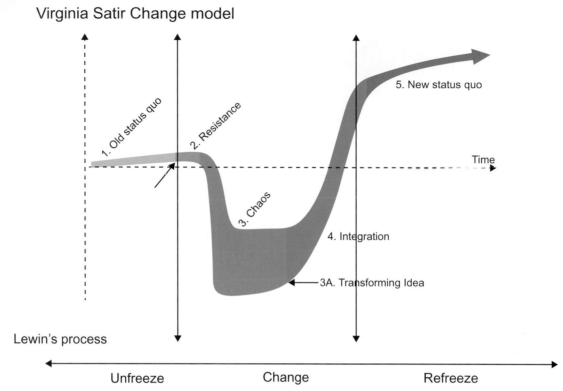

Fig. 13.8 Virginia Satir's model. (Satir, 1994.)

one could confidently assert that 20% of change is in the writing of strategies, policies, plans, operational manuals, evaluations, and system and structure design and 80% of change is reliant on people and their behaviour, interactions, communications, motivations, and relationships.

To lead people through change, leaders require firstly to understand what kind of leadership they can offer, what kind of leadership is required, how others experience their leadership, and how they will need to develop their leadership. Through this leadership analysis, supporting people through the change process can be analysed, critiqued, and reflected upon as part of a leadership learning journey.

We are offered a plethora of theories on leadership, we are surrounded by people who will define themselves as 'transformational leaders', and we are bombarded by interventions from 'project management' through to 'transcendental' transformations and a multitude of positions in between. All of this is to capture the ability to influence other people's thoughts, feelings, and behaviours—to get things done.

The critical component of leadership is understanding how others perceive they are led. To lead requires the ability to move individuals from the 'current' paradigm to the 'desired' paragidm. Without this ability one may have the title that denotes 'leadership' without the requisite skills. This creates organisational and inter / intra-personal challenges.

CONCLUSION

The chapter provided an overview of three change management theories that may be useful with transformation to integrated services. This chapter also provided frameworks and a narrative that reflects the complex nature of systemic change utilising the example of ICS development across the northwest of England.

The chapter demonstrated that change can be viewed through a number of lenses, from the broad conceptual level in the case of CAS, through to the change processes offered by Lewin, and finally as a 'tool' for change management as captured by the Deming wheel.

References

Burns, B. (2020). The origins of Lewin's three-step model of change. *Journal of Applied Behavioral Science*, *56*(1), 32–59. https://doi.org/10.1177/0021886319892685.

Burns, B. (2004). Kurt Lewin and complexity theories: back to the future? *Journal of Change Management*, *4*(4), 309–325. https://doi.org/10.1080/14697010420000303811.

Crosby, G. (2020). *Planned change: Why Kurt Lewin's social science is still best practice for business results, change management, and human progress*. New York: Productivity Press.

Deming E. W, (2012). The Essential Deming: Leadership Principles from the Father of Quality. MrGraw Hill. London

EKR Foundation. (2022). *Kübler-Ross Change Curve®*. https://www.ekrfoundation.org/5-stages-of-grief/change-curve.

Lewin, K. (1942). Field theory and learning in social sciences. In D. Cartwright (Ed.), *Field theory in social science, selected theoretical papers* (pp. 212–230). American Psychological Association.

Miller, C. (2007). *The book of change* (1st ed.). Cambridge: Cambridge Scholars Publishing.

NHS. (2019). *Designing integrated care systems (ICSs) in England*. https://www.england.nhs.uk/wp-content/uploads/2019/06/designing-integrated-care-systems-in-england.pdf

Obolensky, N. (2014). *Complex adaptive leadership: Embracing paradox and uncertainty*. Farnham: Gower Publishing.

Satir, V. (1994). *Helping families to change*. Lanham: Jason Aronson.

14

Co-production and Organisational Challenges (A Framework for Change)

Dr Hayley Bamber, Dr Tracey Williamson, and Dr Elaine Ball

KEY CONCEPTS

- Corporate
- Continuous change
- Power imbalances
- Interface
- Attitudes towards co-production

INTRODUCTION

Previous chapters have considered how integration can occur with consideration of how co-production can be a vehicle for change. Chapter 7 discussed the challenges with defining the concept of co-production and identified the core characteristics which can act as key principles. This chapter aims to consider the challenges which exist when implementing co-production and consider how these can be addressed, culminating in the suggestion of a co-production model. The evidence for the approach advocated is based on a professional doctoral thesis (Bamber, 2020). This study was a descriptive case study of one UK organisation that had implemented co-production.

RESEARCH METHODOLOGY

The methodology used was a descriptive case study as it aimed to investigate a specific phenomenon which had

CASE STUDY

The case study explores the observations and themes identified in the exploration of co-production. The research aimed to determine the understanding of senior managers, middle managers, and clinical leads within community mental health teams (CMHTs) who were key participants in implementing co-production within the organisation.

limited preliminary research, such as co-production (Yin, 2014). A single embedded case study design was selected with sub-divisions of participant groups.

Local Context

The study was conducted in the northwest of England. Knowledge of co-production within the organisation came from senior managers' brief history where they purported that managers and clinical leads would co-produce together to provide cost-effective services. The organisation's co-production model did not include service users or community members. Fig. 14.1 illustrates the Trust's managerial hierarchy, highlighting co-production relationships between network directors and clinical network directors.

Selection of Participants—Inclusion

Senior Managers

Senior managers were individuals who were on the senior leadership team/Trust board. They were individuals who had made the decision to implement co-production and it was anticipated that they could provide context and insight into the facilitators and barriers when implementing the model.

Middle Managers

Middle managers were band 7 and band 8 practitioners with managerial responsibility for the CMHTs. Senior managers identified them as being integral to the implementation of co-production and it was important to gain insight into their understanding of co-production.

Clinical Leads

Clinical leads were consultant psychiatrists within the CMHTs. Senior managers identified them as being crucial to co-production.

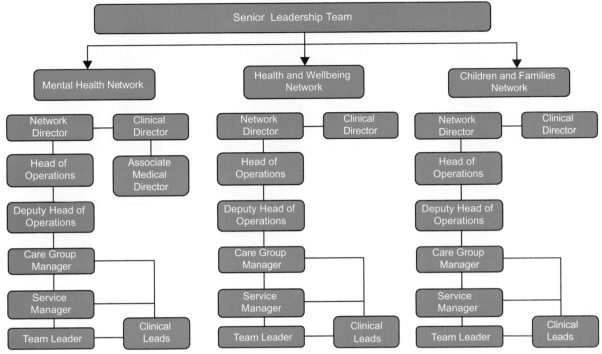

Fig. 14.1 Organisational structure.

As middle managers and clinical leads were responsible for grassroots implementation, they were ideally situated to report on the how the model was operating in practice.

Selection of Participants—Exclusion

Service Users

Service users were highlighted (in the doctoral literature review) as a critical component of co-production. However, due to the design of the organisation's co-production model (not including service users), it was clear that there was a lack of clarity around what co-production meant and how this should be implemented within practice (Bradley, 2015; Clark, 2015). Therefore, the focus of the study needed to be on understanding what key organisational players determined co-production to be, to support considering how to include service users moving forward.

Community

As with service users, whilst essential for co-production, there was a lack of consideration of community within the organisation's model and therefore the community was excluded from this study.

Findings of the Study

Transcripts from 12 one-on-one interviews were analysed and themed using the thematic analysis protocol recommended by Miles and Huberman (1994), identifying five key themes (Fig. 14.2).

Discussion of the Themes

Theme 1—Corporate Machine

'Corporate machine', a term used by a participant to describe the 'disconnect' between corporate and clinical services, was a key theme with many participants. Sub-themes were (1) corporate versus clinical, (2) perceived management attitudes, (3) commitment, and (4) politics (see Fig. 14.3).

Corporate versus clinical. Participants noted a clear 'disconnect' between corporate and clinical services which impacted on understanding roles, organisational drivers, and communication. Financial stability, a key NHS driver (Department of Health and Social Care, 2019), presented subsequent demands, which directly conflicted with co-production as illustrated below:

> 'I think that it is very financially driven, and I think it is very much about pleasing the clinical commissioning groups (CCGs) and meeting what their expectations are, and I think we are moving away from co-production'

(MM2)

The notion of 'disconnect' negatively affecting communication was clear among participants:

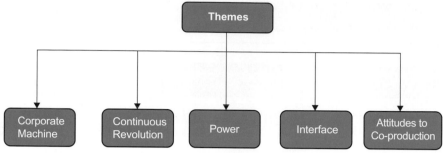

Fig. 14.2 Theme map.

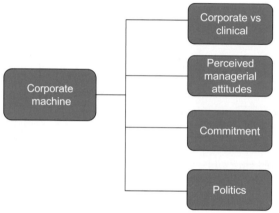

Fig. 14.3 Theme 1—corporate machine.

'I think the top and the bottom just lose, completely lose sight of each other'

(CL1)

With the Trust's 'tick box' mentality of effective communication, as noted by a senior manager:

'And I would recognise the corporate versus clinical, as I think that's driving the senior management versus frontline staff issue, and that would be the order I would put that in, and I will be really honest, I will put that firmly in the camp of nursing and quality, less of an issue I think personally in finance and human resources (HR), but the marking homework mentality, serious untoward incident, investigations, the computer says no, I think firmly sits in that portfolio'

(SM2)

A participant suggested that the promotion of staff into managerial positions could be a possible solution:

'I sincerely hope that there is a bit more connect between senior management and colleagues, and I feel actually we need to step up to the management position, people who are on the frontline'

(CL5)

Role confusion amongst middle managers and clinical leads increased frustrations and the 'disconnect' which was potentially reducing the scope for co-production, as outlined below:

'It never ceases to amaze me now, in this day and age, that there seems to be a lot of people, what I call corporate services, that we never had when I started out, and I am not saying that is a bad thing, but I do sometimes wonder what actually everybody does'

(MM4)

However, clear role definition existed for senior managers, suggesting that co-production could be facilitated with a shared understanding:

'It's interesting when we talk about corporate services, because we have tried to reframe that so support services who are actually there to support the frontline'

(SM1)

Despite challenges, participants felt communication methods existed through which co-production could be communicated:

'I recently attended the ENGAGE day, and that was nice, so have similar events when you talk about different directions that the Trust is going with co-production'

(CL5)

All participants confirmed that, for co-production to be successful, the clear 'disconnect' needed to be addressed. Addressing perceived managerial attitudes within current culture could bridge the divide, as explored below.

Perceived management attitudes. Many participants expressed that organisational culture and managerial attitudes impacts on staff wellbeing, suggesting that a culture of no shared goal setting would pose significant challenges to successful co-production. Some participants noted that managers dismissing concerns undervalued staff:

'I think there is a general dismissiveness of concerns that I see happening to people'

(CL1)

Being dismissed can lead to staff feeling unheard, as outlined below:

'We have whistleblowing at the XXXX (inpatient ward), we have got staff who are saying very clearly that it is an unpleasant environment, yet the Trust chooses to ignore all of these things'

(CL4)

Although managerial attitudes present clear challenges, most noted that the Trust means well and endeavours to provide effective services, as summarised below:

'I think they try their best, and they are basically well-meaning in terms of respect and delivering the service'

(CL2)

Despite being well-meaning, occasions occur where the cultural impacts are negative. The Trust's vision of doing more for the better and for less negatively impacted staff:

'you know this getting away from this amazing and quite amusing notion in a concrete way where you do more, for better, for less…it is sort of well-meaning… but those three things combined, well they can only either say that people are unrealistic, or if it is realistic it's because people have been doing things less well with more, so whichever way you look at it, it is a really invalidating thing to do'

(CL1)

Despite acknowledgement that efforts are made, all felt that more action is required for successful co-production.

Culturally moving towards becoming catalytic and facilitative was deemed as a requirement.

Commitment. As noted, tick-box responses to demands is a core cultural component, with a participant illustrating that achieving targets adds pressure to workloads, reducing the capacity for co-production:

'Documentation is one thing that I am keen about, but it just takes so much time in terms of ensuring that the clinic letters are thorough and address all the areas and they are typed on time and communicated'

(CL5)

Another participant highlighted the need for tick boxes, yet felt that local level decision-making would be beneficial:

'our tick box documentation, I mean I don't want us to get rid of that because it is really important, but if it allowed you to be more flexible with that in the greater good then that could be a real benefit'

(CL1)

The sample recognised co-production's potential but viewed the Trust's implementation as a tick-box exercise for reputational prestige:

'…it was quite clear no co-production was taking place; it was just a tick-box exercise'

(MM1)

Questioning the organisation's commitment:

'I also question if the organisation is fully committed to it or not, because I haven't seen enough evidence of co-production in action'

(MM1)

All middle managers and four clinical leads strongly noted ambiguity around what co-production is and a lack of modelling from senior managers, as illustrated below:

'I think the Trust perspective is very ambiguous in what they believe co-production is'

(MM2)

'They talk about it but it is often not demonstrated from a senior level, and as we know, if things are not demonstrated from above, then it is very difficult for us to then feed that back up'

(MM2)

A senior manager raised the concern that not all board members were fully committed to co-production:

'I think that it is partly about the individuals, partly about the maturity of the relationships, and some of it about people just understanding that, because quite paradoxically, despite the board signing up to that and supporting it, there are individuals around the board table who I think have a more traditional view of how you achieve performance and account-ability'

(SM1)

An organisation's commitment to co-production is essential; however, participants felt that the politicised nature of the NHS was a significant barrier.

Politics. Clinical leads highlight the impact that politics has on clinical practice and effective co-production. Some perceive that political correctness impedes the ability to provide effective services, whilst others view the Trust as behaving 'politically correctly' for competitive advantage.

The following quote summarised the common opinion that political representation does not exemplify the reality experienced by service staff:

'I think the Trust is very good, like big organisations are, at a bit of public relations (PR) sort of model where it is around saying the right thing and the right buzz word, advertising promotions, to just protect their reputation or enhance their reputa-tion, but when you actually go deeper into it, none of that is actually there'

(CL2)

One participant commented on how managers' reluc-tance to share power would be further limited by co-production, with them believing that reputation to acquire business supersedes distributing power:

'There is a big risk in terms of the agenda, which is controlled at the moment by the Trust, in terms of controlling the finances and managing resources and trying to give reputationally, give out a really strong, positive message to people who want to buy our service. I am aware that this is a real challenge in terms of losing services, which is where reputa-tion is important'

(CL1)

Several factors contributed to the 'disconnect', includ-ing the divide between corporate and clinical services, per-ceived managerial attitudes, organisational commitment, and the political landscape which led participants to ques-tion the authenticity of co-production. Continuous change became a major theme, contributing to the 'disconnect'.

Theme 2—Continuous Revolution

Continuous revolution describes participants' experiences of change within the NHS. The sub-themes identified were (1) attitudes to change, (2) clinical concerns, and (3) mul-tiple change (see Fig. 14.4).

Attitudes to change. Views on change were split into two sections: personal experiences and organisational approach. First, all agreed that change was challenging, and that co-production was not actively happening:

'it tends to be difficult and I guess as with a lot of people. I think that changes to services are often quite personally difficult'

(CL1)

However, one participant explored when support was provided to enact change, suggesting that when backing is available, change is manageable:

'I have been able to initiate change within my team, and I think I feel pretty much supported by my team leader whenever I have come up with any sugg-estions'

(CL5)

Participants collectively expressed cynicism about the motives for the implementation of co-production:

'…nobody understands it, and nobody believes it'

(CL4)

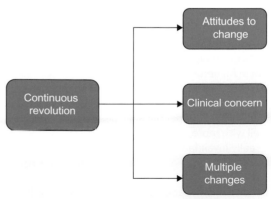

Fig. 14.4 Theme 2—continuous revolution.

As well as mistrust, all participants emphasised that a change in culture is required to empower staff:

'I think culture is hugely, hugely important because I think as a clinical lead, I need to be empowered, and I need to be part of the change rather than being told that this thing is happening to your team'

(CL5)

It was suggested that co-production culture is critical to change management:

'I think there is some inconsistent practices across the Trust, so I think we could definitely do better, and I think it needs to come from the change in culture where we normalise it that it has to be co-production'

(CL5)

Another collective view was the need to embed changes and receive adequate training on co-production skills, as highlighted below:

'So I guess if there was some training and it clearly identified what co-production is or co-production isn't I guess, suppose maybe for me I quite like when an example is given where someone did something and the benefits of using a co-production model'

(MM4)

Irrespective of poor experience of change, collective optimism was noted for truly transformative change, as summarised by the following quote:

'...there is a potential benefit of greater change too, by pushing things to something which is genuinely different'

(CL1)

If change is not organisationally transformational, then service delivery will be affected, impacting on co-production's success. All clinical leads collectively considered this to be a clinical concern.

Clinical concern. Unaddressed clinical concerns can impact on recruitment and retention as highlighted in the following quote when a previous employee publicised their views in public arenas:

'So, one of the most anti-advocates against the Trust...he left the Trust...he is known to be a world class leader in his field, but in his lectures...he calls

us an organisation that is very top down, does not know what it is doing'

(CL4)

Participants expressed that there were issues with maintaining a safe working environment, which has led individuals to take decisive action:

'they are withdrawing services from areas where they don't feel it is safe'

(CL4)

Additionally, participants were concerned that service users were not key to decision-making (a core element of co-production):

'we are known as an organisation that has no regard for its patients. With all your goodwill but your political stance is like this'

(CL4)

A common-held view was that the management of service user complaints was dishonest and counterproductive:

'the NHS is terrified of upsetting people and being straight with people'

(CL1)

Some participants felt that senior managers were not truthful about the drivers for change, as outlined below:

'I think in some cases, sometimes you feel that there is a bit of cheekiness, there is a cost saving sold as a, "right we are doing a service transformation, we are changing the service", but essentially when you look at it, you have a reduction in your care coordinators'

(CL5)

However, if honesty was adopted, addressing the 'disconnect' could strengthen co-production:

'I think more straightforwardness and honesty about things doesn't make things okay, but it might bring people a little closer to a real position'

(CL1)

Whilst participants expressed strong views surrounding attitudes and clinical concerns, they also discussed the volume of changes and the subsequent impact on clinical practice.

Multiple change. All participants highlighted a culture of constant organisational changes affecting staff wellbeing and co-production:

> 'it's just one change after another. It doesn't seem that there has been a period of stability to try and really see what is going on. At the minute, it is so chaotic, that everyone is really confused'
>
> *(CL2)*

Many participants felt that constant management changes continually shifts focus because of individual motivations:

> 'that short termism whereby most managerial posts similar to political posts seem to run often procedurally on a two- to three-year kind of term'
>
> *(CL1)*

Senior managers confirmed the regular changes, noting that the organisation has minimal control:

> 'I think there is something about how do we do change implementation, because the changes are going to stay there, and that's not necessarily in our gift to control; what is in our gift to control is how we develop the models in the first place'
>
> *(SM2)*

Many drivers, which the Trust has no control over, including economic climate, dictate the need for change, as stressed below:

> 'I would like to be able to give people assurances that it's going to stop, but it isn't. I think the problem is, things that are fixed, we have to drive efficiency between 2% and 4% every year. There is nothing to cut now, so we have to do that through transformation and find different ways of doing it'
>
> *(SM1)*

Participants stressed that change is challenging and is more successful when they can 'buy in' to the process; therefore, incentivising co-production is crucial. In addition to change, participants stressed that power has a further impact on change and successful co-production.

Theme 3—Power

The following sub-themes were identified: (1) imbalance, (2) not being heard and done to, (3) emotional response, and (4) what needs to happen to address the power imbalances (Fig. 14.5).

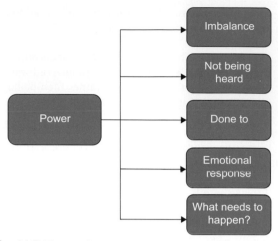

Fig. 14.5 Theme 3—power.

Imbalance. The middle managers and clinical leads strongly voiced that power imbalances existed; however, even senior managers felt powerless:

> 'I suspect most people within the Trust feel that they don't have very much of it, even people who are perceived to have significant amounts of it by people who think that they have less than that person. I suspect that if you ask the people higher up in the Trust, they think about the power that people have over them in terms of commissioners or the Department of Health'
>
> *(CL1)*

Middle managers and clinical leads all felt that power is weighted towards senior management:

> 'I think there is a bit more balance towards management. Perhaps I saw it more because I came from a Trust which was more primarily clinically led. I am not saying that it needs to be driven by the clinicians, but I think it needs to be a little more balanced, and sometimes you are being told this is happening'
>
> *(CL5)*

Conversely, senior managers believed that this was a misconception:

> 'I think people make assumptions of positional power without question'
>
> *(SM2)*

One prominent finding was the disempowerment of clinical leads with participants expressing that they noted a distinct move away from doctors exercising power, which left them deskilled and reluctant to engage actively in change:

'there was a move away from doctors having a certain amount of power within those relationships'

(CL1)

'So, in a way you are sort of deskilled, to be honest with you'

(CL2)

'We are focused too much on offering the clinical care and leaving other systematic issues to someone else; who is that someone else?'

(CL5)

One senior manager recognised the inaction from clinical leads, stating that there was a need to strengthen the medical voice to improve co-production:

'something about mental health particularly in relation to Medics that is really paradoxical because if you were in an acute trust, often the Medics are the most powerful voice, and they exercise it and as a variance depending on what specialty they are in – orthopedics, cardiac surgeons, and neuro surgeons who again are the loudest. Actually, I think one of the challenges we have is that the medical voice is not powerful enough in this organisation'

(SM1)

Power imbalances can impact on engagement in decision-making, with the participants expressing having little choice or control in the decisions made:

'I think we got bullied into it, into this new model'

(CL2)

'sometimes you feel that whatever order comes from the top, we will implement like God will command you to do this, then we do it'

(CL2)

With co-production, a key concept is equally distributed power, and all participants agreed that power should be distributed but recognised this could be challenging:

'I don't see that being feasible or practical in this Trust'

(CL2)

'because you can't even have a microwave or a kettle in your office now, never mind make major changes to the way your organisation works'

(CL2)

'I tried to argue my case, but it wasn't really taken on—we do that in another team, why can't we do it here'

(CL5)

A senior manager suggested that people need to rethink how they perceive power within the Trust so they can be self-empowered:

'so x number of people are considered the senior team; actually, the team are the people who you need to get together to do the job, and it shouldn't matter where or what you are within the organisation, you get the right people together, but that is not in a dominant form as yet'

(SM2)

Despite this lone view, other senior managers discussed how they were enforced to complete tasks, suggesting that self-empowerment alone is not enough:

'I think that a lot of the things that I end up doing are not of my choosing in the sense that there is a decision at a strategic level'

(SM3)

Middle managers and clinical leads described how power imbalances have led to their voices 'not being heard' and feeling 'done to', which they feel is a barrier to co-production.

Not being heard and being done to. Not being heard leads to disempowerment in the workplace (TUC, 2015) as verbalised:

'the other part of the culture that has become really clear to me in the time that I have worked here is that the top don't hear what the reality is, and that is just a recurring theme'

(CL1)

Participants felt that the Trust pays lip service to staff and perceived them as resistant to change, compounding feelings of not being heard impacting on relationships:

'The decisions have already been made, and we might have meetings and consultations, but it is only really paying lip service'

(MM4)

'It's really difficult for people planning changes to hear concerns about changes without dismissing them as people being resistant to change'

(CL1)

Some participants reported their input being dismissed, as strongly emphasised here:

'it was very demoralising. We went ahead with the changes, and soon all of those problems became a reality'

(CL2)

For successful co-production, all participants felt that listening is essential for all involved in the process:

'I think it would be about listening to people and particularly not just at a managerial level but listening to people across the Trust'

(MM2)

Listening and responding to this is essential to avoid powerlessness. One participant reflected on a management restructure where they ended up in a more senior role, despite advocating that they did not want to progress:

'I suppose I felt that it was something more done to me really'

(MM4)

All participants wished to address challenges with a senior manager, suggesting a possible solution:

'if you take something that cuts across the whole of CMHT, you could actually say we would like six reps from CMHT to form a little group as a bit of a think time and work with you, and we want you to connect with different teams and connecting with your teams and asking different teams to be looking at different bits of it and trying to bring it together and synthesising. It would all be more complicated and messy, but when you got the outcome, you can play it back and people will go "oh well, at least they listen"; that's the other thing, co-production doesn't mean you get your own way, but you do get chance to say your piece'

(SM1)

Participants reported feeling powerless, disengaged, and invalidated due to a lack of power distribution. These feelings led to emotional responses, which compounded the notion that a negative organisational culture can impact on co-production.

Emotional response. A negative culture in combination with feeling undervalued can lead to emotional responses that impact on co-production efforts. All participants

noted increased stress levels, especially in delivering high-quality care amidst unhelpful systems:

'I'm just going to do my job and I am happy with that—I don't want to take the stress now of getting involved and not being heard'

(CL2)

'it always feels like you are trying to do the right thing in spite of some processes which are supposed [to] support that'

(CL1)

Stress impacts on work-life balance and wellbeing, subsequently resulting in some people not being able to remain in work, as summarised below:

'we see it day in and day out, staff leaving because they can't cope, and it is too sharp at the front end and you are being told to do yet another thing, and they may not say anything, but they vote with their feet, so I think we need to focus on that'

(CL5)

All participants described challenges with staff retention, recognising that this could impact on co-production due to a loss of skills as experienced staff are replaced with newer staff because of burnout:

'So, it is easy sometimes to recruit but sometimes harder to retain our staff, which is hugely disruptive for our patients and co-production'

(CL5)

'you train someone to the highest level and then they leave, so I think we need to focus on retaining staff and ensuring that they don't burn out, because it is a huge stress'

(CL5)

One participant felt that co-production could address the retention issues:

'If you think about the staff survey, all of the things that were really identified was that we are not effectively co-producing, and the reason that's important fundamentally is if we have a high turnover rate or we are not attractive to recruit, then we actually don't have services, and we don't attract the best people either; we get the people that might have had behaviours that we want to see less of in other organisations coming to us as a result of that, so I think that's fundamental'

(SM2)

Emotional responses were evident and impact on co-production. Power imbalances are impeding staff efforts to co-produce and maintain their own wellbeing. Participants, however, were keen to remain solution-focused and to consider how power could be redistributed. *What needs to happen to distribute power.* Participants highlighted three main areas where power imbalance could be addressed Firstly, happiness:

'The things that aren't considered co-production are...the happiness of staff'

(MM2)

Participants felt they needed to be heard, validated, and involved to be happy. However, they expressed that there were occasions where managerial actions did not do this:

'there is an expectation that people want to be treated in a really quite childish way, where the people in authority protect people from the reality'

(CL1)

Secondly, there was a desire for clear understanding of roles and functions within co-production, as summarised:

'I think there was some mention, thinking back there was some mention of this coming, but it wasn't like, "oh, this is starting now, and this is what the expectations are"'

(CL2)

Participants believed that there is a need to explore what co-production is, what is expected, and how it will work:

'how if our Trust was doing it, that introduction of what the thing is, why the thing is, and what their sense of what it might be and how it might work, with some dialogue and development of that idea to get to a point where the people who there was an expectation to operate that way, had a similar expectation'

(CL1)

Finally, participants highlighted the provision of ownership of team decision-making:

'I think if you give the actual team leader and consultant the message that, "you own this, and we

would not interfere with it", I think that would be more acceptable than well effectively what happens here is that the reality being, where the Trust is telling you what to do'

(CL2)

Power was a significant theme, illustrating how a challenging cultural climate is a barrier to co-production. All participants noted that power misuse impacts on individuals and service provision. Participants felt that an effective interface could support power distribution and the implementation of co-production.

Theme 4—Interface

This theme was broken down into the following sub-themes: (1) discussion, (2) communication methods, and (3) relationships (see Fig. 14.6).

Discussion. The reported concern of 'not being heard' highlighted the requirement for more involvement in process development to avoid barriers to service delivery:

'something which often seems like an intuitively good idea, but the process itself often dilutes the idea to such a degree that people feel the need to make some sort of change, but the bits that might have been most useful get lost along the way'

(CL1)

Participants did note that having these conversations was an issue due to the lack of communication from all parties:

'there isn't really a way of there being a two-way discussion, I think on either side actually'

(CL1)

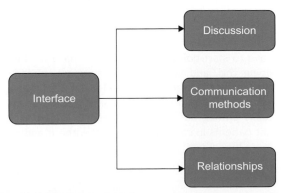

Fig. 14.6 Theme 4—interface.

All participants agreed that a communication strategy needs to be developed to ensure that the model does not become obsolete:

'The initial communication was fine, but I guess the fact that it then just disappeared'

(CL1)

'there should be communication and there should be agreement'

(MM3)

All senior managers noted that their communication on co-production had not been thorough and this had resulted in varied implementation:

'If you believe that communication is about ensuring that people understand, then we have probably been pretty dismal. If communication is about telling people, I think we had a go at telling people, but that is different'

(SM1)

All participants wanted to know more about co-production's origins and the expectation for local implementation:

'there are things we think, "oh well that might not apply or may be unhelpful or detrimental or wasteful"; then you would make the decision not to go along with those things, and ideally share that with people as to your feedback'

(CL1)

Participants made visible the importance of discussion and more robust dissemination.

Communication methods. Communication delivery methods are critical for successful co-production with participants expressing that email communication (the main communication method) is ineffective due to the volume received:

'you get emails at least once a month saying you have to start doing this as well, you have to start doing this, and you know the system is already stretched as it is, and I really feel that it is time that we as a Trust and we as clinicians think about actually putting our focus on areas that would benefit patients in co-production most without adding more bureaucratic layer to our work'

(CL5)

Whilst emails target many people (Baggot, 2007), they are ineffectual for implementing major change as information gets lost:

'the number of emails and number of correspondences you get, you don't get a chance to do justice and read everything in detail. I could do more if I understood better what the Trust's vision of co-production is? I am sure that the Trust would have other ways of engaging their clinical leads and team leaders to make them better informed?'

(CL5)

All participants had heard about co-production via different forums (governance meeting, discussion papers, training); however, they believed that this was not sufficient and considered alternatives:

'maybe there could have been something in the communications bulletin, with a link you could click on'

(MM4)

'they maybe could have used a screensaver'

(MM4)

'if there is co-production, we need to be informed that this is what the Trust is intending to do, and we need you to come here and sit down with us, like with Appreciative Leadership, appreciative kind of dialogue and thinking about how best we could take this forward really, and contributing to the policy and suchlike'

(CL5)

Whilst opinions of the best communication method differed, all confirmed that training sessions would be beneficial:

'if there was some training and it clearly identified what co-production is or co-production isn't'

(MM4)

Some senior managers acknowledged their denial about how well they communicate:

'I'm sure it's probably not been communicated as well as it could have been, and I'm not sure it's been communicated well enough, and again it's the classic dilemma of a leader, like, "am I not being clear enough or are they just not listening?" and it's so easy to go, "oh they're not listening; I've told them

15 times and they still aren't hearing it". Particularly very senior people, you live in a very rarified world, and if all of the people you speak to know about it or wouldn't dare admit that they didn't, you can kid yourself that the rest of the organisation knows about it and understands'

(SM1)

It is clear that the method of communication is critical to successful implementation of co-production and participants also noted that healthy working relationships were equally important.

Relationships. Equitable relationships are essential for co-working and co-production, which was a view shared by middle managers and clinical leads:

'I think relationships are the key, if you have good relationships with your colleagues, with your consultants, with your senior managers, with your team leaders, they will go above and beyond, and they will do anything'

(CL5)

Participants emphasised that effective relationships would increase the probability of addressing the 'disconnect':

'I think the top and bottom completely lose sight of each other. I think that is a real risk'

(CL1)

Participants repeatedly discussed reality and it was clear there were two separate realities within the Trust: frontline staff reality versus senior manager reality:

'there are possibly just two quite distinct cultures within the organisation whereby we just don't communicate well with each other and have a differed sense of things'

(CL1)

With conflicting realities, consideration of how to maintain relationships is critical, especially when differing personalities compete:

'I think that sometimes, certain personality traits might affect as well. There are different people modelling different ego states, where they think they are superior to someone else or better than someone else, so consequently not give the other partner the respect they deserve'

(MM1)

Reciprocal relationships are needed when addressing interface challenges and therefore are vital for co-production. Individuals' attitudes towards co-production are also critical.

Theme 5—Attitudes Towards Co-production

This theme was divided into three sub-themes: (1) knowledge, (2) beliefs, and (3) incentives (see Fig. 14.7).

Knowledge. Participants expressed a lack of co-production knowledge, as summarised below:

'I have not had a great deal of knowledge or experience of co-production'

(MM1)

They felt that clarity about what co-production entails is also needed; however, ambiguity remains which has led to a lack of understanding:

'I think the Trust perspective is very ambiguous in what they believe co-production is'

(MM2)

'I'm not entirely certain of an absolute definition of co-production, but my understanding would be an integrated approach between professionals in the delivery of service'

(MM3)

Despite minimal knowledge among all middle managers and clinical leads, senior managers had a sound understanding:

'But for me, co-production is about getting the right people together to come up with the most effective solution and have that the debate about how you get to that point. Co-production isn't just doctors

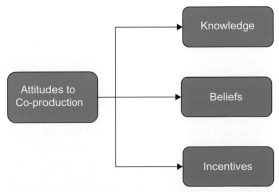

Fig. 14.7 Theme 5—attitudes towards co-production.

and nurses and a manager; it could be a team of service users, it could be two organisations jointly looking at how, so I think we get quite caught up on its got to be a very stereotypical head of operations, clinical director, lead nurse, lead manager, that perhaps co-production at its most naive, I think it can cover a whole range of spheres. I think we shy away from having those conversations; what I think we tend to do is we developed what I describe as unconscious compromise from either one party or the other, as we get caught up in not having a straightforward dialogue and I think we need to support people to do that'

(SM2)

This strengthens the assertion that an effective communication strategy is needed. Despite reported challenges, all participants feel that co-production can enhance service user care:

'it's about how we can come to a decision around what disciplines believe, obviously in the best interests of that service user and how we can effectively move that person's care forward'

(MM2)

While there were varying levels of co-production knowledge, participants felt that having a common understanding would increase success. Participants' beliefs regarding co-production was another identified attitude.

Beliefs. Most participants believed that co-production is viable and focused on the potential benefits of co-production:

'I think co-production, if implemented properly and extensively, it is probably the better model because ultimately the type of work we do in the healthcare component. I think co-production fits in very nicely with that because you have a multidisciplinary team (MDT) approach; you will have a management approach and a clinical approach, which has the potential to be very very good'

(MM1)

It was also noted that there is no better model than co-production for the organisation:

'I think you have to co-produce, and not one model or one discipline of staff will have the answer, so it is really important that we all work together and have our own distinct professions and identities but

come together to discuss issues. So, I don't think there is a better model'

(MM2)

Whilst all participants believed that co-production is a positive model, they also identified that it needs embedding in the culture:

'I don't think co-production should always be about when there is an issue, but I sometimes think that because we are so busy, and we work in the NHS, that sometimes that is how it constantly feels'

(MM4)

Participants did however feel that senior managers need to model co-production behaviours to consolidate their commitment, although co-production at local levels was acknowledged:

'there are some very good examples within team, and I think higher up needs to view this so that they can take this back and reflect on that and how they could embed that higher up'

(MM2)

Some participants commented that service users need to be involved within the process for co-production to be successful:

'I think personally that is the only way to move forward, if you had the service users on board'

(CL2)

Beliefs about co-production are central to engagement, clearly illustrating that staff beliefs can impact on implementation. However, the study findings go further, suggesting that motives for engagement are also essential, as when dishonesty is perceived, engagement decreases. All participants also identified that incentives are needed.

Incentives. All participants identified incentives to engage with co-production. It was considered that increased collaboration with more ownership and shared leadership would support a successful co-production model and rebuild relationships:

'it's that being more of a collaboration than one person saying what we are going to do and everyone thinking that they are being dictated to'

(MM4)

The first incentive discussed was staff happiness:

'the happiness of staff. They feel invested in it, and they can go home and feel like they have done a good job'

(MM2)

Staff wellbeing and happiness results in reduced stress and if co-production is also occurring, then a further reduction in stress levels could be experienced:

'Ultimately, it makes things easier for people, so the incentive will be that it will leave people feeling less anxious in terms of their personal accountability for everything; it's a sense of shared and collective'

(SM1)

The second incentive identified was decision-ownership which most clinical leads believed was critical for 'buy in' to the model:

'I think if you give the actual team leader and consultant the message that, "you own this, and we would not interfere with it"'

(CL2)

The third incentive discussed was using this change process to consider how to amend long-standing practices which would provide local teams with flexibility:

'What we really want is a broad understanding across the Trust of people functioning in a particular way with an allowance for local variation of service variation because the Trust is big and disparate, so you are always going to have some things that work in different ways because of the services. It might be that even within a small location, they have ended up with quite different services if they were much more in the gift of that being a shared decision in terms of direction'

(CL1)

If the Trust allowed this review of practices, then a focus on how service users can benefit from a co-production approach could be considered beneficial to both staff and service users:

'You would hope that there might be some particular benefits in terms of the experience people had coming into services. I think the thing which opening things up might allow people to do much better

TABLE 14.1   Core Components Needed for Implementation of Co-production
Core components required to commence implementation
Inclusion of service users in a co-production model
Positive organisational culture
Equal distribution of power
Effective communication
Effective change management strategies
Identification of incentives to engage staff

is to have more straightforward relationships with some of the patients that we have'

(CL1)

The final incentive noted by one participant was that co-production has the potential to reduce risks associated with mental health settings:

'I think reduced risk—whether it is the risk of poor mental health, risk to other, risk to self—so if you have got patients on the same page as you, I think it works much better that way. I think it is definitely worth it in terms of the long-term benefit, the recovery of the patient, better patient satisfaction, if you invest that time in co-production'

(CL5)

It was commonly agreed that incentive could push forward a co-production agenda.

Descriptive model. Following completion of the findings, a descriptive model of co-production was considered. The first element of the model is identifying the core components required for implementation (Table 14.1) followed by consideration of actions needed and recommendations on how these could be achieved in practice (Table 14.2).

CONCLUSION

The analysis of data identified five themes, with the first four being clearly rooted in the Trust's culture, resulting in 'disconnect' and unsuccessful co-production. The final theme illustrated a hope for the future with some clear consideration of how this could be achieved. The

TABLE 14.2   Actions and How to Implement Them in Co-production

Action	How?
Commit to reviewing their culture	– Attaining feedback from staff – Care Quality Commission reports – -Staff surveys
Consider how power can be distributed where hierarchical structures exist	– Commit to co-production – Honest conversations about power – Work with staff and service users actively
Consider how to convey their co-production vision	– An effective communication strategy – Training
Inform frontline staff about the realities of change	– Honest dialogue – Clear purpose – Ownership
Involve service users	– Don't pay lip service – Listen to their experiences – Ask how things could be done better – Consider how service users can be engaged

subsequent framework developed from Bamber's (2020) study aims to support the implementation of co-production within organisations, highlighting key concepts that could increase success.

References

Baggot, C. (2007). *Email marketing by the numbers: how to use the world's greatest marketing tool to take any organisation to the next level.* New Jersey: John Wiley & Sons.

Bamber, H. M. (2020). *Managers' and clinical leads' perspectives of a co-production model for community mental health service improvement in the NHS: a case study* [Professional Doctorate thesis, University of Salford].

Bradley, E. (2015). Carers and co-production: enabling expertise through experience. *Mental Health Review Journal,* 20(4), 232–241. https://psycnet.apa.org/doi/10.1108/MHRJ-05-2014-0016

Clark, M. (2015). Co-production in mental health. *Mental Health Review Journal,* 20(4), 213–219. https://psycnet.apa.org/doi/10.1108/MHRJ-10-2015-0030

Department of Health and Social Care. (2019). NHS financial stability. London: National Audit Office.

Miles, M. B., & Huberman, A. M. (1994). *Qualitative data analysis: An expanded sourcebook* (2nd ed.). London: Sage Publications.

TUC. (2015). *Mental health and the workplace: A TUC Education workbook.* London: TUC.

Yin, R. K. (2014). *Case study research: Design and methods* (5th ed.). Thousand Oaks, CA: Sage.

15

An Integrated Digital Future: Intelligence, Transformation, and Personalised Care

Dr Hayley Bamber, Samantha Pywell, and Linda Vernon

KEY CONCEPTS

- The concept of an integrated digital future in health and social care
- Challenges with applying the WHO principles within an integrated digital future
- Real-world examples using the case study
- The digital paradigm: transformation post-pandemic
- The importance of partnerships in integrated care and empowering citizens' choice

INTRODUCTION

Previous chapters have focused on conceptualising and contextualising integrated care. This chapter aims to consider this knowledge and how this has been influenced through the rapid rise of digital health and social care. This chapter will aim to define, situate, and explore the contribution of an integrated digital future within integrated care through considering the impact that the COVID-19 pandemic has had on its implementation. A real-life example in a case study will be illustrated to support the contextualisation of this integrated digital future.

THE CONCEPT OF AN INTEGRATED DIGITAL FUTURE IN HEALTH AND SOCIAL CARE

An integrated digital future in health, social care, and beyond is significantly challenging, and cannot be delivered without addressing the fundamental core influencers, including organisational siloes and the associated cultural and technical challenges impacting compatibility of digital integration, workforce upskilling, personal choice, and patient needs (NHS, 2021; NHS Providers, 2022). Digital integration, intelligence, and transformation in the context of person-centred care must therefore be addressed through the lens of an integrated digital future

and end users' needs (clinicians, patients, families, etc.). Yet, without *'the supply of more efficient health services'* (Good Things Foundation, 2018) increasing the population's access to the fundamental right of the Internet and 'basic digital skills' (Good Things Foundation, 2018), there is potential for inequity of digital access directly impacting individuals' health and wellbeing. The contribution of digital technology within integrated care cannot and should not be underestimated, as acknowledged in the *Nine Pillars of Integrated Care* (International Foundation of Integrated Care, 2022), but balanced within the needs of the individuals using and navigating the system. Integrated care (and therefore all things digital within the integrated care system [ICS]) needs to 'cater for everyone' (World Health Organization [WHO], 2016). However, the Internet is not free and neither is the technology (e.g., hardware and software) required to use it for the purpose of integrated care, thus creating and widening inequities in access to content (e.g., public health messaging on social media) (McKee & Stuckler, 2019). A combined strategy of *'digital citizen empowerment'* and use of the health inequities lens is therefore needed for the sustainability of positive outcomes within an integrated digital future (Sharma et al., 2022). To explore this further, we first need to expand upon digital integration (digital interoperability, intelligence, and transformation) as all are critical factors to the future of integrated care (King's Fund, 2022; Transformation Directorate at NHS England, 2022a). Definitions are illustrated first, then placed in context of the case study.

Digital Integration

Digital integration (in the context of integrated care) can be defined though the components of interoperability (King's Fund, 2022), digital intelligence, and transformation (Transformation Directorate at NHS England, 2022a). The digital integration of patient data can be beneficial to increasing the speed of information sharing for clinicians involved in their care, increasing timely assessment and interventions (Transformation Directorate at NHS England, 2022a). Gatekeeping digital information is required in some parts of the ICS (e.g., safeguarding of patient data). However, not making information open-access (e.g., contact details for social prescribing destination providers (Voluntary, Community, Faith and Social Enterprise [VCFSE] organisations) who want to be found) could be seen as an avoidable obstacle to equitable digital integration across an ICS. Those in need of using the data (e.g., community, voluntary, and faith groups; small social enterprises) may not have the funding resources to pay to access information which could significantly benefit citizens (e.g., local destinations of social prescribing). Without digital integration, disharmonious incompatible data can exist (e.g., patient records held on different systems with different and at times incomplete data on each).

Interoperability

'Interoperability is the technical term used to describe the flow of information – about decisions made and care that has been or is being provided – across care settings. Good interoperability facilitates the best care in the best place with decisions made using all available information.'

(King's Fund, 2022)

The four levels of interoperability by the Healthcare Information and Management Systems Society (HIMSS, 2017) in the context of integrated care are illustrated below. These four levels influence strategic direction and policy on integrated care; however, on a practical level, the eternal conundrum of semantic interoperability must be acknowledged. Linguistic professions can analyse where language use changes due to meanings and context (Archer et al., 2022). Incompatibility of systems due to language which significantly impact interoperability are future challenges that will not go away, but rather need continuous reassessment.

1. Foundational—'establishes the inter connectivity requirements needed for one system or application to securely communicate data to and receive data from another'.
2. Structural—'defines the format, syntax, and organisation of data exchange including at the data field level for interpretation'.
3. Semantic—'provides for common underlying models and codification of the data including the use of data elements with standardised definitions from publicly

available value sets and coding vocabularies, providing shared understanding and meaning to the user'.
4. Organisational—'includes governance, policy, social, legal and organisational considerations to facilitate the secure, seamless and timely communication and use of data both within and between organisation, entities and individuals. These components enable shared consent, trust and integrated end-user processes and workflows.' (HIMSS, 2017)

Intelligence

Digital intelligence within an ICS is about systems and the data stored which can make a difference to individuals' present and future care (through improving clinical and wellbeing outcomes), primarily by 'operationalising' or sharing of relevant information for system-level analytics (Combined Intelligence for Population Health Action, 2022; Deloitte Centre for Health Solutions, 2019; Vernon, 2021). The National Institute for Health and Care Research (NIHR, 2022) illustrated this in their 'Whole System Integrated Care' approach, where data intelligence was shared to address the population needs during the pandemic in London. Data intelligence can include intelligence about people (data about patients or those receiving care), services and care provision (such as waiting times, attendance rates, key performance indicators, or audit data), or outcomes (data from patient-recorded outcome measures or patient-recorded experience measures) (Pennucci et al., 2019). Data intelligence is the use of existing data for prediction of future health and care, including predicting when someone may become unwell (with the positive outcome of intervening before a negative outcome happens). Data intelligence supports ICSs in a number of ways: for the provision of direct care (e.g., prediction of future health and care needs), supporting preventative interventions (Vernon, 2021), and avoiding 'unnecessarily wasting resources' (Orlowski et al., 2021); for secondary uses, such as population health management; to support further research into health and care provision, when anonymised or pseudonymised data is held in a trusted research environment; and individually for the patient, when they are given access to data about their biometrics, diagnostic tests, and care provision, and can complement that with data collected outside healthcare such as blood pressure, step count, and information from wearable data (Zhang et al., 2022). Despite the advancements in data intelligence, each ICS must strive toward collecting more data specific to inequities and inequalities impacting citizen health to analyse and address the wider determinants of health in a timely manner through increased accuracy and contextual depth to data intelligence (Marmot et al., 2020; WHO, 2022).

Transformation

Digital transformation is where significant changes occur to improve patient outcomes as a result of digital improvements and influences (both internal and external to the organisation) (Kaehne, 2022). Transformation is much more than converting paper or analogue processes to online or digital processes—transformation is where the implementation of digital tools fundamentally improves the way the service is provided or how people access service in an ICS. An example of digital transformation is the rapid shift to telehealth and telecare adoption as a direct result of the pandemic, allowing people to be monitored and supported with their health or care needs while at home (Kaehne, 2022). Retainable through the rationale of patient preference (reasonable request) or a reasonable adjustment to appointments, online video-call appointments are arguably more accessible and convenient for both clinicians and patients alike (when the clinician and patient have the access and skills to navigate this digital world). Additionally, transformation within the ICS can evolve organically as individuals' own needs change and technology advances. Ultimately, this is dependent upon the capabilities and ceilings of the digital environment (and staff digital skills) in which digital transformation occurs.

Person-Centred Care

Person-centred care is a term that has long been discussed and explored throughout healthcare literature (The Health Foundation, 2016); however, there remains debate about the successful application in practice. All literature identifies the importance of personalised care within ICSs to support ensuring that individuals needs are met through personalised goal setting (Berntsen et al., 2018). (NHS England, 2022b) defined personalised care as when *'people have choice and control over the way their care is planned and delivered. It is based on 'what matters' to them and their individual strengths and needs.'* The Health Foundation (2016) outlined a framework focused on four key principles of person-centred care which can be applied to all aspects of an integrated digital future within an ICS:

1. 'Affording people dignity, compassion, and respect.
2. Offering coordinated care, support, or treatment.
3. Offering personalised care, support, or treatment.
4. Supporting people to recognise and develop their own strengths and abilities to enable them to live an independent and fulfilling life.'

(The Health Foundation, 2016)

CASE STUDY Citizen Empowerment Within Digital Transformation of an ICS

The case study used to support this chapter explores the implementation of 'citizen empowerment' (NHS England, 2021) within the digital transformation in an ICS and a digital directory of service to underpin integrated care (specific to social prescribing) across a commissioning footprint. This system level integration case study by Linda Vernon, the Acting Digital Culture and Transformation Clinical Lead at the Lancashire & South Cumbria ICS, was selected to illustrate the cross-organisational co-ordination required across the Lancashire & South Cumbria ICS for outputs and services, such as a social prescribing directory. Vernon argues, critically, that 'citizen empowerment is needed for positive outcomes within an integrated digital future'.

The ICS has delivered significant support to those who continue to remain digitally excluded, particularly with access to training and skills development via Digital Health Champions (Digital Unite, 2021) (volunteers and existing health and care staff), raising awareness of health apps, and in collaboration with partner organisations in the ICS (particularly VCFSE organisations) with access to devices and connectivity. Developing end users' skills and confidence will potentially improve their experience of using digital health tools and other digital resources to help support the wider determinants of health, along with simultaneously upskilling and developing staff and volunteers in health, care, and VCFSE organisations and improving those champions' employment opportunities.

Providing citizens and patients with the tools and skills to use apps and other digital health tools is one important aspect of digitally activating our population. However, there is much more information and support available online (including awareness of real-world services and support) to empower people and support better health outcomes. In particular, the ICS has been working toward the creation of a single catalogue of supporting VCFSE services, where the information contained can be crowd-sourced from people across all sectors, confirmed by an assurance team, and pushed to interoperable solutions that may be either citizen/patient-facing or professional-facing. The approach is built on the use of an open-data standard, Open Referral UK, now endorsed for use across public sector services (Central Digital & Data Office, 2022) by the UK Data Standards Authority. The model is described in detail by Vernon (2021) and has only been possible to implement due to engagement and a commitment to collaborative working across the health, local government, and VCFSE sectors.

CASE STUDY   The Role and Needs of the Citizen in Integrated Digital Transformation

The citizen has an important role in digital transformation as the digital solutions being delivered in health and care require the citizen or patient to use them to interact and transact with services. Digital solutions have a large part to play in supporting people to stay well (prevention) and/ or manage their illness (use of apps, wearables and remote monitoring devices, access to their health and care records, etc.), providing them with tools and information at the right time, supporting better health and care outcomes. The Lancashire & South Cumbria ICS has taken an inclusive approach to digital transformation (Davies, 2022). Aligned with recommendations from both NHSEI and NHS Digital (Blackstock, 2021), the approach has helped identify insights into the health and care needs of citizens and how digital technology can support some of those needs.

The pandemic accelerated the pace of digital transformation for frontline staff and raised expectations on citizens to adopt digital health technologies. Despite accelerated digital adoption in the last few years (5 years' growth in 1), 5% of our population remains digitally excluded (Lloyds Bank, 2021), and this is likely to be higher among deprived or otherwise challenged communities (Marmot et al., 2020). The very people who are digitally excluded are those who are likely to be at higher risk of health inequalities (Honeyman et al., 2020) and therefore be higher consumers of health and care services. With high levels of health inequalities in our area, we are particularly mindful of the wider determinants of health (Marmot et al., 2020; WHO, 2022) and how digital, whilst potentially increasing the health inequality gap, can also support people with those determinants, such as access to education and employment opportunities, social connection and inclusion, and opportunities.

Ultimately, all the work outlined above is designed to support the people of Lancashire & South Cumbria with digital resources to stay well, find information easily and in a timely manner, participate in shared decision-making about their healthcare, self-manage their illnesses, and interact/transact with healthcare. As digital tools are developed in the post-pandemic period to support patient-initiated follow-ups, remote consultations, remote monitoring and virtual reporting (such as participating in a remote pre operative assessment), and other initiatives, the underpinning foundations of digital inclusion, access to a reliable and complete digital catalogue of services, and user-centred design are imperative to successful deployment.

Integrated care is more than structural changes to digital systems: it is about people and their health, or 'the end users' (Verdoy et al., 2022). Critically, we cannot shift up to a large system approach unless there is an accurate understanding of local individuals' needs through data. Understanding whole-system change influences actions at all levels (NIHR, 2022). At a macro level, the legislation of both patient data and integrated care presents challenges to the compatibility of intelligence locally for patient care. Inequities (not just inequalities) are fundamental to both measure, grow, and develop integrated care at macro, meso, and micro levels, hence the real need to examine local health inequities (Marmot et al., 2020). The consensus is that digital should be embedded in all aspects (International Foundation for Integrated Care, 2022), yet systems are in danger of making the future for citizens and inequities worse if digital integration, intelligence,

and transformation in ICSs is not considered through the lens of personalised health inequalities (and inequities) (Marmot et al., 2020).

CHALLENGES WITH THE WHO DEFINITION

Fundamentally, the WHO (2016) *Core Principles of Integrated Care* (Table 15.1) and subsequent definitions of integrated care highlight the centrality of addressing inequities. However, by instigating a digital world as both the foundations and structure within integrated care, this creates multiple barriers that both staff working in integrated care and individuals receiving care (or need care) can face. Digital heat maps (Leeming & Hurring, 2017), although only of static Wi-Fi and not representative of mobile devices (including contract length or use of mobiles), illustrated some of the complex picture of inequalities surrounding access to the Internet (Good Things Foundation, 2021). An expectation of a patient (and employee outside of the workplace) to email, scan a QR code, or log in to a website can be seen as inequity within integrated care provision (contributing to additional barriers), and yet the structure of the ICS is to be built within the digital world in the UK (Good Things Foundation, 2018). So where is the bridge? How is the digital world of an ICS bridged between the land of those with digital access and skills and those who do not? Seeing digital access, skills, and wellbeing as critical to the wider picture of successful outcomes in an ICS is, although difficult to measure, a reality. Lack of digital access is evidenced to negatively impact an individual's health and wellbeing through lack of access to

TABLE 15.1   Adapted from the World Health Organisation Core Principles of Integrated Care

Principle	Explanation	Real World Digital Experience
Comprehensive	'Care offered in a way that is responsive to the needs and aspirations of the populations and individuals'	Using data to inform intelligent clinical and commissioning decision-making and to anticipate future care needs for individuals and populations
Equitable	Equity of access of care to all	Fundamental crack. Lack of equitable access to digital. Fundamental access (no signal, can't afford, no consistent access). Internet is not free. Devices to access the Internet are not free. Many barriers to getting onto the Internet and then consistent use. Digital has the potential to both increase equitable access to healthcare (for example, video consultations allowing people to receive care at a home or work environment) and increase health inequalities due to the 'digital divide' caused by lack of access to devices, connectivity, or the skills to use them. Wider determinants of health and wellbeing not all recorded (WHO, 2022)
Sustainable	Care should be provided in a way that promotes sustainability	Reduce duplication through shared records (EMIS, NHS Transformation Directorate at NHS England 2022a, etc.)
Coordinated	Care should wrap around the person and be co-ordinated in a way that benefits the person	Personalised care (NHS, 2019)
Continuous	Care should be provided across the life course	Continuous digital health care records (NHS Digital, 2022)
Holistic	All aspects of a person's life need to be considered	Wider determinants of health (Marmot et al., 2020)
Preventative	Prevention and the social determinants of health and ill health need to be central	Long Term Plan (NHS, 2019)
Empowerment	People should have control of their own health	Movements such as the Disability Movement (Disability Rights (2022) and the Mental Health Service User Movement (Wallcraft & Bryant, 2003)) stressed the need for individuals to have an active say in their own care and this must consider the digital aspects of care as well.

(Continued)

TABLE 15.1   Adapted from the World Health Organisation Core Principles of Integrated Care—cont'd

Principle	Explanation	Real World Digital Experience
Respectful	*Care should consider and be sensitive to people's dignity, social situation, and culture*	see Chapter 7 on co-production
Collaborative	*Delivering and planning care to include stakeholders*	How can individuals' give feedback? Rethink if only through digital means—need phone line, accept letters, etc.
Co-produced	*People are active partners at a strategy, organisational, and individual level*	see Chapter 7 on co-production
Governed through shared accountability	*Between care providers and local people to ensure quality care and improved health outcomes*	Potential to achieve through co-production
Evidence-informed	*Best evidence base and assessed through measurable outcomes*	Standard practice for health and social care professionals, yet not all digital interventions or use of digital is evidence-based.
Whole-systems thinking	*Whole system rather than siloes*	Break down communication siloes between organisations to increase innovation and collaboration across integrated care system
Ethical	*Risk–benefit ratio is considered for all interventions*	Challenges with a lack of agreed ethical guidelines for the provision of digital mental health care (Martinez-Martin et al., 2020)

WHO, 2016 p5

fundamental interactions within society (Good Things Foundation, 2018). The illustrative example (Fig. 15.1), from a report by Lloyds Bank (2021) on individuals' reasons for using the Internet, misses the specific contextual detail on how vital these activities are to the individual to maintain and improve their health. What makes an individual well, specific to the interaction of what is contained with the digital world and an ICS, is yet to be researched with the specificity of the real barriers that individuals face.

The Digital Paradigm: Transformation Post-Pandemic

The COVID-19 pandemic of 2020 instigated a tectonic shift in the use of digital technology across health and social care (Rabello et al., 2022). It both created the large-scale international demand for telehealth primarily due to lockdowns and remote working (WHO, 2021), and platform adoption to work in this way; for example, the adoption

of Microsoft Teams by NHSX (Blackstock, 2021). This highlighted the potential for increased choice for individuals who prefer accessing health, social care, and third sector (e.g., appointments) through the Internet (NHS, 2022). The pandemic created an unstable digital paradigm (which we are currently in at the time of writing this book), creating a rapid shift from need for digital innovation through transformation and glimpses of the post-pandemic digital world for integrated care that we hope to eventually find ourselves in.

Microsoft was adopted by NHS Digital as a key provider in 2020, resulting in NHS (social care and wider) organisational adoption of the video-call platform Microsoft Teams (MS Teams) (Blackstock, 2021). Although other platforms (Attend anywhere) were being used, MS Teams resulted in the potential to connect communication across organisations and beyond. This transformation from being heavily dependent upon emails and phone calls to the potential

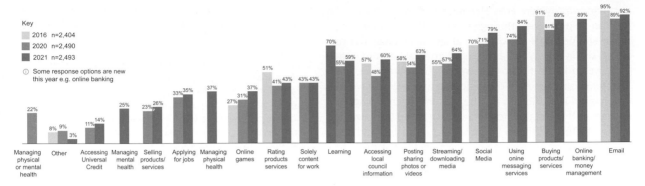

Fig. 15.1 Reasons for using the Internet. (Lloyds Bank, 2021).

for either video or phone calls from anywhere is unlocking an increase in communication speed (e.g., staff do not need to wait at a desk to act on key information).

Unlocking communication potential for ICSs is an essential task, as seen with alternative (and arguably pre-existing) methods to in-person assessment and intervention in the pandemic with patients (telehealth, telecare, text, messaging platforms, phone call, questionnaires, education videos and content sent by email). Pywell (2022) illustrated a proof of concept on connecting the local social prescribing landscape (crossing an ICS footprint containing VCFSE) within an MS Teams call hosted by a university, based on the DigiLearn Sector (#DLS). A Senior Learning Technologist from the University of Central Lancashire (UCLan) identified that creating the #DLS meant understanding the value of connecting beyond one organisation where the benefits outweigh the risks. The intention was to increase the 'community capacity' (Morris et al., 2020) and future potential of the ICS through breaking down traditional communication siloes. Limited only by software capabilities (e.g., number of people within one MS Team), access to Internet and individual digital skills could connect and empower professions and interest-specific groups (e.g., all occupational therapists across health and social care, all colleagues [early adopters] across the social prescribing landscape) with the intent of increasing the speed of communications, fostering innovative environments, and obtaining real-time information on challenges across the ICS impacting social prescribing that could be solved through simple timely knowledge exchange. UCLAn and Jisc (2022) highlighted the benefit to this multiorganisational approach through increased speed of communication across organisations. Translated to the ICS, this example could include health, social care, voluntary sector, private businesses, local council, and infrastructure organisations (e.g., police and ambulance services) working

together. The value of knowledge-sharing is difficult to measure but goes beyond one communication method. The ripples of positive influence within the ICS are reflected in an increased harmony and balance of knowledge.

Although there remains international debate on the exact stage of the COVID-19 pandemic that each country is in, patient care and the means to do so through integrated digital care remains a significant ongoing priority. The reasonable adjustment and reasonable request of a citizen to dial into an appointment is protected both under personalised care through 'citizen empowerment' (NHS Transformation Directorate at NHS England 2022a) and in law (Equality Act, 2010). ICSs must strive to push back from the perception of only being gatekeepers of information within systems to an empowering and collaborative co-production model, understanding their local populations' digital and health needs through creation of more listening and co-production spaces for knowledge exchange despite the instability of digital paradigms, pandemics, and government (and world) influences.

The Importance of Partnerships in Integrated Care Empowering Citizens' Choice

The centrality of personalised care and citizen choice within decisions impacting the digital future of integrated care need to be co-produced to address and reduce potential health inequities (Gold, 2021; Chapter 7 on co-production). Assuming clinicians, families, and individuals themselves have consistent access to the Internet, the financial means to continue to access (both through Internet and device costs), and the requisite digital skills are a set of an assumptions which can unravel the well-meaning intentions of policymakers (McKee & Stuckler, 2019). For integrated care to succeed, it needs integrated digital technology (with open access as seen in social prescribing with understanding where the local destination providers are). However, the practicalities of this can be unravelled through the simple lack of Internet signal and personal choice. Individuals can choose not to access the Internet, and at the fundamental heart of integrated care is the tension between personal choice and a system constructed and developing into a digital world which is not accessible to all. The reasonable choice not to engage with the digital health and care world (however it is constructed within an ICS) must be respected and not vilified, for that pressure to conform could contribute to increasing health inequalities and impact an individual's wellbeing. This choice works for patients but not health and care professionals as the expectations upon all are increasing as systems develop. The fundamental right of citizens to choose whether to use the digital world or not needs respecting, and support for citizens to navigate both digital and non digital worlds needs to remain even in this new age of integrated care. When we start to record and act on citizens' digital preferences and access to the digital world rather than engaging/non engaging with employees within an ICS, we change the narrative to clearer representation of all citizens' digital needs, preferences, and situations rather than the naive and fallacious argument of patients' own digital skills being the only barrier (caused by them) to their care. True digital integration is inherently complex and relies upon individuals' digital access, wellbeing, and skills; hence, a personalised approach to an individual's digital needs is imperative to make the integrated care agenda work.

CONCLUSION

To conclude, this chapter on an integrated digital future included the definition of the concept of an integrated digital future in health and social care. It illustrated the challenges with the application of the WHO principles within an integrated digital future and a case study example from an ICS in the UK. This chapter also included a discussion on the digital paradigm in post-pandemic transformation and finished with the importance of partnerships in integrated care and empowering citizens' choice.

References

Archer, D., Aijmer, K., & Wichmann, A. (2022). *Pragmatics: An advanced resource book for students*. London: Routledge.

Berntsen, G., Høyem, A., Lettrem, I., Ruland, C., Rumpsfeld, M., & Gammon, D. (2018). A person-centered Integrated care quality framework, based on a qualitative study of patients' evaluation of care in light of chronic care ideals. *BMC Health Services Research*, *18*(1), 1–15. https://doi.org/10.1186/s12913-018-3246-z

Blackstock, S. (2021, January 14). *How Microsoft Teams can support your clinical practice during the pandemic*. NHS Digital. https://www.nhsx.nhs.uk/blogs/how-microsoft-teams-can-support-your-clinical-practice-during-the-pandemic/

Central Digital & Data Office. (2002, August 9). *Guidance: Record and share information about public services in local authorities*. https://www.gov.uk/government/publications/open-standards-for-government/record-and-share-information-about-public-services-in-local-authorities

Combined Intelligence for Population Health Action. (2022). *CIPHA*. https://www.cipha.nhs.uk/

Davies, R. (2022). *Inclusive Digital Transformation: what you need to know*. Thrive by Design. https://www.thrivebydesign.org.uk/our-learning/Inclusive-digital-transformation-what-you-need-to-know

Deloitte Centre for Health Solutions. (2019). *The transition to integrated care: population health management in England*. https://www2.deloitte.com/content/dam/Deloitte/uk/Documents/public-sector/deloitte-uk-public-sector-population-health-management.pdf

Digital Unite. (2021). https://www.digitalunite.com/

Disability Rights UK. (2022). *Disability Rights Handbook Edition 47. April 2022—April 2023*. London: Disability Rights UK.

EMIS. https://www.emishealth.com/

Equality Act. (2010). London: Stationery Office.

Gold, R. (2021, December 21). *How NHS Digital is developing user-centred design maturity*. NHS Digital. https://digital.nhs.uk/blog/design-matters/2021/how-nhs-digital-is-developing-user-centred-design-maturity

Good Things Foundation. (2018). *The economic impact of Digital Inclusion in the UK: A report for Good Things Foundation*. https://www.goodthingsfoundation.org/wp-content/uploads/2021/02/the_economic_impact_of_digital_inclusion_in_the_uk_final_submission_stc_0.pdf

Good Things Foundation. (2021). *A blueprint to fix the digital divide*. https://www.goodthingsfoundation.org/insights/a-blueprint-to-fix-the-digital-divide/

HIMSS. (2017). *Dictionary of healthcare information technology terms, acronyms and organizations* (4th ed.). London: HIMSS.

Honeyman, M., Maguire, D., Evans, H., & Davies, A. (2020). *Digital technology and health inequalities: a scoping review (2020)*. Cardiff: Public Health Wales NHS Trust.

International Foundation for Integrated Care. (2022). *Nine Pillars of Integrated Care*. https://integratedcarefoundation.org/nine-pillars-of-integrated-care#1589446997093-e458b4d0-6308

Jisc. (2022). *DigiLearn Sector*. https://www.jisc.ac.uk/get-involved/digilearn-sector

Kaehne, A. (2022). *Integrated care: Reflections on change in health services*. Bingley: Emerald Group Publishing.

King's Fund. (2022). *Digital technologies and interoperability: enabling the future of integrated care*. https://www.kingsfund.org.uk/projects/interoperability-digital-enabling-integrated-care

Leeming, S., & Hurring, C. (2017, August 23). *Heatmapping digital exclusion*. Department for Digital, Culture, Media

& Sport. https://digitalinclusion.blog.gov.uk/2017/08/23/heatmapping-digital-exclusion/

Lloyds Bank. (2021). *UK Consumer Digital Index 2021: The UK's largest study of digital and financial lives*. https://www.lloydsbank.com/assets/media/pdfs/banking_with_us/whats-happening/210513-lloyds-consumer-digital-index-2021-report.pdf

Marmot, M., Allen, J., Boyce, T., Goldblatt, P., & Morrison, J. (2020). *Health equity in England: The Marmot review 10 years on*. London: The Institute of Health Equity, The Health Foundation.

Martinez-Martin, N., Dasgupta, I., Carter, A., Chandler, J. A., Kellmeyer, P., Kreitmair, K., Weiss, A., & Cabrera, L. Y. (2020). Ethics of digital mental health during COVID-19: crisis and opportunities. *JMIR Mental Health*, 7(12), e23776. https://doi.org/10.2196/23776

McKee, M., & Stuckler, D. (2019). How the Internet risks widening health inequalities. *American Journal of Public Health*, 108(9), 1178–1179. https://doi.org/10.2105/AJPH.2018.304616

Morris, D., Thomas, P., Ridley, J., & Webber, M. (2020). Community-enhanced social prescribing: integrating community in policy and practice. *International Journal of Community Well being*, 5, 179–195. https://doi.org/10.1007/s42413-020-00080-9

NHS. (2019). *The NHS long term plan*. https://www.longterm-plan.nhs.uk/

NHS. (2022). Making the case for a more personalised care approach. https://www.england.nhs.uk/personalisedcare/making-the-case-for-a-more-personalised-care-approach/

NHS Digital. (2022). Offering patients access to their future health information. https://digital.nhs.uk/services/nhs-app/nhs-app-guidance-for-gp-practices/guidance-on-nhs-app-features/accelerating-patient-access-to-their-record/offering-patients-access-to-their-future-health-information#:~:text=On%201%20November%202022%2C%20patients,to%20create%20the%20same%20functionality.

NHS England. (2021, October 4). *What Good Looks Like framework*. https://transform.england.nhs.uk/digitise-connect-transform/what-good-looks-like/what-good-looks-like-publication/

NHS England. (2022a). *NHS England—Transformation Directorate*. https://www.nhsx.nhs.uk/

NHS England. (2022b). *What is personalised care?* https://www.england.nhs.uk/personalisedcare/what-is-personalised-care/

NHS Providers. (2022). *Building a digital strategy: understanding the system context*. https://nhsproviders.org/building-a-digital-strategy/understand-the-system-context

NIHR. (2022). WSIC Whole System Integrated Care, London. https://www.nwlondonics.nhs.uk/professionals/whole-systems-integrated-care-wsic

Orlowski, A., Snow, S., Humphreys, H., Smith, W., Jones, R. S., Ashton, R., & Bottle, A. (2021). Bridging the impactibility gap in population health management: a systematic review.

BMJ Open, 11(12), e052455. https://doi.org/10.1136/bmjopen-2021-052455

Pennucci, F., De Rosis, S., & Nuti, S. (2019). Can the jointly collection of PROMs and PREMs improve integrated care? The changing process of the assessment system for the hearth failure path in Tuscany Region. *International Journal of Integrated Care*, 19(4), 421. https://doi.org/10.5334/ijic.s3421

Pywell, S. (2022). *Connecting local social prescribing communities through an online community of practice* [Conference presentation]. 4th International Social Prescribing Network Conference, online.

Rabello, G. M., Pêgo-Fernandes, P. M., & Jatene, F. B. (2022). Are we preparing for the digital healthcare era. *Sao Paulo Medical Journal*, 140(2), 161–162. https://doi.org/10.1590/2F1516-3180.2022.140225112021

Sharma, S., Kar, A. K., Gupta, M. P., Dwivedi, Y. K., & Janssen, M. (2022). Digital citizen empowerment: a systematic literature review of theories and development models. *Information Technology for Development*, 28(4), 660–687. https://doi.org/10.1080/02681102.2022.2046533

The Health Foundation. (2016). *Person-centred care made simple. What everyone should know about patient centred care*. London: The Health Foundation.

Verdoy, D., Gil, A. O., Lilja, M., Isaksson, J., Vergara, I., de la Higuera, L., Udby, S., Sorknæs, A. D., McCann, L., Zwiefka, A., Blömeke, J., Arndt, F., Kaye, R., Khan, O., Erturkmen, G. B. L., Cámara, A., Kalra, D., & de Manuel, E. (2022). Integrated personalized care for patients with advanced chronic diseases to improve health and quality of life (ADLIFE Project). *International journal of Integrated Care*, 22(S1), 122. https://doi.org/10.5334/ijic.ICIC21068

Vernon, L. (2021). Healthier Lancashire and South Cumbria—a digital catalogue of service information to improve health management. https://openreferraluk.org/community/case-studies/lancs-south-cumbria

Wallcraft, J., & Bryant, M. (2003). *The mental health service user movement in England*. London: Sainsbury Centre for Mental Health.

World Health Organization. (2016). *Technical series on primary health care: Integrating health services*. Geneva: WHO Press.

World Health Organization. (2021). *Global strategy on digital health 2020-2025*. Geneva: WHO Press.

World Health Organization. (2022). *Social determinants of health*. https://www.who.int/health-topics/social-determinants-of-health#tab=tab_1

Zhang, J., Yang, M., Ge, Y., Ivers, R., Webster, R., & Tian, M. (2022). The role of digital health for post-surgery care of older patients with hip fracture: a scoping review. *International Journal of Medical Informatics*, 160, 104790. https://doi.org/10.1016/j.ijmedinf.2022.104709

Further Reading

HSJ. (2021, May 18). *Digital priorities for integrated care systems*. https://www.hsj.co.uk/technology-and-innovation/digital-priorities-for-integrated-care-systems/7030068.article

International Foundation for Integrated Care. (2019). *Digital health enabling integrated care: The interoperability challenge*. https://integratedcarefoundation.org/wp-content/uploads/2019/10/Digital-health-SIG-5-12-2019-ver-1.pdf

International Foundation for Integrated Care. (2021). *Digital Health Enabling Integrated Care Webinar Series*. https://integratedcarefoundation.org/events/digital-health-enabling-integrated-care-webinar-series-2#1485246030073-5e90f1df-668a

Lancashire & South Cumbria Health and Care Partnership. (2022, July 29). *Our Digital Future – a strategy for Lancashire and South Cumbria*. https://www.healthierlsc.co.uk/digitalfuture

16

Development of Neighbourhood Teams: A Framework for Preparedness

Dr Kirsty Marshall

KEY CONCEPTS

- Leadership
- Team development
- Neighbourhood and place
- Team development

INTRODUCTION

The preceding chapters have explored the *'how'* of integrated care, including transformation approaches and the vital inclusion of co-production as an enabler in shifting the health and social care context. Chapter 5 discussed the central role that neighbourhood working has played in the development of place-based and population-focused integrated care. Within this chapter, we build on these themes and explore the practical and cultural requirements to prepare teams that are adopting neighbourhood working. The evidence for the approach advocated is based on a professional doctoral thesis (Marshall, 2020). This study was an ethnographic narrative on the early stages of a neighbourhood team, as part of a wider organisational and system-integrated care

---

CASE STUDY

The following case study explores the observations and themes identified in the formation of a neighbourhood team. The research aimed to understand the experiences of the team members and followed the journey of an adult social care team and nursing team for 9 months from before co-location, through their early stages of integration, and the formation of the neighbourhood team.

Research Methodology

The methodology used was institutional ethnography. This approach was adopted as it aimed to understand the external influencing factors that exist within institutions, from the standpoint of the people within them (Smith, 2005).

Local Context

The study was located in the northwest of England. The borough (UK geographical district with an administrative unit 'borough council') in which the neighbourhood team was based had been moving towards an integrated care approach since 2016 and this included local authority, health, and other services coming together at macro, meso, and micro levels. The new integrated system held the vision to:

'Significantly raise healthy life expectancy in Tameside and Glossop through a place-based approach to better prosperity, health and wellbeing'

It was within this backdrop that the neighbourhood team was formed. While the team included a range of professionals, the two main teams coming together were the adult community nursing service (District Nursing) and the adult social care team. The new team had a targeted care approach focusing on adults (over 16) with complex health and social care needs.

(Continued)

The author would like to acknowledge and thank Kerry Williams and Julie Moore who helped with the original research in this chapter.

CASE STUDY—cont'd

Over the 9-month study period, the team went through a process of transformation in their approach to service delivery, working with their client groups and professional working relationships. It is important to acknowledge that the case presented here does not claim to be the whole story of integration for this team. However, the narrative reflects a segment of an ongoing journey, exploring external influences that existed in the pivotal period just prior to and during the initial stages of the team's transition. Their journey is presented as themes.

Findings of the Study

Fieldnotes from across the 9 months of observation, discussions, and exploration were themed using Braun and Clarke's (2006) thematic analysis method. The following key themes were identified (Fig. 16.1):

Discussion of the Themes

During the study, there was a process of convergence and separation within team structure and relationships. This involved both the adult social care and community nursing teams moving from their traditional team structures into the integrated neighbourhood team, although it is important to note that this was not a linear progression—the teams became closer and retracted from each other multiple times over the early stages of team development. The transition was a practical, structural, and cultural one. Each element progressed at a different pace;

however, there was a clear interdependency between each element. Fig. 16.2 highlights some core observed changes in the early stages of adoption.

A significant structural change was the co-location, which commenced early and involved very practical challenges in information technology (IT) and car parking which impacted the daily working lives of the teams. The cultural change was far more nuanced as the team members adopted facets of the other team's culture (symbols, language, norms, values, and artifacts) while simultaneously holding on to their own deeply held values and norms. As individuals came together as a new team, they constructed and changed the meaning and identity of the team through a process of testing different ideas. One example of the shifting culture was the adoption of language common to each professional group: social care team members mentioned utilising medical language in hospital settings and community nursing teams discussed the psychosocial aspects of people's care. The following field note demonstrates that the movement of the team involved the building of trust and reflected underlying principles held by each professional group (Marshall, 2020):

'We work together now…we have gained a trust and understanding of each other—this makes it easier to support people…and ensure that they have the patients, people get the right level of support.'
                              (Social worker – feedback meeting).

Theme 1—Convergence and separation in the creation of the integrated team

Reimagining of the team and creation of team vision

Metamorphosis of role and task

We are the neighbourhood—Space and integration

Theme 2—The complexity of hopefulness in reimagining the integrated space

Expression of the desired but uncertain future

Hope as a reflection of dissatisfaction with the current situation

The counterbalancing of challenges faced within the transition

Theme 3—Continuity and change the making of an integrated team member

Marginalised professional groups and collective endeavour

Organic development of integrated leadership 'Professional me', 'team me'

Fig. 16.1 Theme map.

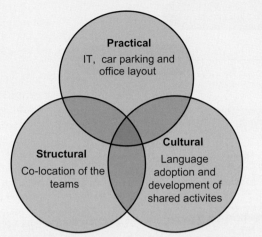

Fig. 16.2 Changes in the early stages of adoption. *IT*, Information technology.

Underlying the formation of the neighbourhood team were extrinsic and intrinsic factors including wider government policy, local demographic challenges, and existing team and professional cultures. These factors could be seen as influencing one of the strongest drivers observed with the team: hopefulness. Hopefulness was present throughout the study and the sense of hope felt by the team acted as a complex and powerful influence for cultural change.

Hope impacted the team in three distinct ways:

- An expression of a desired but uncertain future
- A reflection of dissatisfaction with the present
- A counterbalance to challenges of transformation

Team members were not simply optimistic. They were involved in a dialogue together throughout the change process about what a potential future would look like. Even when faced with issues and problems within the process of becoming integrated team members, they used hope to continue the change and support the transformation.

Prior to co-location, the two teams communicated predominately via emails and referrals rather than face-to-face. Co-location was a structural change that enabled joint working but also acted as a facilitator for a cultural transformation. However, it is important to recognise that the cultural shift needed more than simply co-locating the teams. This shift was enabled and encouraged by the leadership of the teams. Both leaders collaborated, engaging with each other in sharing work, attending joint meetings, and making joint decisions. The leadership behaviours were then mirrored across the teams, resulting in joint leadership becoming viewed as a core facet of the developing team identity. During this transition, an interesting feature of the team development was their ability to maintain a sense of their own professional identity. The different identities co-existed within the burgeoning team, which appeared as an important feature within this development as professional identity is often cited as a challenge to the development of integrated care. Professional groups often collaborated but were careful during interactions to support the other's professional standing. In one observation between a community nurse and a social worker, the nurse and the social worker referred to each other's specific professional identity: '…you are the nurse so shall you complete this section…', 'Can you help as you are the social worker and this is your field…'.

The study ended at what remained the start of the team's journey, but the learning extracted supported the development of the framework. The framework was co-produced with participants to ensure it reflected the key areas that the team felt were important during the transition to neighbourhood working—moving through the structural changes into a deeper cultural shift and creating a team that embodied the principles of integrated care and neighbourhood working.

development. The study recommended the use of a framework to assess and prepare teams prior to commencement of neighbourhood working.

THE MAKING OF A NEIGHBOURHOOD TEAM—A FRAMEWORK FOR PREPARATION

The following section will outline the application of the framework in relation to the development of neighbourhood teams. The study did not aim to be generalisable and the framework is based on the experiences of only one case. However, the findings of the study reflect previous studies, and these will be drawn on to support the individual elements of the framework.

The framework (Fig. 16.3) describes key activities to be considered prior to the commencement of developing the neighbourhood teams and includes organisation-level and team-level requirements. The framework aims to structure conversation and support the development of activities that will enhance each section across the organisational and team levels.

Level 1—Organisational Preparedness

Organisational preparedness relates to developing an environment in which integrated neighbourhood teams can flourish. The study identified that there were three areas at an organisational level which were important to the creating of a positive environment for integration: a

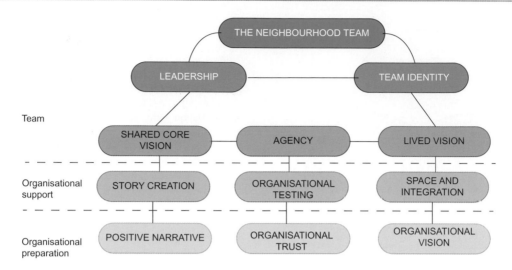

Fig. 16.3 Neighbourhood team development.

positive narrative, organisational trust, and organisational vision. As discussed in the case study, the process of integration was not a linear one but one where teams move through a process of converging and separating from each other. The analysis of the findings identified several key factors in how teams experienced integration structurally, practically, and culturally. These included an imperative of a local narrative for integration, the place of hope and hopefulness in uniting teams, the importance of 'bottom-up' action, and the imperative of joint leadership (Marshall, 2020).

Positive Narrative

Organisational leaders need to consider how an integrated care and neighbourhood team narrative is created. The narrative should consider external text (policy, think tank, media), be linked to the core values of teams, and embed a sense of positivity and hope throughout. Foot (2012), Foot and Hopkins (2010), Greater Manchester Combined Authority (2015), Shaw et al. (2011), Wood et al. (2016), and the all support the creation of strategic narratives that privilege empowering people and communities in the development of integrated care.

Within the case study, the adult social care and community nursing teams both expressed improving patient and service user outcomes as motivational drivers for integration. The joining of external, organisational, and local narratives to professional values enhanced the feeling of hope within the team, which led to a greater support for integration. A positive narrative, which can engage and motivate team members during the early transition to integrated working, was viewed as essential, and is

reflected in previous studies by RAND Europe and Ernst and Young LLP (2012), who found that staff believed it was important that integrated care should be about improving patient experience and access to services. Finally, the narrative needs to be authentic, as the importance of the narrative is that, if successful, it will reflect the core value set and align these to the integration agenda, fostering hopefulness within the team (Marshall, 2020).

Organisational Trust

It has been known for decades that organisational trust in healthcare has a beneficial impact in relationships not only between patients and clinicians but also between colleagues and managers (Gustafsson et al., 2021). Trust is a stalwart of the clinician/patient relationship and is vital for successful interactions and positive patient outcomes. However, research has demonstrated that trust is also important within organisational relationships. Healthcare organisations that foster trusting relationships often benefit from improved staff morale, job satisfaction, and patient safety and experience (Firth-Cozen, 2004; Gustafsson et al., 2021).

When reflecting on the journey towards integrated care and the development of neighbourhood teams, organisational trust is a key element to consider. During any large organisational change, trust is important. However, if the adoption of neighbourhood teams is to truly reflect the principles of integrated care (Chapter 5), it requires a leap of faith on the part of the teams, managers, and service users. This is because not only do the structure of the teams need to be addressed, but also the relationships between people, clinicians, and organisations need to be considered.

Organisational trust is strongly linked to acceptance and involvement in neighbourhood development (Marshall, 2020). Goodwin et al. (2012) explain that in successful examples of integrated care, managers and clinicians created a unifying narrative which encapsulated the purpose of integrated care, underpinned the design of new services, and acted as a clear point of reference. Edgren and Barnard (2012) further explain that, in the development of integrated care, it is important to foster the capacity for self-organisation, improvisation, and flexibility. It was observed within the case study that narrative, self-organisation, and flexibility enabled the team to develop their neighbourhood model and, importantly, the new team felt that the organisation trusted them to do this through the provision of space and a flexible and adaptive approach. The organisation is a vital catalyst in the process, as they are required to provide permission (trust) and relinquish centrally held power (Marshall, 2020).

Neighbourhood working often involves both inter- and intraorganisational integration. Commonly, this involves health and social care coming together (as in this case), but in more complex integrated care, neighbourhood approaches can include a whole spectrum of formal and informal partnerships from across a geographical locality (Behavioural Insights Team, 2018). One solution to supporting these complex multiorganisational requirements was put forward by Edgren and Barnard (2012), who argue that the use of complex adaptive systems (CAS) methodology as a model for integration enables organisational structures that are not rigid or supervised. CAS has a long history, with versions of the theory stretching back to the 19th century (The Health Foundation, 2010). As a methodology, CAS challenges assumptions of cause and effect, seeing healthcare as a dynamic process, where interactions and relationships simultaneously affect and are shaped by each other and the system (Edgren & Barnard, 2012). Radermacher et al's (2011) qualitative study explored the experiences of existing partnerships between organisations and small community groups and advocated for careful consideration of a selection implementation approach, stating that stringent top-down implementation preserves the notion of 'one model of partnership', which could impose superfluous restrictions, hindering creativity and leading to disempowerment at the team level.

Across integrated care, leadership is a core component (Chapter 9) and one way an organisation can demonstrate trust is by the inclusion of key leadership roles within the neighbourhood team. Within this case study, that role was the neighbourhood manager. The role of the neighbourhood manager was important to the change as they provided strategic leadership, translating organisational vision and providing two-way communication between the team and the wider organisation. The neighbourhood manager did not operationalise the changes; the manager's role was seen as encouraging the team to take ownership of the change within the organisational framework and guiding and inspiring the team towards achieving integration. The umbrella review by Winters et al. (2016) found that effective leadership is an integral element of cross-sector service provision, a view supported by Mackie and Darvill (2016), whose systematic review stated that leaders and managers play a key role when implementing integrated care. Bryson et al. (2006) further highlighted that cross-sector collaborations have a greater chance of success if there is one or more linking mechanism between the partners, including the use of powerful sponsors or high-level leadership.

Vision

The importance of vision is well documented in organisational management text; however, it takes on an increasingly important role within neighbourhood team development due to the complex organisational and professional relationships. Drennan et al. (2005) state that when there is a lack of a shared vision, even teams that are committed to a partnership could struggle with the complexity of multiple divergent agendas, aspirations, and knowledge. Winters et al. (2016) noted that there is a need in cross-sector service provision to provide a strong shared vision to strengthen connections between sectors. The creation of vision can act as a powerful beacon and control—vision inspires organisational members towards ideals and goals (Ginter et al., 2018). Interestingly, in the case study, team members did not discuss the organisational vision or interact closely with it, but they did deconstruct and construct it to create an internal team vision with meaning to them. Therefore, when developing a vision for integrated care, it should be clear and concise but also flexible so that individual teams can construct local meaning to the wider vision and develop local ownership.

Level 2—Organisational Support

Organisations entering into a neighbourhood approach need to not only consider how they prepare at a strategic and operational level, but also how they will create an environment in which the neighbourhood team can flourish. Level two of the framework is centred around this environment building.

Story Creation

Organisations can be viewed as socially constructed and complex, and it has been long understood that stories and narratives are utilised by people within organisations as a means of understanding and sense-making (Brown &

Humphreys, 2003; Weick, 1995). Stories are one of the prime means from which people construct their social reality and are a powerful catalyst for action in the context of change (Reissner et al., 2011). Reissner et al. (2011) state that when applied to change, stories have a dual purpose. Firstly, they are a powerful sense-making tool in which those experiencing change make change meaningful, and secondly, they can be a mechanism to challenge official accounts of change. The study from which the preparedness framework was developed was an institutional ethnography and therefore was interested in bringing to the fore multiple stories of change, especially the stories of those who felt marginalised within the organisation. As the analysis progressed, the importance of the stories became more apparent, as they were used by the neighbourhood team members not only for the aforementioned reasons, but additionally as mechanisms for testing, adopting, or rejecting change. Positive stories led often to adoption of a change, and negative stories led to rejection of changes by the wider team. Therefore, using stories as part of the change process can lead to creative solutions, in line with bottom-up change management theories (Duffield & Whitty, 2016). An example of how stories supported both structural and cultural adoption of change within this neighbourhood development was the use of the social prescribing team by the nursing team. Social prescribing has been adopted in the UK as a method of providing nonmedical interventions to support individuals within the community (more detail on social prescribing can be found in Chapters 12 and 18). The nursing team introduced and spread the adoption of using social prescribers through passing stories between each other about experiences with the new service. These stories were in informal (lunch conversations) and formal settings (handovers). Interestingly, as the stories developed, they led to deeper discussion on the nurse's role in preventative and social interventions. Also, the stories began to move from talking about a structural change (the introduction of the social prescribing team) to a more cultural change, as the nursing team explored the purpose of their role and the role of the newly forming team.

Organisational Testing

As previously alluded to within the case study, the development of organisational testing was very reliant on organisational trust. Rapid testing approaches are common within information technology, product development, and other fast-developing services (Chang & Taylor, 2016). However, the findings within the case study suggested that the approach can also be used in the development of integration. The teams in this study gradually developed a method of testing their ideas and

using stories to spread changes and encourage adoption of successful change and rejection of change that did not provide positive outcomes. This case study was mainly centred on two professional groups (nurses and social workers). In more complex neighbourhood developments, consideration would need to be given to the wider power dynamics at play. These include considering the communication between multi- and intersector partners, which is, by its very nature, a complex process involving multiple negotiations and constructions (Cairns & Harris, 2011; Freeman & Peck, 2006; Øvretveit et al., 2010). Cairns and Harris (2011) additionally state that power within integration is often unequal and problematic: there can be conflict about who determines or enforces the norms of communication and how these communication norms affect and integration.

Space and Integration

Providing the space for change is a complex concept and requires careful consideration. The seminal work of Lefebvre (1991) identifies space not merely as geographical but also as a social construct: as lived/physical space, a conceived or conceptualised space, and the perceived space. When considering the new integrated teams, leaders need to consider not just the physical elements of space (offices, desks, storage), but also how team members construct and deconstruct space within their world. Integrated care requires complex changes in how space is conceived, with the shift being geographical, cultural, conceptual, or all three. The exploration of space is a vital part of the adoption of integrated care, as this case demonstrated. If insufficient attention is paid to how space is experienced, even the most practical of elements (car parking, IT, desks) can potentially become powerful symbols of dissatisfaction that can potentially derail the integration process, as individuals and teams disengage with the organisation.

Level 3—Team

The team section of the framework relates to key elements that need to be present to support neighbourhood teams' early success.

Shared Core Values

Within the case study, the shared vision supported the sense of hope and helped manage conflicts based on professional difference. Mitchell et al's (2020) UK study described the 'social care vs. health service issue'. Their study demonstrated that there was a perception among social care staff that they were dominated by the much larger NHS (health) sector, and this impacted how they felt about their role in integration. This is important, as

Beacon (2015) states that shared vision is necessary to establish a common need amongst partners. This includes the establishment of shared risk and recognition of shared benefits across the system and for the wider community. The building of a shared vision of care across sectors is integral to the success of integration, as those engaged in the change need to agree there is a need for change. An example of the development of shared vision can be seen in Heenan and Birrell (2009) and Curry and Ham (2010), who both discuss the well-established integrated system in Northern Ireland (NI), highlighting practical methods for increasing interdisciplinary trust, respect, and shared vision, such as shared leadership. Work in NI identified methods that support shared vision such as leadership roles which are not limited to single professional groups, managers who are not constrained by artificial boundaries between health and social care, and professional identity, changing behaviours as teams develop understanding of each other's roles.

As neighbourhood working expands and neighbourhoods become more complex structures with wider partners, it is important to consider what this means for the development of a shared vision. Beacon (2015) cautions that shared purpose needs to support core professionals to develop trusted relationships and work together; however, they must also acknowledge that the role of the community and volunteer sector has been undervalued. This is especially important if integrated care is to truly reflect its aim on centring care around people, place, and community. Shaw et al. (2011), Rosen et al. (2011), and RAND Europe and Ernst and Young LLP (2012) express the need for inclusion of service users, as the view of the community is integral to integrated care, stating that any shared vision needs to include their perspective, and that inclusion of the service user will help build staff commitment and a strong sense that integration is doing the right thing. Marshall (2020) further supports this view stating that a team's acceptance of integrated care may be linked to how closely it aligns with the shared and common values held by each group. These values include empowerment of people, community, person-centredness, and promotion of independence. Building a strong sense of shared values enables professionals to work closely together and reduces friction points and professional barriers (Marshall 2020).

Agency

In the case study, the hope that neighbourhood working would transform the service provision was a central driver for the teams. Snyder (2002) states that there is a distinction between hope and optimism. Optimism requires a faith that things will turn out well, whereas hope is a positive motivational state which includes a determination to achieve those goals through a person's agency. For the team to deliver the cultural and structural change to become a neighbourhood team, they needed not just hope but also the agency to deliver the required changes (Marshall, 2020). Therefore, transformation requires active players in change and those active players require the agency to act within the space of the integrated neighbourhood team. While agency is important, it does not negate the need to consider and remove the wider limitations of the social, organisational, and professional structures.

Lived Vision

As previously discussed, narrative and clear vision are significant in developing an environment where local-level teams feel empowered to be involved in change. For the integration to lead to transformation, these macro visions and narratives need to be matched by the teams being provided with the space to transform the vision into something that is lived within their actualities, since it is through the living of the vision of integration within everyday actions that the required change takes place. It is important for organisations to consider how to support teams to make those connections.

Leadership

Leadership in integrated care settings is discussed in depth in Chapter 9. Leadership is fundamental to any transformation process, and an ability to lead across a range of professionals and services is a core part of integrated leadership (Mitchell et al., 2020). The framework stipulates that local leadership is an essential component to neighbourhood working. The development of neighbourhood teams requires formal leadership roles, but also requires the fostering of self-determination within teams and leadership to be present in a range of roles. The development of leadership across the team strongly interlinks with the creation of agency within the team and therefore the ability to drive forward an integrated care agenda (Mitchell et al., 2015).

Team Identity

Tajfel's (1974) theory of social identity considers how people's sense of who they are is influenced by the groups they belong to (i.e., their group membership). The theory discusses how people get a sense of pride and self-esteem from their groups and a sense of belonging to the social world. However, there is also a process of social categorisation and a creation of a 'them and us'. The stories the team members told after the co-location demonstrated a need to relay and reinforce group membership in the formal work, talk, and the social aspect of the group. There needs to be a recognition during transformation of the influence of groups. It is also important to consider the work of the sociologist Freidson (1973), who states that professions have distinctive conventions and institutions which differentiate them from other types of occupations and from each other. For integration to be successful, the teams are required to create a new identity; however, the creation of new team identity is complex and multi-faceted, as it includes multiple different professional groups. Therefore, team identity is included, as, during the building of this new identity, those groups will be required to explore how their professional values align to the principles of integrated care and challenge long-held assumptions of the relationships that professionals have with each other and the communities and individuals they work with. During this process, team members will need space to converge and separate from each other as they test out the new identities.

IMPACT ON PEOPLE

The development of a neighbourhood approach should not be simply viewed as adoption of a new model of care or a co-location of staff. For neighbourhood working to reach its potential, it requires a radical rethink of relationships between systems, people, and place, including how professional groups see themselves and each other (Marshall, 2020). In the case study, the impact on people was not fully realised, due to the early stage of the implementation and the impact of COVID-19 on joint working practices. However, evidence from previous research highlights that neighbourhood working can transform outcomes for local communities. The Dutch Buurtzorg model remains one of the most significant neighbourhood working developments and its influence can be seen across the world (Chapter 6). In the UK, Drennan et al. (2018) found that the introduction of neighbourhood nursing led to more proactive and responsive care and enhanced experience of both staff and service users. Furthermore, an evaluation by RAND Europe and Ernst and Young LLP (2012) reported positive feedback from patients through letters, phone calls, and on websites. These findings are reflected by NHS England (2014), which found that many pioneer sites were able to demonstrate that they had improved patient experience of care through the integration of services. In other research, an international perspective can be seen in Nandram and Koster's (2014) study in the Netherlands which found that the Buurtzorg model enhanced patient experience by changing the paradigm of nursing care from one based on targets and predetermined time slots to a more patient-centred approach.

CONCLUSION

In contrast to traditional 'deficit' services, integrated care, including neighbourhood working, aims to provide seamless care which is responsive to people's needs rather than being designed to serve providers (Ham et al., 2013; Suter et al., 2009). The framework developed from Marshall's (2020) study aims to support those developing a neighbourhood team to consider key elements that will impact the team's journey. The study found three themes which were then further developed into the framework to act as a usable tool for practitioners. As the study was qualitative in nature, it is not generalisable, nor did it aim to be. Rather, it is the narrative of one point in the story of one team and, through that narrative, the framework grew to provide a transferable tool for teams.

References

Beacon, A. (2015). Practice-integrated care teams–learning for a better future. *Journal of Integrated Care*, *23*(2), 74–87. https://doi.org/10.1108/JICA-01-2015-0005

Behavioural Insights Team. (2018). *Applying behavioural insights to health and social care integration in Greater Manchester*. https://www.greatermanchester-ca.gov.uk/media/1878/integrated-neighbourhood-teams.pdf

Braun, V., & Clarke, V. (2006). Using thematic analysis in psychology. *Qualitative Research in Psychology*, *3*(2), 77–101. https://doi.org/10.1191/1478088706qp063oa

Brown, A. D., & Humphreys, M. (2003). Epic and tragic tales: making sense of change. *Journal of Applied Behavioral Science*, *39*(2), 121–144. https://doi.org/10.1177/0021886303255557

Bryson, J., Crosby, B., & Middleton Stone, M. (2006). The design and implementation of cross-sector collaborations: propositions from the literature. *Public Administration Review*, *66*(s1), 44–55. https://doi.org/10.1111/j.1540-6210.2006.00665.x

Cairns, A., & Harris, M. (2011). Local cross-sector partnerships: tackling the challenges collaboratively. *Nonprofit Management and Leadership*, *21*(3), 311–321. https://doi.org/10.1002/nml.20027

Chang, W., & Taylor, S. A. (2016). The effectiveness of customer participation in new product development: a meta-analysis. *Journal of Marketing*, *80*(1), 47–64. https://doi.org/10.1509/jm.14.0057

Curry, N., & Ham, C. (2010). *Clinical and service integration: the route to improved outcomes*. London: King's Fund.

Drennan, V., Iliffe, S., Haworth, D., Tai, S., Lenihan, P., & Deave, T. (2005). The feasibility and acceptability of a specialist health and social care team for the promotion of health and independence in 'at risk' older adults. *Health and Social Care in the Community*, *13*(2), 136–144. https://doi.org/10.1111/j.1365-2524.2005.00541.x

Drennan, V. M., Calestani, M., Ross, F., Saunders, M., & West, P. (2018). Tackling the workforce crisis in district nursing: can the Dutch Buurtzorg model offer a solution and a better patient experience? A mixed methods case study. *BMJ Open*, *8*(6), e021931. https://doi.org/10.1136/bmjopen-2018-021931

Duffield, S., & Whitty, S. J. (2016). How to apply the Systemic Lessons Learned Knowledge model to wire an organisation for the capability of storytelling. *International Journal of Project Management*, *34*(3), 429–443. https://doi.org/10.1016/j.ijproman.2015.11.004

Edgren, L., & Barnard, K. (2012). Complex adaptive systems for the management of integrated care. *Leadership in Health Services*, *25*(1), 39–51. https://doi.org/10.1108/17511871211198061

Firth-Cozens, J. (2004). Organisational trust: the keystone to patient safety. *BMJ Quality & Safety*, *13*(1), 56–61. https://doi.org/10.1136/qshc.2003.007971

Foot, J. (2012). *What makes us healthy? The asset approach in practice: evidence, action, evaluation.* http://janefoot.com/downloads/files/healthy%20FINAL%20FINAL.pdf

Foot, J., & Hopkins, T. (2010). *A glass half-full: how an asset approach can improve community health and well-being.* https://www.local.gov.uk/sites/default/files/documents/glass-half-full-how-asset-3db.pdf

Freeman, T., & Peck, E. (2006). Evaluating partnerships: a case study of integrated specialist mental health services. *Health & Social Care in the Community*, *14*(5), 408–417. https://doi.org/10.1111/j.1365-2524.2006.00658.x

Freidson, E. (1973). *The professions and their prospects.* Beverly Hills: Sage Publications.

Ginter, P. M., Duncan, W. J., & Swayne, L. E. (2018). *The strategic management of health care organizations.* Hoboken: John Wiley & Sons.

Goodwin, N., Smith, J., Davies, A., Perry, C., Rosen, R., Dixon, A., Dixon, J., & Ham, C. (2012). *Integrated care for patients and populations: improving outcomes by working together.* London: King's Fund, Nuffield Trust.

Greater Manchester Combined Authority. (2015). *Taking Charge of Our Health and Social Care in Greater Manchester.* https://www.greatermanchester-ca.gov.uk/media/1120/taking-charge-of-our-health-and-social-care-plan.pdf

Gustafsson, S., Gillespie, N., Searle, R., Hope Hailey, V., & Dietz, G. (2021). Preserving organizational trust during disruption. *Organization Studies*, *42*(9), 1409–1433. https://doi.org/10.1177/0170840620912705

Ham, C., Heenan, D., Longley, M., & Steel, D. R. (2013). *Integrated care in Northern Ireland, Scotland and Wales: Lessons for England.* London: King's Fund.

Heenan, D., & Birrell, D. (2009). Organisational integration in health and social care: some reflections on the Northern Ireland experience. *Journal of Integrated Care*, *17*(5), 3–12. https://doi.org/10.1108/14769018200900032

Lefebvre, H. (1991). *Critique of Everyday Life, Vol. 2: Foundations for a sociology of the everyday.* New York: Verso.

Mackie, S., & Darvill, A. (2016). Factors enabling implementation of integrated health and social care: a systematic review. *British Journal of Community Nursing*, *21*(2), 82–87. https://doi.org/10.12968/bjcn.2016.21.2.82

Marshall, K. (2020). *An exploration of neighbourhood team members experiences of the transition from traditional health and social care teams to integrated care systems, within a defined health and social care economy* (Publication No. 59618) [Professional Doctorate thesis, University of Salford]. https://usir.salford.ac.uk/id/eprint/59618

Mitchell, C., Tazzyman, A., Howard, S. J., & Hodgson, D. (2020). More that unites us than divides us? A qualitative study of integration of community health and social care services. *BMC Family Practice*, *21*(1), 1–10. https://doi.org/10.1186/s12875-020-01168-z

Mitchell, R., Boyle, B., Parker, V., Giles, M., Chiang, V., & Joyce, P. (2015). Managing inclusiveness and diversity in teams: how leader inclusiveness affects performance through status and team identity. *Human Resource Management*, *54*(2), 217–239. https://doi.org/10.1002/hrm.21658

Nandram, S., & Koster, N. (2014). Organizational innovation and integrated care: lessons from Buurtzorg. *Journal of Integrated Care*, *22*(4), 174–184. https://doi.org/10.1108/JICA-06-2014-0024

NHS England. (2014). *Integrated care and support pioneer programme.* London: Stationery Office.

Øvretveit, J., Hansson, J., & Brommels, M. (2010). An integrated health and social care organisation in Sweden: Creation and structure of a unique local public health and social care system. *Health Policy*, *97*(2), 113–121. https://doi.org/10.1016/j.healthpol.2010.05.012

Radermacher, H., Karunarathna, Y., Grace, N., & Feldman, S. (2011). Partner or perish? Exploring inter-organisational partnerships. *Health Social Care Community*, *19*(5), 550–560. https://doi.org/10.1111/j.1365-2524.2011.01007.x

RAND Europe, Ernst & Young, LLP. (2012). *National evaluation of the Department of Health's integrated care pilot.* London: Ernst & Young LLP.

Reissner, S. C., Pagan, V., & Smith, C. (2011). 'Our iceberg is melting': story, metaphor and the management of organisational change. *Culture and Organization*, *17*(5), 417–433. https://doi.org/10.1080/14759551.2011.622908

Rosen, R., Mountford, J., Lewis, G., Lewis, R., Shand, J., & Shaw, S. (2011). *Integration in action: four international case studies.* London: Nuffield Trust.

Shaw, S., Rosen, R., & Rumbold, B. (2011). *What is integrated care? An overview of integrated care in the NHS.* London: Nuffield Trust.

Smith, D. E. (2005). *Institutional ethnography: A sociology for people.* Lanham: Alta-Mira Press.

Snyder, C. R. (2002). Hope theory: rainbows in the mind. *Psychological Inquiry*, *13*(4), 249–275. https://doi.org/10.1207/S15327965PLI1304-01

Suter, E., Oelke, N. D., Adair, C. E., & Armitage, G. D. (2009). Ten key principles for successful health systems integration. *Healthcare Quarterly*, *13*, 16–23. https://doi.org/10.12927/hcq.2009.21092

Tajfel, H. (1974). Social identity and intergroup behaviour. *Social Science Information*, *13*(2), 65–93. https://doi.org/10.1177/053901847401300204

The Health Foundation. (2010). *Complex adaptive systems*. Retrieved from. https://www.health.org.uk/publications/complex-adaptive-systems?gclid=CjwKCAjwhJukBhBPEiwAniIcNdFtwOH6blrEl1N3HMI4BH1P-EfafPK0l_F1CyX6kJ-M1n_PV_0ZuBoCOwoQAvD_BwE

Weick, K. E. (1995). *Sensemaking in organizations*. Thousand Oaks, CA: Sage Publications

Winters, S., Magalhaes, L., Kinsella, E., & Kothari, A. (2016). Cross-sector service provision in health and social care: An umbrella review. *International Journal of Integrated Care*, *16*(1), 10. https://doi.org/10.5334/ijic.2460

Wood, S., Finnis, A., Khan, H., & Ejbye, J. (2016). *At the heart of health: Realising the value of people and communities*. https://www.health.org.uk/publications/at-the-heart-of-health-realising-the-value-of-people-and-communities

Further Reading

Article

Mitchell, C., Tazzyman, A., Howard, S. J., & Hodgson, D. (2020). More that unites us than divides us? A qualitative study of integration of community health and social care services. *BMC Family Practice*, *21*(1), 1–10. https://doi.org/10.1186/s12875-020-01168-z

Nandram, S., & Koster, N. (2014). Organizational innovation and integrated care: lessons from Buurtzorg. *Journal of Integrated Care*, *22*(4), 174–184. https://doi.org/10.1108/JICA-06-2014-0024

Report

Behavioural Insights Team. (2018). *Applying behavioural insights to health and social care integration in Greater Manchester*. https://www.greatermanchester-ca.gov.uk/media/1878/integrated-neighbourhood-teams.pdf

17

Understanding How People Move Through the System: Dementia Care

Dr Sarah Kate Smith and Chris Sewards

KEY CONCEPTS

- **Dementia care**—can encompass care at home, in day centres, and in residential and respite care
- **Service user and carer perspectives**—the opinions and perspectives of those using the service and their care partners are paramount and need to be heard over and above other perspectives.
- **Person-centred care**—requires individualising a person's care to their interests, abilities, history, and personality.
- **Comorbidities**—the presence of one or more additional conditions often co-occurring with a primary condition, like dementia.

INTRODUCTION

Within the UK, the adult social care sector is a key part of our health and care system, supporting some of society's most vulnerable, including people living with dementia. Although the sector has historically been considered as the poor relation in comparison to the NHS, the COVID-19 pandemic continues to highlight the essential role of adult social care and the importance of a fully integrated health and social care system in the future. Nevertheless, full integration between health and social care cannot be realised until the experiences of people who use these services are placed front and centre. If 'organisational influences' continue to make decisions based on what is assumed people need, then people living with dementia are going to continue experiencing less than satisfactory outcomes.

'People living with dementia need to know what help is available to them … we have been forgotten and ignored for too long. People are not being given the support they need to plan for their futures. The system is too complicated … and services don't reflect what users need or want.'

(Alzheimer's Society, 2021)

It is time to shift the focus from organisations and processes to people and outcomes, and a truly integrated health and social care system has the capacity to improve outcomes and experiences of care for people living with dementia.

DEMENTIA CARE AND INTEGRATION

Consistency and continuity of care and support have been identified worldwide as crucial due to increasing multimorbidity and ageing populations. This has led to the introduction of integrated care models to deliver initiatives and person-centred co-ordinated care (Damarell et al., 2020). Integrated care is an approach to organising health and care services, particularly for older people, yet recent findings suggest that the structures involved in integrated care are deficient when compensating for changes in individual ability to draw on the resources that sustained them at home (Hughes et al., 2022). However, there is an opportunity for innovation to take place as reforms progress. Integrated care is currently viewed as an approach for health and social care professionals to utilise when organising care rather than a practical resource for people to access in changing circumstances. One of the early implementers of integrating health and social care in north Manchester was the Manchester Community Response Team North. The impact of this was positive in healthcare but replicating throughout the health and social care systems presents new challenges. There may be tension between statutory health provision and tiered social care provision, putting pressure on councils; ensuring adequate funding will overcome this to overcome

CASE STUDY

Aspire operates services for older people and people with a learning disability in four hubs within Salford, with the main hubs for people living with dementia being the Poppy Day Centre and Humphrey Booth Resource Centre (HBRC). Combined with the day and resource centres, there is a respite unit with four available beds. Aspire is currently funded by Salford City Council and the Clinical Commissioning Group and is part of the voluntary, community, and social enterprise (VCSE) sector, which is well supported in the city. The dementia services offered are from a single location, with the community mental health team (CMHT) on the same site.

All of the services form part of the Aspire 'Older Person's Pathway', with a 'step up, step down' approach to service provision. This involves maintaining wellbeing for people living with dementia and carers in Salford from when they attend the resource centre as a member of a social gathering to possibly requiring respite, home care, and day care: the service adapts to the person rather than the person adapting to the service on offer. Poppy Day Care, HBRC, and Poppy Complex Care Respite are unique offers in Greater Manchester's 10 boroughs and could be a solution to fragmented care across the region. However, greater partnership agreements between often competing VCSE organisations within the integrated care system (ICS) would be required to 'demystify' what is available. The approach by Aspire and the 'step up, step down' approach is not unique (https://integratedcarefoundation.org/):

'It is the familiarity of the service … our day care centre with our respite unit where people are coming in all the time … to see the same faces. It is not unfamiliar, daunting or strange.'

(Woolrych & Sixsmith, 2013)

Across all services within Aspire, the importance of lived experience and the voices of service users are the greatest source of stakeholder involvement. The pioneer of person-centred care stressed a focus on the bringing together of ideas and ways of working to emphasise communication and relationships (Kitwood, 1997). The term 'person-centred care' is used widely in dementia care settings, resulting in the concept becoming synonymous with good quality care, although what lies behind the rhetoric in terms of practice may of course vary (Brooker, 2004). Aspire strives to shape services according to what people would like to be available rather than be passive recipients of services that we think may be acceptable. Peer support and co-ordinated care is essential to how people navigate their dementia experience. This lived experience is often the user of the service and the secondary user, the carer, care partner, or family support mechanism.

Good integrated dementia care can reduce confusion, repetition, delay, gaps in service delivery, and people getting lost in the system. Tension arises between the needs of the person living with dementia and existing, standardised services and the need to focus on preventative, wellbeing-focused psychosocial interventions in addition to medical interventions targeting dementia and comorbidities. The perspective of Aspire service users is at the heart of any discussion about integrated care. This is because achieving integrated care requires those involved with planning and providing services to involve and include the person's perspective as the centre of service delivery development and delivery.

general health inequalities in addition to those living with dementia in the UK and worldwide.

People living with dementia and carers require ongoing support and care from individuals and teams which is coupled with an increasing pressure to deliver savings in line with the Health and Social Care Act (Glover-Thomas, 2013) and subsequent 'austerity' funding cuts. Future-proofing services has also had a high profile, against a backdrop of the COVID-19 pandemic and already worsening deficits being experienced by health and social care organisations (King's Fund, 2021). Demand for health and social care has increased even under normal circumstances, and this is intensified further by difficulties recruiting to the social care workforce (among other sectors during and in the aftermath of COVID-19 and leaving the EU).

Integrated dementia care, dementia care pathways, and local arrangements around diagnosis and immediately following diagnosis are quite standardised across England. Memory Assessment Teams have seen funding increases in the wake of the Prime Minister's Challenge on Dementia 2020 (Department of Health and Social Care, 2020). Immediately following diagnosis, a local organisation will signpost support groups for both people living with dementia and carers. Contact will be maintained if the person living with dementia is taking medication but will cease otherwise. This can lead to the next contact being in times of crisis, although GP appointments for review are yearly or as required. However, people living with dementia and their carers and families often have a number of 'touch-points' to navigate from the initial GP appointment onwards. This can be psychological, health-related, or psychosocial, creating a structure of support, although existing health and social care divides may mean that boundaries across roles may be challenging to navigate. It is here that Aspire services, using the integrated care umbrella, could provide psychosocial, health, and other assistance at HBRC (as part of a wider VCSE provision), Poppy Day Centre, and the respite unit.

Approaches that seek to address fragmentation of care are common across many health systems, and the need to do so is increasing as more people live longer and with complex comorbidities. Integrated care does not appear to evolve as a natural response to emerging care needs in any system of care, whether planned or market-driven. The COVID-19 pandemic and subsequent lockdowns have highlighted that our social care system is not integrated and is not delivering what is needed for those who need it. The barriers to overcome are multiple and include staff shortages, postcode variations in access to care, unfair means tests, and a lack of personalised support (HM Government, 2022). ICSs are being established in all areas of the country to drive improvements in population health by integrating services to provide better, more joined-up care for patients and users (Charles, 2022). However, there is a danger that the new ICSs will exacerbate differences in care systems, creating further variation around access, funding, decision-making, and geography.

The trend in UK health and social care policy over the last 15 years has been toward early diagnosis, prevention/modifiable risk factors (Livingston et al., 2020), and reducing dependence on pharmacological interventions (Banerjee, 2009) and residential and hospital care. This facilitates people living with dementia to live at home for longer and proactive community approaches are key to preventing unnecessary hospital admissions (Office for Health Improvement and Disparities, 2022). The integration of adult health and social care provides an opportunity to co-ordinate the interventions required to support people with dementia and their carers in the community. Now is the time to ensure that the proposed integrated health and social care partnership budgets can facilitate seamless support to ensure the range of support needs of people with dementia and that their carers are not overlooked. Caring for carers has been a repeated trope since the UK's first Dementia Strategy (Department of Health, 2009). The move towards community capacity building and proportionately fewer resources for institutional care requires a co-ordinated approach to support people with dementia in the community. However, integrated care for a person living with dementia and their care support mechanisms may mean the dementia and non pharmacological interventions are secondary to comorbidity and pharmacological issues.

In a review of integrated care studies, González-Ortiz et al. (2018) identified recommendations related only to a small number of influencing aspects, including delivery system design, community resources and policies, and performance and quality. These were often derived from specific contexts and settings or with a defined target population rather than the needs of the wider health and social care population. There were also few studies to propose frameworks indicating key areas of intervention in order to foster care integration. Instead, lists of possible necessary steps to integrated care were set out locally (De Syllas, 2015) and world-wide (WHO Regional Office for Europe, 2016). It may be, then, that experts view care integration as primarily a systemic or organisational activity rather than an approach that co-ordinates care with and around people's needs at the clinical and service level. Integrated care has the fundamental aim of improving outcomes and tackling inequalities, to enhance productivity, make best use of resources, and to strengthen local communities (NHS England, 2021); this is perhaps where larger community interest companies like Aspire could act as a conduit for services and signposting, in this case across Salford. Therefore, in the UK, we consider integrated care to be achieved at various levels. At the macro level, there are legal, regulatory, and economic barriers and enablers. The meso level concerns local health service and community factors, such as attitudes and support from managers and patients. The micro level relates to day-to-day practice of individual health and social care professionals and patients. The micro level is often the focus in integrated care in practice (Briggs et al., 2018) with the meso and macro levels less developed or simply not working (Hughes et al., 2022). Role clarity is of considerable importance, as is overcoming embedded professional hierarchies and traditional role expectations influencing interactions between individual colleagues or professional groups, like the NHS or health and social care staff.

The Greater Manchester ICS will include NHS organisations, councils, the Greater Manchester Combined Authority, VCSE sector colleagues, and others, all working together to help achieve the common vision of improving people's health and wellbeing. This system will operate on (at least) three levels: Greater Manchester, locality, and neighbourhood. The importance of working with communities has been identified and connecting with a range of partners such as Healthwatch, the VCSE sector, and experts by experience will all ensure that public, patient, and carer voices are heard. The importance of places and place-based support are an important component of ICS structures, as they typically cover the area, neighbourhood, and services with which most residents identify. Place-level citizens' panel inputs (e.g., listening to the people with lived experience in a locality rather than assuming all localities are the same) in addition to this can help to reinforce the granular level of information required for each individual neighbourhood to benefit as seamlessly and effectively as possible.

A clear example is Dementia United, which was initiated in 2015 to undertake a review of the dementia health and care services of Greater Manchester to standardise provision, improve the lived experience of people living with dementia, and to reduce pressure on the health and social care system. Dementia United co-designed and co-produced areas to be prioritised and the focus of support using the devolved Greater Manchester budget. In Greater Manchester, we have been working as an informal ICS for the last 5 years through VOCAL, which is the voice and influence model of the VCSE sector in Salford, and the Health and Care Bill (2021) will formalise the arrangements already in place. There will continue to be team working in neighbourhoods, localities, and at the Greater Manchester level, just as there is now. It will mean continuing to build upon and improve partnership working across organisation boundaries, working together with VCSE colleagues and our communities.

Providing services in this way is also seen as less daunting for the older person, allowing the preservation of 'face to face care' and continuity in care delivery.

It does makes sense for health and social care to be integrated and working collaboratively, although for this to be successful and to make a difference to other services for people living with dementia who access the service, communication is key. All those involved in the person's care and treatment should have access on a need-to-know basis with the person living with dementia and their carer knowing fully who is involved and what is happening each step of the way. Nevertheless, the picture both nationally and internationally represents a landscape full of uncertainty for people living with dementia (Van Wijngaarden et al., 2018). Even where numerous services exist, people living with dementia and carers are unsure of how to approach any non-health-related offer of support, as navigating this is reliant on how the information is conveyed in a timely manner.

IMPACT ON PEOPLE

'The patient's perspective is at the heart of any discussion about integrated care. Achieving integrated care requires those involved with planning and providing services to impose the patient's perspective as the organising principle of service delivery.'

(Oldham, 2013)

If people living with dementia are to feel the benefit of ICSs, the boundaries of mental health services, health services, social care, and psychosocial interventions leading to increased wellbeing need to be navigated at all stages of the process. Social care is particularly important as this is tiered according to perceived need and according to individual council criteria. The voices of people living with dementia and their carers and families has increased substantially in the preceding 20 years and it is to be hoped that this citizen-level progress is maintained. The lived experience is particularly important in the case of dementia as a condition, as many now consider dementia to be the most feared condition for those over 55. It is essential to view the dementia experience both individually and holistically and to understand there is more to treatment than integrated care records, frameworks, and strategies. Of the people living with dementia in the UK, 91.8% have another health condition, with 16.9% having six or more (Scrutton & Brancati, 2016); hence, integrated care will benefit the vast majority of people living with dementia but may be considered secondary beyond other immediate health issues. The potential impact of an effective integrated health and social care system will have positive repercussions for people living with dementia, their carers, families, and friends, and will also have the potential to increase wellbeing across this whole network.

CONCLUSION

The *Integrated Care Systems: Design Framework* (NHS England, 2021) highlights broad outcomes for ICSs around improving outcomes in population health and healthcare, from tackling widening inequalities in outcomes, experience, and access and enhancing productivity and value for money. There are many common factors regarding the application of integrated care, and many to consider specifically around the experiences of people living with dementia. We have found within Aspire services that relationships and feedback mechanisms are key to establishing requirements for people 'ageing in place' with clarity and using accessible language is essential. However, ageing in place can also lead to loneliness and isolation, another consideration for true integration of care and support. The factors to consider may apply at various times during the experience of dementia, from early interventions at the time of diagnosis and Aspire's proposed 'step up, step down' care and support arrangements, to the need to have communication between systems, like preventing spending more time awaiting discharge from hospital, thus increasing the prospect of returning home being unsuccessful.

The hierarchy between people and organisations and between health and social care, with social care being viewed with a different lens from healthcare and it not being as politically volatile, continues to present challenges around equity of approach and real intersectionality of health and social care services. The pandemic has restored the balance somewhat as emphasis has changed from the NHS solely as 'heroes' to 'essential workers' and the social care workforce is seen in a more positive light. The Aspire social care workforce has similarly seen their roles recast as essential workers and a part of a whole-system approach. Nevertheless, the differences between commercialised social care and healthcare remain, but hopefully ICSs will acknowledge this. If a truly integrated care system is to be effective, then leadership, co-ordination, and advocacy within an ICS must attempt to remove the potential organisation boundary conflicts, as the design of the ICS relies on the system and the people within it working collaboratively.

References

Alzheimer's Society. (2021). *Stabilise, energise, realise: a long-term plan for social care*. https://www.alzheimers.org.uk/sites/default/files/2021-08/stabilise-energise-realise-report.pdf

Banerjee, S. (2009). *The use of antipsychotic medication for people with dementia: Time for action*. https://www.aph.gov.au/DocumentStore.ashx?id=48340346-1dbd-4e37-920b-0e724229047b

Briggs, A. M., Valentijn, P. P., Thiyagarajan, J. A., & Araujo De Carvalho, I. (2018). Elements of integrated care approaches for older people: a review of reviews. *BMJ Open, 8*(4), e021194. https://doi.org/10.1136/bmjopen-2017-021194

Brooker, D. (2004). What is person-centred care in dementia? *Reviews in Clinical Gerontology, 13*(3), 215–222. https://doi.org/10.1017/S095925980400108X

Charles, A. (2022). *Integrated care systems explained: making sense of systems, places and neighbourhoods*. https://www.kingsfund.org.uk/publications/integrated-care-systems-explained

Damarell, R. A., Lewis, S., Trenerry, C., & Tieman, J. J. (2020). Integrated Care Search: development and validation of a PubMed search filter for retrieving the integrated care research evidence. *BMC Medical Research Methodology, 20*(1), 1–16. https://doi.org/10.1186/s12874-020-0901-y

De Syllas, J. (2015). *Integrating care: The architecture of the comprehensive health centre*. London: Routledge.

Department of Health. (2009). *Policy paper: Living Well With Dementia: a national dementia strategy*. https://www.gov.uk/government/publications/living-well-with-dementia-a-national-dementia-strategy

Department of Health and Social Care. (2020). *Prime Minister's challenge on dementia 2020*. https://www.gov.uk/government/publications/prime-ministers-challenge-on-dementia-2020/prime-ministers-challenge-on-dementia-2020

Glover-Thomas, N. (2013). The Health and Social Care Act 2012: the emergence of equal treatment for mental health care or another false dawn. *Medical Law International, 13*(4), 279–297. https://doi.org/10.1177/0968533214521090

González-Ortiz, L. G., Calciolari, S., Goodwin, N., & Stein, V. (2018). The core dimensions of integrated care: a literature review to support the development of a comprehensive framework for implementing integrated care. *International Journal of Integrated Care, 18*(3), 1–12. https://doi.org/10.5334/ijic.4198

HM Government. (2022). *COVID-19 response: living with COVID-19*. https://assets.publishing.service.gov.uk/government/uploads/system/uploads/attachment_data/file/1056229/COVID-19_Response_-_Living_with_COVID-19.pdf

Hughes, G., Shaw, S. E., & Greenhalgh, T. (2022). Why doesn't integrated care work? Using Strong Structuration Theory to explain the limitations of an English case. *Sociology of Health and Illness, 44*(1), 113–129. https://doi.org/10.1111/1467-9566.13398

Kitwood, T. (1997). Dementia reconsidered: the person comes first. *British Medical Journal, 318*, 880. https://doi.org/10.1136/bmj.318.7187.880a

Livingston, G., Huntley, J., Sommerlad, A., Ames, D., Ballard, C., Banerjee, S., Brayne, C., Burns, A., Cohen-Mansfield, J., Cooper, C., Costafreda, S. G., Dias, A., Fox, N., Gitlin, L. N., Howard, R., Kales, H. C., Kivimäki, M., Larson, E. B., Ogunniyi, A., ... Mukadam, N. (2020). Dementia prevention, intervention, and care: 2020 report of the Lancet Commission. *The Lancet, 396*(10248), 413–446. https://doi.org/10.1016/S0140-6736(20)30367-6

NHS England. (2021). *Integrated care systems: design framework. Version 1, June 2021*. https://www.england.nhs.uk/wp-content/uploads/2021/06/B0642-ics-design-framework-june-2021.pdf

Office for Health Improvement and Disparities. (2022). *Dementia Profile*. https://fingertips.phe.org.uk/profile-group/mental-health/profile/dementia

Oldham, J. (2013). Integrated care. *Journal of Psychiatric Practice, 19*(5), 343. https://doi.org/10.1097/01.pra.0000435033.37685.00

Scrutton, J., & Brancati, C. U. (2016). *Dementia and comorbidities: Ensuring parity of care*. London: ILC-UK.

The King's Fund. (2021). *NHS trusts in deficit*. https://www.kingsfund.org.uk/projects/nhs-in-a-nutshell/trusts-deficit

UK Government. (2021). *Health and Care Bill*. https://bills.parliament.uk/publications/45209/documents/1397

Van Wijngaarden, E., Van Der Wedden, H., Henning, Z., Komen, R., & The, A.-M. (2018). Entangled in uncertainty: the experience of living with dementia from the perspective of family caregivers. *PLoS One*, *13*(6), e0198034. https://doi. org/10.1371/journal.pone.0198034

WHO Regional Office for Europe. (2016). *Integrated care models: an overview*. https://www.euro.who.int/__data/assets/ pdf_file/0005/322475/Integrated-care-models-overview.pdf

Woolrych, R., & Sixsmith, J. (2013). Toward integrated services for dementia: a formal carer perspective. *Journal of Integrated Care*, *21*(4), 208–220. https://doi.org/10.1108/ JICA-02-2013-0006

Further Reading

Charles, A., Ewbank, L., Naylor, C., Walsh, N., & Murray, R. (2021). *Developing place-based partnerships: The foundation of effective integrated care systems*. London: King's Fund.

Department of Health & Social Care. (2021, February 11). *Policy paper: Integration and innovation: working together to improve health and social care for all (HTML version)*. https://www.gov.uk/government/publications/ working-together-to-improve-health-and-social-care-for-all/ integration-and-innovation-working-together-to-improve- health-and-social-care-for-all-html-version

NHS Clinical Commissioners. (2021). *Our action for you on the proposals outlined in the Integration and Innovation white paper (2021)*. https://www.nhsconfed.org/system/ files/2021-06/Actions-integration-and-innovation.pdf

NHS England. (2021). *Integrating care: Next steps to building strong and effective integrated care systems across England.* https://www.england.nhs.uk/wp-content/uploads/2021/01/ integrating-care-next-steps-to-building-strong-and-effective- integrated-care-systems.pdf

NHS England. (2021). Guidance on the employment commitment: Supporting the development and transition towards statutory Integrated Care Systems. Version 1.0. https:// www.england.nhs.uk/wp-content/uploads/2021/06/B0724- employment-commitment-guidance-supporting-ics-v1.pdf

18

Understanding Social Value as a Basis for Integrated Care

*Professor Julian Manley**

KEY CONCEPTS

- Social value
- Place-based approaches
- Strategic approaches
- Partnership working

INTRODUCTION

Integrated care systems (ICSs) were established in July 2022 in England through an initial 42 integrated care network designs as a result of the Health and Care Act (2022). These have been planned as partnerships for different organisations to jointly plan and deliver health and care for local populations in a holistic way which is sensitive to local needs and issues by tapping into the expertise, skills, and knowledge that may already exist in communities, but which have not yet been sufficiently embraced and brought together in order to improve health outcomes and reduce health inequalities. The ICSs will specifically include 'local authorities in the ICS area, which are responsible for social care and public health functions as well as other vital services for local people and businesses' and 'community and voluntary organisations, local residents, people who use services, their carers and representatives and other community partners with a role in supporting the health and wellbeing of the population'. It is in the context of this specified remit that social value has a vital part to play. This chapter will explore the part that social value plays in a system of integrated health care, both as an intrinsic value for citizens and workers—a value for life—and as applied through legislation (Public Services (Social Value) Act, 2012).

ORGANISING SOCIAL VALUE: AN EXAMPLE FROM LANCASHIRE

In Lancashire (a county in the northwest of England), the Lancashire Teaching Hospitals NHS Foundation Trust (LTHTR) has embarked upon a systematic review and networking project that brings together local actors and stakeholders, 'champions', to develop a Social Value Framework (Our Central Lancashire, 2022). In the case of this particular region, the initiative moves forward against a supportive background of ICS development nationwide, but also the Preston Model (PM) of community wealth building (CWB). CWB in its developed PM form (Manley & Whyman, 2021) potentially provides Lancashire with a head start in developing such a strategy.

In July 2021, the Lancashire and South Cumbria ICS Board approved a shared approach to social value. The domains were adopted from the Health Foundation's work on anchor institutions (AIs) (Reed et al., 2019). These domains were adapted to incorporate a wider partnership approach; that is to say, the networked framework strategy ('place-based partnership') that has been developed and was started in November 2021.

The initial definition of social value for the purposes of the network was taken from Preston City Council's definition of the term from their second iteration of the strategic plan for CWB in Preston:

'Social value is the wider benefit gained by a local community from the delivery of public contracts or services. These benefits include employment, training,

***Disclaimer:** Julian Manley is funded by the National Institute for Health Research (NIHR) Public Health Research programme, Grant Reference Number NIHR130808. The views expressed in this publication are those of the author and not necessarily those of the National Institute for Health Research or the Department of Health and Social Care.

a strengthened civil society, improvements to the local environment and mitigation of the climate risk'

(Preston City Council, 2021)

Clearly, however, the LTHTR's Social Value Framework will focus especially on health outcomes that emerge from these (e.g., the mental health benefits of securing quality employment, the physical benefits of reduced pollution in the air through strategies to deal with the climate emergency, etc.). Action on social value is framed in the context of the population intervention triangle as described in a Public Health England document on place-based interventions (Public Health England, 2021). This model describes three levels of intervention: civic-led, community-centred, and service-based. To be effective, system leadership and planning are needed to implement action on civic, service, and community interventions. Of these, civic intervention is recognised by the organisers of the LTHTR's framework as having the greatest reach and therefore highlights the vital role that local authorities have to play. In the case of Preston and the Lancashire region, this makes the connection to the PM instantly advantageous. However, the overall key to success is acknowledged as being the way all interventions are weaved together into a systemic whole: this is the networking challenge of the LTHTR framework and its 'champions'.

Five social value domains have been identified: people, purchasing, property, climate, and partners. Of these, only purchasing is directly connected to the economic aspects of CWB. Most of the potential benefit of such a network resides in the network itself (i.e., in collaboration), which is especially emphasised in the 'partners' domain and covers more than a single strand, being dominant in the sense that partnerships provide the essence of the network as a whole. This is why the LTHTR's leadership of the network emphasises a conversationalist approach to the network's development, which one could describe as a 'social' approach that is apposite to a social value strategy. In the context of the PM, the social value behind the term 'collaboration' clearly resonates with the principle of 'cooperation before competition', which is a pillar of the PM (Manley et al., 2022). In this way, it becomes clear that the Social Value Framework in Lancashire works hand in hand with the PM.

The network has set itself a target of bringing together representatives from stakeholder organisations, along with academics and any other interested party to meet on a regular basis in 2022–23, to measure outcomes and to consider future developments. In other words, there are ambitions to make the network long-term and sustainable.

SOCIAL VALUE, CWB, AND THE IMPLICATIONS FOR HEALTH

What is Social Value?

The Social Value Portal (2022), which was designed to support an understanding of the Social Value Act of 2012 and the measurement of social value nationally, describes five social value themes as part of its Themes—Measurement—Outcomes (TOMS) design. These are: (1) jobs (supporting the promotion of local skills and employment), (2) growth (the promotion of responsible regional business), (3) social (healthier, safer, and more resilient communities), (4) environment (decarbonising and safeguarding our planet), and (5) innovation (social innovation). However, different organisations will choose a different focus depending on that organisation's primary business, public service, or charitable task. The Social Value Portal (2022) definitions provide a useful tool to begin thinking about social value, especially in the context of the Social Value Act, but care should be exercised in accepting all these definitions at face value. Indeed, the 'social' in social value points to attention to the authentic needs of place, and these may vary somewhat from place to place. Social value is felt to be important but is often difficult to judge or measure, indicating that more research needs to be conducted in this field. Nevertheless, Manley et al. (2022) have provided some evidence that consolidates the view that social value is supportive of better health outcomes and therefore, ultimately, greater health equality and social justice.

The Preston Model

The PM encourages the generation and retention of economic wealth through principles of social value, recognising how economics and social progress are inextricably linked. The connection between health outcomes and socioeconomic regeneration is becoming a focus of public health developments in the UK (in addition to the PM, Scottish public health policy is being designed along these lines; Tod et al., 2022). There is still a tendency to emphasise the economic successes of the PM, even in relation to the NHS as an AI. AIs are large institutions in the local area that are 'rooted' or anchored to place; hospitals and universities are obvious examples (Reed et al., 2019). Despite this tendency, there is an increasing realisation that Pearce's model of the economic system (Tod et al., 2022), divided equally three ways into (1) market-driven, (2) publicly funded services, and (3) mutual, social, and charity, is no longer an obvious model. Trebeck and Williams (2019), among others, suggest that the new economics are the 'economics of arrival', meaning that the previously accepted norms of constant economic growth are unsustainable and that society has 'arrived' at a stage of having to consider alternative forms of growth to the economic version. Others suggest the future is in 'degrowth' (Vandeventer & Lloveras 2021) or 'post-growth' (Banerjee et al., 2021; Pansera & Fressoli, 2021). Although this chapter is focussed on social value and integrated health care, it is important to note that the context for a turn to social value should not be just narrowly envisaged in terms of improving health, but that this aim is framed by a wider sense of social and economic change. Behind this thinking lies the logic of a social value approach to the economy, as proposed by CWB projects.

Social Value, ICSs, and the Complete Care Community Programme

The drive towards giving social value strategies greater prominence than before in public health initiatives in the UK arises from the acute need to deal with health inequalities in Britain. One the one hand, these are socially unjust, and on the other hand, economically detrimental in terms of the pressure on hospital beds and various clinical interventions that result from such health inequalities. England experiences some of the largest spatial health inequalities in Europe. In poorer areas, life expectancy is, on average, 9 years less than in more affluent areas. People in disadvantaged areas can expect to live for 19 more years in poor health (Whitehead et al., 2014). While there have been several place-based initiatives in recent years seeking to address these inequalities, problems of inequality and health outcomes stubbornly persist (Popay et al., 2015; Stafford et al., 2008). The COVID-19 pandemic further emphasised the interconnectivity between economic, social, environmental, and community inequalities and poor indices of health outcomes.

The ICS is intended to tackle health inequalities and to support broader social and economic development. The LTHTR's development of a Social Value Framework and the recent emphasis on the ICS and primary care networks (PCNs) all point in the direction of establishing more formal networks for the common good, and it is hoped that they will lead to reducing national health inequalities, all of which resonate with the idea that such systemic networks create a whole that is more than the sum of its parts.

Within the ICS that seeks to place a more holistic vision of healthcare in the UK, the Complete Care Community Programme (CCCP) (Arden & GEM, 2022; Hacker, 2021) is an initiative in progress that is well placed to learn from previous experiences of place-based initiatives and from recent developments in thinking directly influenced by the pandemic, which may represent a pivotal moment of social and community transformation (Ahmad et al., 2020; Blakely, 2020).

By the time of the CCCP, there had already been pre-pandemic legislation and shifts in policy towards recognising the potential impact of proactive social policies on health and economic outcomes and a drawing together of the areas of economic wealth, social capital, and health outcomes as a holistic approach to improving population health and reducing the effects of regional inequalities (Health and Social Care Act 2012; Public Services (Social Value) Act 2012).

The Social Value Act requires public sector procurement to actively consider local and/or regional social and environmental wellbeing that might benefit the surrounding communities. Implicit in this greater demand of the public sector is a sea-change of attitude towards shifting perspectives related to value, from the economic to the social. In business terms, this is what Carroll (2021) calls the 'stakeholder' focus in new business models, or moving away from shareholders and a focus on financial profit, towards the idea that any citizen is a stakeholder who is connected to or affected by the business, including socially affected, and that businesses have a primary responsibility to those stakeholders. It would not be credible to assume that attention to social value should be limited to the public sector, a fact that is recognised by the LTHTR's Social Value Framework in its collaborative approach. When considering the role of stakeholders and their collaboration, this also places social value in the framework of increased citizen participation and engagement with democracy (Manley et al., 2022).

By emphasising the potential role of the NHS in coordinating AIs beyond its own role as an AI, it is possible to envisage the NHS taking on a socioeconomic plan for communities through an increase in attention to social value criteria (Reed et al., 2019). While opportunities exist, the Health Foundation (2017) reports that '[in] England, a 2017 analysis of CCG Freedom of Information Act requests revealed that only 13% of clinical commissioners actively considered social value as part of decision making, and 43% had no policy in place.' Therefore, there is a need for a change of mindset as well as a change in legislation if social value is to be activated as a lever to promote health equalities nationally. The connection between social value and the perception of an institution as an AI also has implicit benefits beyond procurement. If the reason for applying social value criteria to procurement is to benefit communities and ultimately health outcomes, then there are many potential health benefits that accompany such a re-imagining of the AI. A simple example would be that the greater procurement of goods and services locally would, in theory, lead to a lower carbon footprint and reduced pollution, congruent with wider environmental policies and emergent NHS commitments. Such an approach—an understanding and application of social value to procurement, but also beyond procurement, and especially as a means of encouraging local networks—forms part of the experiments in the CCCP.

In this context, the purpose of the CCCP is to encourage systems of change through a population health management approach to support PCNs to work together with communities, voluntary groups, and local councils to address regional health inequalities through networking stakeholders from diverse backgrounds. This approach co-exists with the delivery of integrated care to provide overall care and attention to populations as a whole, in ways that will subsequently benefit groups and individuals who belong to communities.

IMPACT ON PEOPLE

The direct impact of social value initiatives on people, communities, and health is difficult to evaluate, since both social value itself and the possible wellbeing benefits associated to social value are inherently subject to personal assessment and a large number of 'feel-good' factors. More research into this area will be necessary for a clearer measurement of impact on health. However, there is some evidence that social value initiatives do favourably impact on public health. For example, quality employment opportunities and improvements in working conditions and remuneration have been linked to direct health benefits (Bambra et al., 2009). There is also evidence to indicate that a greater sense of control at work may reduce the risk of cardiovascular disease (Marmot et al., 2010). Placing 'community' at the heart of economic development initiatives seems to give residents a greater sense of control over their lives (Whitehead et al., 2016), a more developed sense of collective identity and, with that, a more positive feeling about place (Halliday et al., 2021).

CONCLUSION

The reasoning behind the promotion of social value for the benefit of improved public health outcomes is much the same as the growing support for social prescribing. As Dr Michelle Howarth (Chapter 12) says, 'according to McManus et al. (2014), long-term conditions (LTCs) often manifest in increased GP attendance for social rather than clinical issues.' In both cases, there is a concern to reduce the need for clinical intervention when social enhancement could provide either prevention of the sociomedical problem carried by an individual (through an improved social environment, fruit of the implementation of social value policies), or a 'cure' of sorts through the prescription of social events, tasks, or activities via a GP and/or a link worker. Social value

policies and social prescribing are therefore very much part of the thinking behind ICSs and within the CCCP.

As the example of the Social Value Framework project in Lancashire shows, social value in the context of improving health outcomes and reducing health inequality is very much a proactive project in the northwest of England. This chapter argues that this work has been influenced by the presence of the model of CWB, which has been and is being developed in Preston since around 2012. One of the early achievements of the PM was to change the procurement practices of AIs in the Preston region, generating and retaining significantly more wealth in the area (Manley & Whyman, 2021). Linking the PM project with the movement within public health to connect social value with improved health outcomes was one of the motivations behind the 2019 report by Reed et al., 'Building healthier communities: the role of the NHS as an anchor institution', even though this report still tends to locate social value as limited to the economy and the ability of AIs to generate local wealth (Manley et al., 2022). This chapter argues for a wider interpretation of social value, perhaps closer to that described by Abrams et al. (2021), who make the deeper connection between public health and the potential for a 'Green New Deal'. In such a 'Deal', the economy is transformed from one based on individual wealth and profit to one that attends to the social. Tellingly, in the foreword to this textbook, the authors begin by citing Nye Bevan's 1952 *In Place of Fear*, which champions social health and identifies this with the collective, as opposed to the individual championing of wealth: 'Preventive medicine … is merely another way of saying health by collective action.' (Abrams et al., 2021). It seems, then, that maybe social value is not so new, but had merely slipped out of fashion in the most recent iterations of the NHS. The time is clearly ripe for a reassessment and a rebalancing of the role of social value policies in public health.

References

Abrams, R., Adhikari, R., Aked, H., Angharad, L., Barker, R., Collins, F., Eder, B., Elliott, T., Göpfert, A., Hadley, D., Harmer, A., O'Neill, E., Page, B., Saleh, A., Sharman, M., Stanford, V., van Schalkwyk, M., Wardrope, A., Whitaker, B., & Wood, E. (2021). *The public health case for a green new deal*. London: Medact. https://stat.medact.org/uploads/2021/04/The-public-health-case-for-a-Green-New-Deal-MEDACT-April-2021.pdf

Ahmad, A., Mueller, C., & Tsamakis, K. (2020). Covid-19 pandemic: a public and global mental health opportunity for social transformation. *British Medical Journal, 369*, m1383. https://doi.org/10.1136/bmj.m1383

Arden & G.E.M. *Complete care community*. https://www.ardengemcsu.nhs.uk/complete-care-community/

Bambra, C., Gibson, M., Sowden, A. J., Wright, K., Whitehead, M., & Petticrew, M. (2009). Working for health? Evidence from systematic reviews on the effects on health and health inequalities of organisational changes to the psychosocial work environment. *Preventive Medicine, 48*(5), 454–461. https://doi.org/10.1016/j.ypmed.2008.12.018

Banerjee, S. B., City, M., Jermier, J. M., Peredo, A. M., Perey, R., & Reichel, A. (2021). Theoretical perspectives on organizations and organizing in a post-growth era. *Organization, 28*(3), 337–357. https://doi.org/10.1177/1350508420973629

Blakeley, G. (2020). *The corona crash: How the pandemic will change capitalism*. London: Verso.

Carroll, A. B. (2021). Corporate social responsibility: perspectives on the CSR construct's development and future. *Business & Society, 60*(6), 1258–1278. https://doi.org/10.1177/00076503211001765

Hacker, J. (2021, June 8). *Professor Kingsland: Complete Care Community programme to create 'national learning network' on health inequalities*. Healthcare Leader. https://healthcareleadernews.com/professor-kingsland-complete-care-community-programme-to-create-national-learning-network-on-health-inequalities/

Halliday, E., Brennan, L., Bambra, C., & Popay, J. (2021). 'It is surprising how much nonsense you hear': How residents experience and react to living in a stigmatised place. A narrative synthesis of the qualitative evidence. *Health & Place, 68*, 102525. https://doi.org/10.1016/j.healthplace.2021.102525

Health and Care Act. (2022). London: Stationery Office.

Health and Social Care Act. (2012). London: Stationery Office.

Manley, J., & Whyman, P. B. (2021). *The Preston Model and Community Wealth Building: Creating a socio-economic democracy for the future*. London: Routledge.

Manley, J. Y., Mckeown, M., & Prinos, I. (2022). Saving lives and minds: Understanding social value and the role of anchor institutions in supporting community and public health before and after Covid19. In S. O. Idowu, M. T. Idowu, & A. O. Idowu. (Eds.), *Corporate social responsibility and covid-19 pandemic in global health services*. Springer.

Marmot, M., Allen, J., Goldblatt, P., Boyce, T., McNeish, D., Grady, M., & Geddes, I. (2010). *Fair Society, Healthy Lives: The Marmot review*. London: Strategic Review of Health Inequalities in England Post-2010.

Mcmanus, S., Bebbington, P., Jenkins, R. & Brugha T. (Eds.) (2016) Mental Health And Wellbeing In England: Adult Psychiatric Morbidity Survey 2014. [Online] Available at: https://Content.Digital.Nhs.Uk/Catalogue/ Pub21748/Apms-2014-Full-Rpt.Pdf [Accessed 7 August 2017]

Our Central Lancashire. (2022). *Our Central Lancashire Partnership*. https://www.healthierlsc.co.uk/central-lancs

Pansera, M., & Fressoli, M. (2021). Innovation without growth: frameworks for understanding technological change in a postgrowth era. *Organization, 28*(3), 380–404. https://doi.org/10.1177/1350508420973631

Popay, J., Whitehead, M., Carr-Hill, R., Dibben, C., Dixon, P., Halliday, E., Nazroo, J., Peart, E., Povall, S., Stafford, M., Turner, J., & Walthery, P. (2015). The impact of New Deal for Communities approaches to community engagement: within-person changes in social and health outcomes in New Deal for Communities areas. In J. Popay, M. Whitehead, R. Carr-Hill, C. Dibben, P. Dixon, E. Halliday, J. Nazroo, E. Peart, S. Povall, M. Stafford, J. Turner, & P. Walthery (Eds.), *The impact on health inequalities of approaches to community engagement in the New Deal for Communities regeneration initiative: a mixed methods evaluation*. Southampton: NIHR Journals Library. https://www.ncbi.nlm.nih.gov/books/NBK321023/

Preston City Council. (2021). *Community wealth building 2.0: Leading resilience and recovery in Preston*. https://www.preston.gov.uk/media/5367/Community-Wealth-Building-2-0-Leading-Resilience-and-Recovery-in-Preston-Strategy/pdf/CommWealth-ShowcaseDoc_web.pdf?m=637498454035670000 (accessed 01.07.22)

Public Health England. (2021, September 28). *Guidance: Place-based approaches for reducing health inequalities: main report*. https://www.gov.uk/government/publications/health-inequalities-place-based-approaches-to-reduce-inequalities/place-based-approaches-for-reducing-health-inequalities-main-report

Public Services (Social Value) Act. (2012). London: Stationery Office.

Reed, S., Gopfert, A., Wood, S., Allwood, D., & Warburton, W. (2019). *Building healthier communities: the role of the NHS as an anchor institution*. London: The Health Foundation.

Social Value Portal. (2022). https://socialvalueportal.com/

Stafford, M., Nazroo, J., Popay, J. M., & Whitehead, M. (2008). Tackling inequalities in health: evaluating the New Deal for Communities initiative. *Journal of Epidemiology & Community Health, 62*(4), 298–304. https://doi.org/10.1136/jech.2006.058628

The Health Foundation (2017). Social and Economic Value of Health: Individuals (2017). https://www.health.org.uk/what-we-do/a-healthier-uk-population/health-as-an-asset/the-social-and-economic-value-of-health-2017-individuals.

Tod, E., Shipton, D., McCartney, G., Sarica, S., Scobie, G., Parkinson, J., Bagnall, A.-M., Manley, J., Cumbers, A., Deas, S., & de le Vingne, J. (2022). What is the potential for plural ownership to support a more inclusive economy? A systematic review protocol. *Systematic Reviews, 11*, 76. https://doi.org/10.1186/s13643-022-01955-y

Trebeck, K., & Williams, J. (2019). *The economics of arrival*. Bristol: Policy.

Vandeventer, J. S., & Lloveras, J. (2021). Organizing degrowth: the ontological politics of enacting degrowth in OMS. *Organization, 28*(3), 358–379. https://doi.org/10.1177/1350508420975662

Whitehead, M., Bambra, C., Barr, B., Bowles, J., Caulfield, R., Doran, T., Harrison, D., Lynch, A., McInroy, N., Pleasant, S., & Weldon, J. (2014). *Due North: The report of the Inquiry on Health Equity for the North*. Liverpool: University of Liverpool and the Centre for Economic Strategies.

Whitehead, M., Pennington, A., Orton, L., Nayak, S., Petticrew, M., Sowden, A., & White, M. (2016). How could differences in 'control over destiny' lead to socioeconomic inequalities in health? A synthesis of theories and pathways in the living environment. *Health & Place, 39*, 51–61. https://doi.org/10.1016/j.healthplace.2016.02.00

PART IV

Integrated Care and the Workforce and Community

19

Learning From, With, and About Each Other—The Role of Interprofessional Education

Lydia Hubbard, Dr Amanda Miller, and Dr Melanie Stephens

KEY CONCEPTS

- What is IPE and what is it not, using the IPE scheme at the University of Salford as a case study
- How the IPE scheme has influenced government policy and frameworks of multiprofessional and integrated learning
- Describes the types of IPE activities and how the teaching/learning experiences impact students and staff of the IPE setting, addressing parity-of-esteem concerns
- Identifies how the COVID-19 pandemic developed opportunities for virtual learning within IPE schemes

INTRODUCTION

Lindqvist et al. (2018) identify that effective interprofessional collaborative practice relies on multiple professions working together to achieve a shared goal. Further, interprofessional education (IPE) is a strategy that enables the delivery of quality care through interprofessional collaboration and practice (Reeves et al., 2013). According to the World Health Organization (WHO) (2010), IPE occurs when *'students from two or more professions learn about, from, and with each other'*. The UK's Centre for Advancement of Interprofessional Education (CAIPE) (2002) provides a similar context to the WHO's globally renowned definition, adding that IPE aims to improve collaboration and quality of care. Thus, the principle aim of IPE is to improve the effectiveness of working collaboratively in practice and strengthen the quality of person-centred care. CAIPE (2002) suggests that IPE is integral to all academic and practice-based education. Participating in IPE enables professional and personal development, with facilitators feeling appreciated and valued through their preparation of the future collaborative workforce (El-Awaisi et al., 2021). Moreover, Barr and Low (2011) purport that IPE is a continuum of learning and should be embedded throughout pre- and post-registration studies; thus, a structured and meaningful delivery approach is essential.

CASE STUDY

Interprofessional simulation (IPS) is described as an experiential learning opportunity to increase knowledge and understanding of the roles of other disciplines (Failla & Macauley, 2014). The benefits of IPS have been widely discussed in the literature. Research has identified that students report increased confidence, improved preparedness for practice, better teamworking, improved communication, and a deeper understanding about the roles of other professionals following participation in IPS (Granheim et al., 2018; Kaldheim et al., 2021; Labrague et al., 2018).

Third-year undergraduate students at the University of Salford are offered the opportunity to engage in multiple IPSs. Undergraduates studying diagnostic radiography, nursing (adult, mental health, child and learning disabilities), physiotherapy, midwifery, occupational therapy, and social work are invited to participate. Academics from each of the disciplines take the lead on designing an IPS scenario and students rotate round the various scenarios within interprofessional student groups. An example of such a scenario is identified in Box 19.1.

In 2019, a small evaluative study was conducted exploring the experiences of students following their participation in five IPSs (Miller et al., 2017). The key themes generated from the qualitative data indicated that students gained an understanding of the team role of others, felt that they were more ready for interprofessional working, and had a positive attitude towards IPS. Such themes are consistent with what has been reported previously in the literature.

BOX 19.1 Neonate with an Impaired Neurological Status

Scenario Outline

Maisie (10 days old) attended A&E with her mother with a history of lethargy and irritability. The midwife rang an ambulance following a sign-off home visit in which she had concerns regarding Maisie's current health. Maisie arrived in A&E and required a triage assessment. After this, a CT scan was arranged due to decreased consciousness. Bruising was evident on Maisie's upper body.

Background to Scenario

Born at term, normal vaginal delivery. No significant medical history. Maisie lives with her mother (Nicola). Previous history of domestic violence between Nicola and Maisie's father (Darren) is noted on Maisie's medical record. Nicola and Darren's relationship ended when Nicola became pregnant. She informs the medical staff that she has not had contact with Darren and does not want to discuss the matter any further.

Aim

To enable an interprofessional team of students to liaise and be involved in the assessment of a neonate with an impaired neurological status

Learning Outcomes

To assist in the holistic assessment of a neonate with impaired neurological status

To liaise with other members of the interprofessional team to enable a holistic assessment of needs

To observe the role of other professions in the care of a neonate with impaired neurological status

Suggested Student Roles/Input (Under Supervision as Required)

Nurse: Triage assessment, management of seizure, escalation of concerns

Radiographer: To perform CT scan/liaise with Maisie's mother re: reason for scan and escalation of result

Midwife: Phone call consultation re: referral to A&E

Social worker: Context, communication re: domestic violence

Key Debriefing Points

1. The need for a CT scan; discussion around reduced level of consciousness and significance

2. Issues around radiation, mother's concerns—explanation about what happens during a CT scan

3. Presence of social worker and significance; discussion about background, domestic violence

4. Results of CT scan—cause for concern, how to escalate

5. Bruising on neonate; discussion around significance and safeguarding concerns

HISTORY OF IPE

Throughout history, health and social care professionals have always shared knowledge and experiences to improve patient and service user care. However, it was not until the 1960s in the UK when IPE learning opportunities were envisioned and commenced (Barr, 2007). Fundamentally linked with political change and social growth, IPE was to be used to improve collaboration and interprofessional practice, borne out of the findings of inquiries into tragic failures of care delivery (Department of Health [DH], 1991, 2012; Francis, 2013; Laming, 2003, 2009) and fragmented services working in isolation.

In the UK in 1987, a charitable organisation was created to focus action on matters arising in primary care. The Centre for the Advancement of Interprofessional Education (CAIPE) was established but the trustees and members quite quickly increased their activities to attend to common IPE concerns across local government, higher education, and professional associations.

Shortly after, the WHO issued a statement which reported that if health and social care professionals learned to collaborate as students, these skills would translate to the workplace, facilitating effective clinical or professional teamworking. From this came a series of shared learning workshops funded by the Health Education Authority (HEA) across England and Wales. The workshops focused on specific patient groups and their problems (Spratley, 1990).

In 1989, the DH gave weight to the concept of 'multiprofessional training' in the government white paper '*Community Care in the Next Decade and Beyond*'. The concept then lay the foundations for 'joint training' to be included in the 1990 NHS and Community Care Act (DH, 1991) within community care plans and training strategies (Barr, 2007; DH, 1991).

By 2001, a DH strategic framework was developed that was to be a coordinated approach to professional development. The government white paper '*Working Together, Learning Together: A Framework for Lifelong Learning for the NHS*' (DH, 2001) asserted that opportunities for shared learning across professions should be provided in both theory and practice settings as early as possible.

Primary and community care initiated some of the first IPE activities with small workshops and courses (Barr, 2007). Interest swelled and educational activities increased as professional bodies committed their support. Since then, IPE has firmly established itself in higher-education institutions and the practice and workplace arena, embedding into undergraduate curricula and extending into continuing professional practice. IPE is a regular feature within health and social care policy, professional codes of conduct, and independent bodies' qualification frameworks, providing a clear directive to facilitate IPE and practice that contributes to high-quality service delivery (Thistlethwaite et al., 2014).

WHAT IS HAPPENING NATIONALLY AND INTERNATIONALLY

Since the publication of a WHO report in 1988 which advised that 'students should learn together during certain periods of their education to acquire the skills necessary for solving the priority health problems of individuals and communities known to be particularly amendable to teamwork' (Barr, 2009), academics, researchers, and practitioners globally have been motivated to deliver IPE. In response to national and global policy issues, IPE has been used as a vehicle to reduce patient errors in healthcare in the United States (Ragucci et al., 2009), patient-centred primary care in Canada (Health Canada, 2003), and quality of life in Japan (Takahashi, 2009), to name but a few. Known as the 'quadruple aim', IPE is considered a route to improving the quality of healthcare experience, improving the health of communities and populations, reducing costs of healthcare delivery, whilst improving providers' work experience (Berwick et al., 2008; Brandt et al., 2014). In 2001/2002 in England, the DH made funding available to support the development of IPE within all pre-registration programmes by 2003. Four universities (University of Newcastle, University of South London, University of Sheffield, and a partnership between University of Southampton and University of Portsmouth) and local health and social care providers were chosen. The project was to expose students to IPE during their undergraduate programmes. Since then, other universities have developed their own programmes, either embedded within the pre- or post-qualifying curricula or as 'extracurricular' activities (Humphris, 2011).

By 2010, the WHO had documented examples of IPE from across 42 countries, and in 2017 they developed the National Health Workforce Accords (WHO, 2017),

identifying accreditation of IPE as a standard indicator for undergraduate programmes. Countries such as Australia, Canada, the United States, and the UK are considered the early adopters of IPE with nursing conducting the most studies, mainly at the undergraduate level (Herath et al., 2017).

Despite all the investment to change policy, opinion, and practice and access to a plethora of manuscripts pertaining to the delivery and evaluation of IPE activities, common issues were being highlighted in literature and systematic reviews (Abu-Rish et al., 2012; Brandt et al., 2014; Institute of Medicine, 2015; McNaughton, 2018). This included a lack of robust longitudinal IPE studies guided by theoretical frameworks that are easily replicable and identify enduring outcomes for patients and students. In 2019, a special interest group published a discussion paper that aimed to provide guidance on conducting research related to IPE and collaborative practice (IPECP) (Interprofessional Research Global Partnership, 2019). The group's recommendations included developing innovative and evidence-informed strategies that address the complexity of IPE along the continuum from IPE to collaborative practice.

The advent of the COVID-19 pandemic led to online learning becoming the new normal. Academics and researchers who developed and delivered IPE programmes were required to redesign face-to-face delivery strategies using alternative methods, such as online learning (LeBlanc, 2020). Decision-making had to focus on whether IPE was asynchronous or synchronous and activities had to be developed to ensure students felt connected with the university, their peers, and the materials being studied (Khalili, 2020). IPE activities had to have 'meaningful discourse' where learners share, discuss, and reflect on different perspectives and ideas to co-construct new knowledge (Gilbert & Dabbagh, 2005). They also should create a 'community of inquiry' requiring the presence of social, cognitive, and teaching lives of students and staff to develop deeper rather than surface learning. A variety of teaching and learning strategies and approaches were required.

TYPES OF IPE ACTIVITIES

Since the inception of IPE, educators have used a variety of IPE teaching/learning activities to support students' achievement of competencies to prepare them for collaborative interprofessional and interagency working. The setting of the IPE activity can vary from the use of clinical practice environments in primary, secondary, or tertiary care to simulation laboratories and classrooms in higher-education institutions. The components of IPE activities often have an element of preparatory work for the students to complete prior to the activity, followed by some experiential learning and, on occasions, debriefing. The experiential learning activity is developed to either enable participating students to learn side by side when learning from, with, and about each other, or be immersed in the activity. In a scoping review of the literature on published teaching and learning activities in undergraduate nursing programmes, Murdoch et al. (2017) identified that students experienced IPE during the use of high-fidelity simulation, case studies, small group discussions, and clinical placement experience. Other types of IPE activities can include more sophisticated opportunities, such as student-led clinics, patient shadowing, interprofessional shadowing, and interprofessional student-led training wards.

PARITY OF ESTEEM

Parity of esteem is a definition used in policy *'to refer to an equality in status between routes of study'* (Oxford Reference, 2020). Founded from the Education act (1944) to describe the difference between secondary modern and grammar school education, its use within healthcare is often synonymously linked to the need to value mental health equally to physical health (Royal College of Nursing, 2021). It became enshrined in law by the Health and Social Care Act (2012) and was embedded in health and social care programmes to ensure that attention was paid to develop knowledge and skills of students of the physical health needs of people with serious and complex mental health conditions.

Within IPE, however, it appears that a parity of esteem has become synonymous with recommendations to avoid professionally unbalanced groups of learners within IPE teaching and learning activities; for example, having more nurses than other professions. According to some academics, this means that unbalanced learners may *'disengage from IPE'* (Morehead et al., 2019:13), thus creating a perceived inequality in status of the smaller numbers of allied health professionals within a group to that of the nursing students and becoming a barrier to implementation. However, it can be argued that IPE creates parity of esteem in that professional identities develop through socialisation with each other (Haugland et al., 2019). By learning from, with, and about each other, students develop understanding about each other's roles and responsibilities. Within health and social care specialties, this can be seen in integrated teams that function effectively and cohesively, creating intraprofessional identities where professions not only align with their own registered profession but that of the group they work with (Joynes, 2018).

IMPACT ON PEOPLE

The benefits of IPE for students have been reported extensively, including learning more about each other's roles (Lawlis et al., 2016; Naumann et al., 2021), improving teamwork through collaboration (Koplow et al., 2020), improved professional identity (Spaulding et al., 2021), and increased knowledge regarding referrals to other team members (Birks & Ridley, 2021). Furthermore, IPE helps to increase autonomy and perceived competence (Spaulding et al., 2021), which ultimately has an impact on patient care. Oosterom et al. (2019) found that the use of interprofessional training wards had a positive effect on patient satisfaction rates. Interprofessional training wards have also been reported as being cost-effective (Hansen et al., 2009). The improvement of patient care is a key objective of IPE. Research has shown that IPE improves patient- and family-centred care (Zaudke et al., 2016). Thus, IPE has positive outcomes on both the patient and the organisation.

Anderson et al. (2017) identified that the 'professional' within the context of IPE is not limited to those working in health and social care, and the inclusion of service users, families, and carers is crucial in delivering a holistic learning experience. Involving service users and carers in IPE has been reported as a positive experience for students, facilitators, and the service user/carer (Cooper & Spence-Daw, 2006). Whilst students identify that service user involvement enhances person-centred care and the holistic provision of care, service users feel that their input helps bring the IPE activity to life (Cooper & Spence-Dawe, 2006). A further study found that service users feel empowered and valued through their involvement in IPE (Worsick et al., 2015). Thus, there are distinct, meaningful benefits for all those involved, and it is vital that service users, families, and carers are included in the planning, implementation, and evaluation of IPE.

CONCLUSION

IPE occurs when two or more students from different disciplines learn from, with, and about each other and aims to improve collaborative working and strengthen the quality of person-centred care. IPE is thought to be a continuum of learning, providing professional and personal development for all IPE participants; students pre- and post-registration studies, service users, families, and carers. Confidence, teamworking, and communication were identified as key skills that students gain from IPE. The case study's qualitative data reinforces the students' readiness for interprofessional working and gaining an understanding of the team role of others. Whilst the gains of IPE for students are readily available in the literature, the *'quadruple aim'* of the benefits towards quality of healthcare experience, health of communities and populations, and reducing costs of healthcare delivery (Berwick et al., 2008; Brandt et al., 2014) are less well known.

During the 1960s, IPE was to be used to improve collaboration and interprofessional practice to overcome the tragic failures of care delivery caused from political change and social growth. The history of IPE demonstrates that it is a regular feature within health and social care policy, professional codes of conduct, and independent bodies' qualification frameworks. The first IPE schemes implemented in Australia, Canada, the United States, and the UK classify these countries as early adopters of IPE for undergraduate-level nursing. As more countries included IPE into their pre-registration programmes, it became an accredited standard indicator for undergraduate education. However, there is a gap in research for robust longitudinal IPE studies identifying the sustained outcomes for patients and students against theoretical frameworks.

The setting of IPE activities can vary, ranging from clinical practice environments to the classrooms of higher-education institutions. The structure of IPE activities often requires students to complete an element of preparation work prior to the IPE activity, followed by experiential learning and debriefing, enabling students to experience side-by-side learning. Activities can be extended to include more sophisticated opportunities, like interprofessional student-led training wards and simulations. Despite this, concerns of parity of esteem are raised, expressing how an unbalanced profession within IPE teaching or activities can cause learners to *'disengage from IPE'* (Morehead et al., 2019). The COVID-19 pandemic has created opportunities to re-design face-to-face IPE activities into the virtual setting. This chapter emphasises that adapted IPE activities must provide a *'community of inquiry'* and *'meaningful discourse'* for learners to share, discuss, and reflect on different perspectives and co-construct new knowledge (Gilbert & Dabbagh, 2005).

WHAT IS NEXT?

The COVID-19 pandemic and waves of new variants have highlighted the crucial role of collaboration in the delivery of health and social care during major global emergencies. As IPE is a means of fostering a collaborative culture, the opportunities this brings to education and practice are significant. Telehealth has transformed primary care access and visits virtually overnight. Clinicians have been rapidly equipped for roles they would not ordinarily perform.

Virtual platforms have moved face-to-face teaching online. The future for IPE, therefore, is to robustly design and evaluate virtual spaces and activities to continue to provide opportunities for students to learn from, with, and about each other in order to deliver high-quality evidence-based services and care.

References

Abu-Rish, E., Kim, S., Choe, L., Varpio, L., Malik, E., White, A. A., Craddick, K., Blondon, K., Robins, L., Nagasawa, P., Thigpen, A., Chen, L.-L., Rich, J., & Zierler, B. (2012). Current trends in interprofessional education of health sciences students: a literature review. *Journal of Interprofessional Care*, *26*(6), 444–451. https://doi.org/10.3109/13561820.2012.715604

Anderson, E. S., Gray, R., & Price, K. (2017). Patient safety and interprofessional education: a report of key issues from two interprofessional workshops. *Journal of Interprofessional Care*, *31*(2), 154–163. https://doi.org/10.1080/13561820.2016.1261816

Barr, H. (2007). *OCC 9: Interprofessional education in the United Kingdom 1966 to 1997*. London: The Higher Education Academy.

Barr, H. (2009). An anatomy of continuing interprofessional education. *Journal of Continuing Education in the Health Professions*, *29*(3), 147–150. https://doi.org/10.1002/chp.20027

Barr, H., & Low, H. (2011). *Principles of interprofessional education*. Fareham: CAIPE.

Berwick, D. M., Nolan, T. W., & Whittington, J. (2008). The triple aim: care, health, and cost reproduced. *Health Affairs*, *27*(3), 759–769. https://doi.org/10.1377/hlthaff.27.3.759

Birks, E., & Ridley, A. (2021). Evaluating student knowledge about sexual exploitation using an interprofessional approach to teaching and learning. *British Journal of Nursing*, *30*(10), 600–607. https://doi.org/10.12968/bjon.2021.30.10.600

Brandt, B., Lutfiyya, M. N., King, J. A., & Chioreso, C. (2014). A scoping review of interprofessional collaborative practice and education using the lens of the Triple Aim. *Journal of Interprofessional Care*, *28*(5), 393–399. https://doi.org/10.3109/13561820.2014.906391

CAIPE. (2002). *About CAIPE*. https://www.caipe.org/about

Cooper, H., & Spencer-Dawe, E. (2006). Involving service users in interprofessional education narrowing the gap between theory and practice. *Journal of Interprofessional Care*, *20*(6), 603–617. https://doi.org/10.1080/13561820601029767

Department of Health. (1991). *Working together: A guide to arrangements for inter-agency co-operation for the protection of children from abuse*. London: Department of Health.

Department of Health. (2012). *Transforming care: A national response to Winterbourne View Hospital*. London: Department of Health.

Education Act. (1944).

El-Awaisi, A., Sheikh Ali, S., Abu Nada, A., Rainkie, D., & Awaisu, A. (2021). Insights from healthcare academics on facilitating interprofessional education activities. *Journal of*

Interprofessional Care, 35(5), 760–770. https://doi.org/10.1080/13561820.2020.1811212

Failla, K. R., & McCauley, K. (2014). Interprofessional simulation: a concept analysis. *Clinical Simulation in Nursing, 10*(11), 574–580. https://doi.org/10.1016/j.ecns.2014.07.006

Francis, R. (2013). *Report of the Mid Staffordshire NHS Foundation Trust Public Inquiry*. London: Stationery Office.

Gilbert, P. K., & Dabbagh, N. (2005). How to structure online discussions for meaningful discourse: a case study. *British Journal of Educational Technology, 36*(1), 5–18. https://doi.org/10.1111/j.1467-8535.2005.00434.x

Granheim, B. M., Shaw, J. M., & Mansah, M. (2018). The use of interprofessional learning and simulation in undergraduate nursing programs to address interprofessional communication and collaboration: an integrative review of the literature. *Nurse Education Today, 62*, 118–127. https://doi.org/10.1016/j.nedt.2017.12.021

Hansen, T. B., Jacobsen, F., & Larsen, K. (2009). Cost effective interprofessional training: an evaluation of a training unit in Denmark. *Journal of Interprofessional Care, 23*(3), 234–241. https://doi.org/10.1080/13561820802602420

Haugland, M., Brenna, S. J., & Aanes, M. M. (2019). Interprofessional education as a contributor to professional and interprofessional identities. *Journal of Interprofessional Care*, 1–7. https://doi.org/10.1080/13561820.2019.1693354

Health Canada. (2003). *First Ministers' accord on health care renewal*. http://www.hc-sc.gc.ca/hcs-sss/delivery-prestation/fptcollab/2003accord/index-eng.php

Health and Social Care Act. (2012).

Herath, C., Zhou, Y., Gan, Y., Nakandawire, N., Gong, Y., & Lu, Z. (2017). A comparative study of interprofessional education in global health care: a systematic review. *Medicine (Baltimore), 96*(38), e7336. https://doi.org/10.1097/md.0000000000007336

Humphris, D. (2011). Interprofessional education: a UK perspective. *13th International Health Workforce Collaborative 2011, Brisbane, Australia*. 24-26 October 2011.

Institute of Medicine. (2015). *Measuring the impact of interprofessional education on collaborative practice and patient outcomes*. Washington, DC: The National Academies Press.

Interprofessional Research Global Partnership (2019). IPECP in Post-COVID Healthcare Education and Practice Transformation Era - Joint Discussion Paper. https://interprofessionalresearch.global/.

Joynes, V. C. (2018). Defining and understanding the relationship between professional identity and interprofessional responsibility: implications for educating health and social care students. *Advances in Health Sciences Education, 23*(1), 133–149. https://doi.org/10.1007/s10459-017-9778-x

Kaldheim, H. K. A., Fossum, M., Munday, J., Johnsen, K. M. F., & Slettebø, Å. (2021). A qualitative study of perioperative nursing students' experiences of interprofessional simulation-based learning. *Journal of Clinal Nursing, 30*(1-2), 174–178. https://doi.org/10.1111/jocn.15535

Khalili, H. (2020). Online interprofessional education during and post the COVID-19 pandemic: a commentary. *Journal of Interprofessional Care, 34*(5), 687–690. https://doi.org/10.1080/13561820.2020.1792424

Koplow, S., Morris, M., Rone-Adams, S., Hettrick, H., Litwin, B., Soontupe, L. B., & Vatwani, A. (2020). Student experiences with engagement in a nursing and physical therapy interprofessional education simulation. *Internet Journal of Allied Health Sciences & Practice, 18*(1), 1–9. https://doi.org/10.46743/1540-580X/2020.1842

Labrague, L. J., McEnroe, P. D. M., Fronda, D. C., & Obeidat, A. A. (2018). Interprofessional simulation in undergraduate nursing program: an integrative review. *Nurse Education Today, 67*, 46–55. https://doi.org/10.1016/j.nedt.2018.05.001.

Laming, H. (2003). *The Victoria Climbie inquiry*. London: Stationery Office.

Laming, H. (2009). *The Protection of Children in England: A Progress Report*. London: Stationery Office.

Lawlis, T., Wicks, A., Jamieson, M., Haughey, A., & Grealish, L. (2016). Interprofessional education in practice: evaluation of a work integrated aged care program. *Nurse Education in Practice, 17*, 161–166. https://doi.org/10.1016/j.nepr.2015.11.010

LeBlanc, P. (2020, March 30). *COVID-19 has thrust universities into online learning—how should they adapt*. Brookings. https://www.brookings.edu/blog/education-plus-development/2020/03/30/covid-19-has-thrust-universities-into-online-learning%E2%81%A0-how-should-they-adapt/

Lindqvist, S., Anderson, E., Diack, L., & Reeves, S. (2018). *(2017) CAIPE Fellows statement on integrative care*. https://www.caipe.org/resources/publications/caipe-publications/lindqvist-s-anderson-e-diack-l-reeves-s-2017-caipe-fellows-statement-integrative-care

McNaughton, S. (2018). The long-term impact of undergraduate interprofessional education on graduate interprofessional practice: a scoping review. *Journal of Interprofessional Care, 32*(4), 426–435. https://doi.org/10.1080/13561820.2017.1417239

Miller, A., Henstock, L., Leyland, A., & Carruthers, H. (2017). *Simulation experiences with undergraduate health and social care students: an interprofessional approach*. https://s3.eu-west-2.amazonaws.com/assets.creode.advancehe-document-manager/documents/hea/private/hub/download/d2st5s1_amanda_miller_1568037557.pdf

Morehead, E. K., Gurbutt, D., Keeling, J., & Gordon, M. (2019). 12 tips for developing inter-professional education (IPE) in healthcare. *MedEdPublish, 8*(1).

Murdoch, N. L., Epp, S., & Vinek, J. (2017). Teaching and learning activities to educate nursing students for interprofessional collaboration: a scoping review. *Journal of Interprofessional Care, 31*(6), 744–753. https://doi.org/10.1080/13561820.2017.1356807

Naumann, F. L., Nash, R., Schumacher, U., Taylor, J., & Cottrell, N. (2021). Interprofessional education clinical placement program: a qualitative case study approach. *Journal of Interprofessional Care, 35*(6), 899–906. https://doi.org/10.1080/13561820.2020.1832448

Oosterom, N., Floren, L. C., Ten Cate, O., & Westerveld, H. E. (2019). A review of interprofessional training wards:

enhancing student learning and patient outcomes. *Medical Teacher, 41*(5), 547–554. https://doi.org/10.1080/01421 59x.2018.1503410

Oxford Reference. (2020). *Parity of esteem.* https://www.oxfordreference.com/view/10.1093/oi/authority/.20110803100306642

Ragucci, K. R., Steyer, T., Wager, K. A., West, V. T., & Zoller, J. S. (2009). The Presidential Scholars Program at the Medical University of South Carolina: an extracurricular approach to interprofessional education. *Journal of Interprofessional Care, 23*(2), 134–147. https://doi.org/10.1080/13561820802432430

Reeves, S., Perrier, L., Goldman, J., Freeth, D., & Zwarenstein, M. (2013). Interprofessional education: effects on professional practice and health care outcomes (update). *Cochrane Database of Systematic Reviews, 2013*(3), CD002213. https://doi.org/10.1002/14651858.cd002213.pub3

Royal College of Nursing. (2021). *Parity of esteem – Delivering Physical Health Equality for those with Serious Mental Health Needs.* https://www.rcn.org.uk/Professional-Development/publications/pub-007618

Spaulding, E. M., Marvel, F. A., Jacob, E., Rahman, A., Hansen, B. R., Hanyok, L. A., Martin, S. S., & Han, H.-R. (2021). Interprofessional education and collaboration among healthcare students and professionals: a systematic review and call for action. *Journal of Interprofessional Care, 35*(4), 612–621. https://doi.org/10.1080/13561820.2019.1697214

Spratley, J. (1990). *Disease prevention and health promotion in primary care.* London: Health Education Council.

Takahashi, H. E. (2009). Establishment of the Japan Association for Interprofessional Education and perspectives. *Journal of Interprofessional Care, 23*(6), 554–555. https://doi.org/10.3109/13561820903328750

Thistlethwaite, J., Forman, D., Matthews, L., Rogers, G., Steketee, C., & Yassine, T. (2014). Competencies and frameworks in interprofessional education: a comparative analysis. *Academic Medicine, 89*(6), 869–875. https://doi.org/10.1097/ACM.0000000000000249

World Health Organization. (2010). *Framework for action on interprofessional education and collaborative practice.* Geneva: WHO Press.

World Health Organization. (2017). *National health workforce accounts: A handbook.* Geneva: WHO Press.

Worsick, L., Little, C., Ryan, K., & Carr, E. (2015). Interprofessional learning in primary care: An exploration of the service user experience leads to a new model for co-learning. *Nurse Education Today, 35*, 283–287. https://doi.org/10.1016/j.nedt.2014.05.007

Zaudke, J. K., Paolo, A., Kleoppel, J., Phillips, C., & Shrader, S. (2016). The impact of an interprofessional practice experience on readiness for interprofessional learning. *Family Medicine, 48*(5), 371–376.

Further Reading

The following resources will provide insight into building effective IPE programs and how the field of IPE is advancing.

Book

Waldman, S. D., & Bowlin, S. (2020). *Building a patient-centered interprofessional education program.* Hershey: IGI Global.

Webpage

Centre for the Advancement of Interprofessional Education. https://www.caipe.org

Twitter

'Global Confederation for Interprofessional Education and Collaborative Practice' via @InterprofGlobal

The following resources will provide a greater understanding of the impacts of IPE schemes in various clinical practice environments.

Articles

Svensberg, K., Kalleberg, B. G., Rosvold, E. O., Mathiesen, L., Wøien, H., Hove, L. H., Andersen, R., Waaktaar, T., Schultz, H., Sveaass, N., & Hellesö, R. (2021). Interprofessional education on complex patients in nursing homes: a focus group study. *BMC Medical Education, 21*(1), 504. https://doi.org/10.1186/s12909-021-02867-6

Ivarson, J., Zelic, L., Sondén, A., Samnegård, E., & Bolander Laksov, K. (2020). Call the On-Call: a study of student learning on an interprofessional training ward. *Journal of Interprofessional Care, 35*(2), 275–283. https://doi.org/10.1080/13561820.2020.1725452

Video Playlist

'Student Experiences in Interprofessional Education' https://salford.kanopy.com/video/student-experiences-interprofessional-education-0

The following resources will provide insight into the impacts and influencing factors of healthcare IPE within policy and law.

Article

Girard, M.-A. (2021). Interprofessional education and collaborative practice policies and law: an international review and reflective questions. *Human Resources for Health, 19*, 9. https://doi.org/10.1186/s12960-020-00549-w

Webpage

King's Fund. https://www.kingsfund.org.uk

White Paper

NHS. (2020, November 26). *Integrating care: Next steps to building strong and effective integrated care systems across England.* https://www.england.nhs.uk/publication/integrating-care-next-steps-to-building-strong-and-effective-integrated-care-systems-across-england/

The future for IPE schemes is to re-design and adapt the activities into a virtual setting to expand learning opportunities. Stickley and Gibbs' (2020) study lends a greater understanding of the perceptions of an online IPE experience from physical therapy and health information management students.

Article

Stickley, L., & Gibbs, D. (2020). Physical therapy and health information management students: perceptions of an online interprofessional education experience. *Perspectives in Health Information Management, 18* (Winter), 1f.

20

Using Research Capacity Building in Integrated Care to Grow Leadership Potential

Dr Kirsty Marshall and Dr Hayley Bamber

KEY CONCEPTS

- Research
- Leadership development
- Integrated leadership
- Co-production

INTRODUCTION

The importance of research in health and social care is undeniable, as research evidence has progressed health and social care delivery from unproven practices to treatments based on rigorous research, which in turn has improved outcomes for people (Gifford et al., 2018). Despite the acknowledgement of the importance of research in improving outcomes, there remains a challenge for leaders in research finding and putting evidence bases into practice across several professions and settings (Gifford et al., 2018). It is also widely known that clinical research activity within hospital settings is linked to reduced mortality. Jonker et al. (2020) demonstrated that there appears to be a link between clinical research activity levels and improved patient information, better patient experience, and improved staff experience within hospital settings. This supports previous findings that found that patients who are research participants demonstrate higher levels of satisfaction and reported improved outcomes (Ozdemir et al., 2015).

While the benefits are acknowledged, the distribution of research capacity and opportunities to engage in research is not evenly distributed. For example, a report produced by Henshall et al. (2020) on the National Institute for Health Research 70@70 Senior Nurse Research Leader Programme reported that nurses and midwives are less embedded within the current agenda than other multidisciplinary colleagues. This had an impact on their wider contribution to policy and practice innovation. As integrated care grows, so does the need to embed research capacity within the workforce to ensure that there is robust evidence on which to base practice developments. A bibliometric study by Xu et al. (2017) into global research landscapes and knowledge gaps in multimorbidity concluded that there remain substantial gaps in the research agenda on multimorbidity which need to be addressed. Here lies a challenge and an opportunity for leaders in integrated care about the potential for research capacity building across the integrated setting, supporting knowledge creation, leadership development, and ultimately delivering better experiences and outcomes for people and communities. Within the case study, the integrated care organisation recognised that they needed to provide leadership and opportunities for team members to become engaged in activities. Community nurses have identified barriers as being at both personal (motivation, experience, confidence, professional capacity, training, and emphasis), and organisational levels (cullture, practice capacity, opportunities, and ambition) (Chen et al., 2019; Segrott et al., 2006).

LINKING RESEARCH CAPACITY BUILDING, EVIDENCE-BASED PRACTICE, AND LEADERSHIP

There is an important distinction to be clarified at this stage between the subtle difference between research capacity building, which is the processes of developing the infrastructure, environment, culture, and credibility in which disciplines, professionals, and community groups undertake high-quality research (Segrott et al., 2006), and the process of 'doing research' or a process of sustainable skills development for individuals and organisations to conduct high-quality research (Matus et al., 2018). The project within the case study was primarily focused on capacity building and removing the barriers to engagement with

CASE STUDY

The case study for this chapter is unusual, as in many ways it remains in the foothills of its development. However, it is intrinsically linked to the development of this book and sets out to demonstrate both the importance of leadership and research capacity within an integrated setting. Several chapters within the book are based on amazing projects that have supported the development of integrated care: while some have gone on to be part of research development and many have been disseminated locally, others have remained as local knowledge only. This is a missed opportunity to build the empirical evidence base that will support the growth of integrated care and enable systems, organisations, and services to have a strong evidence base that will support better patient outcomes. It also limits opportunities for practitioners to be engaged in research activity.

During the development of a larger integrated care research project, it was recognised that many nurses, allied health professionals, social care staff, and voluntary sector teams did not have the same access to engagement in research development as their acute sector colleagues. While primary care attracted more research,

there remained room to increase opportunity into how current changes across the system are impacting on patient outcomes.

This project aims to support non-medical staff to engage with research and build research capacity across the neighbourhood with a secondary aim of increasing leadership within integrated care teams. A joint role was developed for 12 months across the University of Salford and the NHS Trust. The secondee had responsibility for being a link across several projects and generating a core set of activities, including mapping current opportunities to engage in research studies, development of training for staff, growing links across stakeholders and with universities, and linking with wider research bodies to promote further opportunities.

One of the first activities to be developed was a writing group. In this group, Trust staff were supported to write journal articles within their field of practice to encourage reflection and to consider evidence-based practice and research (Boud et al., 1994). The writing group was very popular and led to the publication of articles and opportunities for team members to then develop their ideas further.

research. Early in the development of the project, it was clear that there were links between the desire to build a research-positive integrated system and the wider organisational aims to increase and enhance leadership within the newly formed neighbourhoods. One area was building research into the fabric of the newly formed teams supported by the use of evidence-based practice. Johnston et al. (2016) explain that nurses often have difficulty transporting research into practice, citing factors such as a lack of time, training, and mentoring. Similar challenges have been cited in allied healthcare professionals (AHPs) and voluntary sector literature. For example, Matus et al., (2018) reported that AHPs have high levels of motivation to engage in research; however, they face organisational and professional barriers such as lack of time, funding, work demands, a lack of skills, and insufficient support from managers and colleagues.

Several skills have been attributed to heightened research capacity. These include critical thinking, utilisation of evidence-based practice, project management, organisational management and time management, problem-based learning, leadership, quality improvement, and public involvement (Matus et al., 2018). These skills cross over with several required leadership attributes to lead in a complex health and social care system. This enhanced

the project in the case study as it has the potential to provide multiple benefits to the teams.

Research, Leadership, and Change

When considering the moves towards an integrated service, it is important that organisations review their current leadership provisions and put strategies in place to support leaders to develop their own confidence and skills to enhance collaboration (Amanchukwu et al., 2015). Through emboldening our leaders, we can maximise workforce engagement and thus improve organisational and service user outcomes. Successful integration through the vehicle of co-production is more likely to be achieved through facilitation as opposed to direction.

In the case study, we see how the integrated care organisation linked the two important agendas of increasing research capacity and development of leadership skills that would support wider organisational development. The Trust took a proactive approach to research capacity building with an acknowledgement that there needed to be a systematic approach to ensure that opportunities were not missed to develop evidence. The Trust recognised that alongside building research capacity, engaging community teams in research activities could improve staff satisfaction and retention and wellbeing

(Jonker et al., 2020), which would have wider impacts in patient care and quality outcomes.

Change management literature further suggests that individuals endeavouring to work towards a change should present as enthusiastic and inclusive, as this is likely to enable co-production (Bamber, 2020; Bradley, 2015; Krummaker & Vogel, 2012). Such catalysts (as defined in Chapter 7), accompanied by co-production's aims for power distribution and reciprocal relationships, point strongly to the potential benefits of a transformational leadership approach (Krummaker & Vogel, 2012). This style requires leaders to collaborate to determine what change is needed, thus developing a shared vision (Seltzer & Bass, 1990). Through a transformational approach, it is likely that followers' dedication to the change process will be maintained, which in turn can support the development of confidence for leaders in dealing with potential outliers. It is critical, however, to consider that co-production and an integrated approach involve more than working with people; they require fundamental culture changes, where all parties are equal participants (Bamber, 2020; Marshall, 2020). Whilst this is a promising leadership style, literature has warned that challenges exist for transformational leaders when organisations have predetermined targets which do not meet with the group's desired approach to change (Currie & Lockett, 2007). Therefore, we must support our leaders to develop the skills to align organisational priorities to the community's needs through power distribution and active engagement.

Here we see another positive link between research capacity building and leadership capacity. Good ethical research is built on positive engagement with service users. In the UK, the National Institute for Health Care Research (NHIR) has set six standards for public involvement in research:

1. Inclusive opportunities
2. Working together
3. Support and learning
4. Communications
5. Impact
6. Governance
   (nihr.ac.uk, 2019.)

The act of increasing research capacity has the potential to bring issues of public involvement into the consciousness of teams, encouraging them to consider patients and the public as partners. This in turn aligns with current healthcare policy in the UK and many other countries, which promotes patient-centred care and personalisation as well as public involvement across all levels of organisations.

Research Capacity Building and Satisfaction With Wider Work Environment

As stated earlier in this chapter, there is clear evidence that building research capacity and engaging staff in research can increase wider satisfaction with job roles and within the work environment. Equality environment factions are cited as being limiting factors for clinicians to engage in research activity. Bamber (2020) found that there is a need to empower staff who may currently feel unheard. Engaging them actively in research projects can help to provide them with a sense of contribution and help them to identify as agents of change. Doing so may maximise their impact on practice as they will feel their work is transformative and beneficial. Through engagement in research, we are likely to form allies for the integration agenda which is going to increase the chances of success.

Secondly, considering the six standards for public involvement in research, it is important to not only focus on having service users as participants but actively co-producing with service users so they become part of the research team. The richness which these individuals can add to the process is critical, as is their differing lens. It would be imprudent to ignore the evident challenges which exist in progressing this agenda, including engagement of hard-to-reach people, relapse in condition, increased time for the research process, and the distribution of power, to name but a few, which has led some to view co-production in research as not being beneficial (Oliver et al., 2019). Whilst these challenges need thought, planning, and consideration to overcome them, the benefits of service user involvement is tenfold, adding credibility and authenticity to the findings (Conklin et al., 2015). Therefore, it is key that power is distributed, reciprocal relationships developed, and honest conversations held to support the inclusion of service users in co-producing research. It is not enough for researchers to tokenistically consult a few service users from accessible areas to guide their research; concerted efforts to promote wider representation must occur. If this philosophy is embedded within services, it will support wider activities. Greig (2015) warns that the process of integration can lead to people becoming obsessed with process or structure. If this occurs, there will be a limit to the potential for integrated services, which co-production needs to stay true to so the principles and set outcomes are meaningful to communities. This chapter has shown that the skills developed in research are very transferable to the wider aims of integrated care.

CONCLUSION

Increasing research capacity has a huge potential within integrated care services, primarily to build and enhance the evidence base and capture best practice. However, there is a wider potential within the workforce, as studies have shown that teams who engage in research have a higher satisfaction, confidence, and knowledge in the application of evidence-based practice. These advantages are furthered still when considering the development of co-production skills, which would support both research and the delivery of an integrated approach that places the needs of people and communities at its centre.

REFLECTIONS OF PROFESSIONAL DOCTORATE—HOW ENGAGING IN COMMUNITY RESEARCH CAN SUPPORT SERVICE

Finally, in this chapter, Hayley and I wanted to reflect on our own research journeys. We both commenced professional doctorates while working in the NHS and the processes of engaging in research had profound and far-reaching learning for ourself as practitioners and for those we engaged in research with. For the reflection, we have used Gibbs' (1988) reflective cycle.

Reflection: Dr Kirsty Marshall

Description

My professional doctorate study explored the lived experiences of teams as they came together as a neighbourhood in 2018.

Feelings

Turning to a practice setting to conduct an institutional ethnography was a daunting prospect, being unsure of how I would be perceived, and as a novice researcher I was very concerned about ensuring I was methodologically and ethically sound in my practice. I was also worried as I wasn't at that time 'an academic'; rather, I was a district nurse and NHS manager—it is fair to say I had a touch of imposter syndrome.

Evaluation

My understanding of how to work with people was transformed during this period. Through the research processes, I conducted regular supervision and reflexivity sessions. These processes enabled me to understand myself better, my views and biases, and overall, I was able to challenge myself and gain more of an understanding of how I interact and work with others.

Analysis

The research methodology I used was institutional ethnography as defined by Smith (2005). Smith (2005) holds the view that research needs to be conducted using methods that are sensitive to people and is based in their lives. There is also a focus on representing those who are marginalised. The rationale for focussing on marginalised groups is that they provide a unique insight into organisational behaviour and the relations of ruling, giving a voice to the seldom heard.

This approach was very influential for my thinking at the time and has influenced my leadership approach since. Conducting the research enabled me to gain a deepening understanding of how organisations are influenced by external sources and how it is important to enable a wide range of voices to be heard in a range of settings.

An important part of the research was providing feedback to the teams as the knowledge developed was their knowledge and they had been kind enough to share it with me. This was a very impactful event as they discussed the research and their experience of being participants. There was a feeling that they had a story to tell and a narrative of value. It was an amazing journey to have completed with them.

Conclusion

Considering my journey in the context of research capacity building and leadership, completing a doctorate was a massive personal journey, but it was also a journey that made me a more compassionate and thoughtful leader.

Action

I am still a researcher and senior lecturer in the field of integrated care and the training I received in my doctorate studies have been embedded as a skill set from which to grow and develop. I am eternally grateful to those people who participated in my research, I owe them a great deal and I will hopefully pay this back by supporting others to develop their research potential.

Reflection: Dr Hayley Bamber

Description

As part of the professional doctorate process, I completed a piece of community-based research to support managers and clinical leads understanding of a co-production model within community mental health services.

Feelings

I was excited to undertake this project but also concerned about how new the topic was and how undefined co-production was at the time. I was upset and at times felt hopeless hearing some of the comments which staff members were making about how they felt treated within the organisation when it came to change, but I felt hopeful that my research could support a positive change in practice.

Evaluation

What didn't go too well was my underestimation of how people were feeling within the organisation. They were reporting feeling 'done to' and 'unheard' and provided examples of where their views and concerns had been dismissed. However, using a clear interview, including guided questions, navigated people towards positive thoughts for the future. What did become apparent within the study was that people were hopeful that a truly community- and service user-focused approach could have a positive outcome for the people they worked with, and they believed that this was the only way services could proceed to provide good-quality care.

Analysis

Whilst underestimating people's feelings did not have a detrimental impact on the study, it is important to consider how organisational change can impact and influence staff's wellbeing and job satisfaction Hennink et al. (2020). If they do not feel heard or trusted, then they are likely to disengage from the process, which can impede a leader's ability to successfully make the desired change Hiatt and Creasey (2003). Additionally, without ownership over local processes, participants felt there was no way successful change could be achieved Wilcox and Jenkins (2015). Essential in this process is the service user (who within the studied organisation were not included within their co-production model), which participants strongly felt was missing.

The guidance of questions to look at the future supported participants to not dwell on the negative experiences that they had Keele (2015). They were able to recognise that if co-production was adopted in its truest form (with service user and community involvement), with leaders clearly communicating their vision and expectations, then there was a real chance that culture within the organisation could shift, and service users could receive better support (Bamber, 2020).

Conclusion

There were clear strengths and limitations within my research study and underestimating the strength of people's feelings made some interviews challenging (due to my positionality within the organisation). However, a clear strength was the use of the interview guide which provided a focus to the future, which appears to be hopeful.

References

Amanchukwu, R. N., Stanley, G. J., & Ololube, N. P. (2015). A review of leadership theories, principles and styles and their relevance to educational management. *Management*, 5(1), 6–14. https://doi.org/10.5923/j.mm.20150501.02

Bamber, H. (2020) *Managers' and clinical leads' perspectives of a co-production model for community mental health service improvement in the NHS: A case study* [Professional Doctorate thesis, University of Salford]. https://usir.salford.ac.uk/id/eprint/57907/3/Hayley%20Bamber%20Final%20Thesis%20amendments%20for%20external.pdf

Boud, D., Keogh, R., & Walker, D. (1994). *Reflection: Turning experience into learning* (3rd ed.). New York: Routledge Falmer.

Bradley, E. (2015). Carers and co-production: Enabling expertise through experience. *Mental Health Review Journal*, 20(4), 232–241. https://doi.org/10.1108/MHRJ-05-2014-0016

Chen, Q., Sun, M., Tang, S., & Castro, A. R. (2019). Research capacity in nursing: A concept analysis based on a scoping review. *BMJ Open*, 9(11), e032356. https://doi.org/10.1136/bmjopen-2019-032356

Conklin, A., Morris, Z., & Nolte, E. (2015). What is the evidence base for public involvement in health-care policy? Results of a systematic scoping review. *Health Expectations*, 18(2), 153–165. https://doi.org/10.1111/hex.12038

Currie, G., & Lockett, A. (2007). A critique of transformational leadership: Moral, professional and contingent dimensions of leadership within public services organization. *Human Relations*, 60(2), 341–370. https://doi.org/10.1177/0018726707075884

Gibbs, G. (1988). *Learning by doing: A guide to teaching and learning methods* (1st ed.). Oxford: Oxford Polytechnic.

Gifford, W. A., Squires, J. E., Angus, D. E., Ashley, L. A., Brosseau, L., Craik, J. M., Domecq, M.-C., Egan, M., Holyoke, P., Juergensen, L., Wallin, L., Wazni, L., & Graham, I. D. (2018). Managerial leadership for research use in nursing and allied health care professions: A systematic review. *Implementation Science*, 13(1), 1–23. https://doi.org/10.1186/s13012-018-0817-7

Greig, R. (2015). *Co-production – the missing link in integration*. https://www.scie.org.uk/co-production/blogs/co-production-and-integration

Hennink, M., Hutter, I., & Bailey, A. (2020). *Qualitative research methods*. London: SAGE Publications Limited.

Henshall, C., Greenfield, D. M., Jarman, H., Rostron, H., Jones, H., & Barrett, S. (2020). A nationwide initiative to increase nursing and midwifery research leadership: Overview of year one programme development, implementation and evaluation. *Journal of Clinical Nursing*. https://doi.org/10.1111/jocn.15558

Hiatt, J., & Creasey, T. J. (2003). Change management: The people side of change. Prosci.

Johnston, B., Coole, C., Narayanasamy, M., Feakes, R., Whitworth, G., Tyrell, T., & Hardy, B. (2016). Exploring the barriers to and facilitators of implementing research into practice. *British Journal of Community Nursing*, 21(8), 392–398. https://doi.org/10.12968/bjcn.2016.21.8.392

Jonker, L., Fisher, S. J., & Dagnan, D. (2020). Patients admitted to more research-active hospitals have more confidence in staff and are better informed about their condition and medication: Results from a retrospective cross-sectional study. *Journal of Evaluation in Clinical Practice*, *26*(1), 203–208. https://doi.org/10.1111/jep.13118

Keele, R. (2011). *Nursing research and evidence-based practice.* Jones & Bartlett Learning.

Krummaker, S., & Vogel, B. (2012). An in-depth view of the facets, antecedents and effects of leaders' change competency: Lessons from a case study. *Journal of Applied Behavioral Science*, *49*(3), 279–307. https://doi.org/10.1177/0021886312469442

Marshall, K. (2020). *An exploration of neighbourhood team members experiences of the transition from traditional health and social care teams to integrated care systems, within a defined health and social care economy* (Publication No.: 595618) [Professional Doctorate thesis, University of Salford].

Matus, J., Walker, A., & Mickan, S. (2018). Research capacity building frameworks for allied health professionals - a systematic review. BMC health services research, 18(1), 716. https://doi.org/10.1186/s12913-018-3518-7

NIHR (2019, December 18) PPI (Patient and Public involvement) resourses for applicants to NIHR research programmes. https://www.nihr.ac.uk/documents/ppi-patient-and-public-involvement-resources-for-applicants-to-nihr-research-programmes/23437

Oliver, K., Kothari, A., & Mays, N. (2019). The dark side of co-production: Do the costs outweigh the benefits for health research? *Health Research Policy and Systems*, *17*(1), 33. https://doi.org/10.1186/s12961-019-0432-3

Ozdemir, B. A., Karthikesalingam, A., Sinha, S., Poloniecki, J. D., Hinchliffe, R. J., Thompson, M. M., Grower, J., Boaz, A., & Holt, P. J. (2015). Research activity and the association with mortality. *PloS One*, *10*(2), e0118253. https://doi.org/10.1371/journal.pone.0118253

Segrott, J., McIvor, M., & Green, B. (2006). Challenges and strategies in developing nursing research capacity: A review of the literature. *International Journal of Nursing Studies*, *43*(5), 637–651. https://doi.org/10.1016/j.ijnurstu.2005.07.011

Seltzer, J., & Bass, B. M. (1990). Transformational leadership: Beyond initiation and consideration. *Journal of Management*, *16*(4), 693–703. https://doi.org/10.1177/014920639001600403

Smith, D. E. (2005). *Institutional ethnography: A sociology for people*. Rowman Altamira.

Wilcox, M., & Jenkins, M. (2015). *Engaging change: A people-centred approach to business transformation*. Kogan Page, Limited.

Xu, X., Mishra, G. D., & Jones, M. (2017). Mapping the global research landscape and knowledge gaps on multimorbidity: A bibliometric study. *Journal of Global Health*, *7*(1), 010414. https://doi.org/10.7189/jogh.07.01041

21

Transforming Culture and Values Through Integrated Practice

Dr Lorna Chesterton, Siobhán Kelly, Dr Melanie Stephens, Professor Andrew Clark, and Professor Anya Ahmed

KEY CONCEPTS

- Integrated practice
- Workforce
- Organisational culture
- Multidisciplinary teams
- Education

OVERVIEW OF CHAPTER

Integrated practice describes the collaborative process of utilising the combined resources of health and social care systems to meet the needs of the population. This chapter outlines the ways in which integrated practice might be transformed by and, in turn, transform individual and organisational cultures and values in the provision of social care. It draws on a case study of a student placement scheme that provided training placements for multidisciplinary teams of health and social care and allied health professional students in care homes. The opportunities and challenges afforded by such an initiative are considered in the wider context of the complexities of integrated care policies and practices.

INTRODUCTION

Evidence suggests that integrated practice facilitates a change in culture and values within a practice environment (NHS England, 2020). Culture is a complex and often contested concept, and space precludes a detailed discussion of the term; however, briefly, culture might be conceptualised as representing a collective set of shared values, goals, attitudes, and behaviours of a group, which is established and maintained through a process of socialisation (du Toit, 1995). Values are interlinked with culture and are the beliefs which underpin behaviour and decision-making (Chitty & Black, 2007). In bringing together different organisations with differing cultures, an ambition in the NHS People Plan (NHS England, 2020:6) is to embrace a new, shared culture of inclusion and belonging, where different disciplines can work more effectively together to deliver person-centred care (NHS England, 2020).

Successful integrated practice demands collaboration between health and social care services. Whilst structural issues such as resourcing, policy frameworks, and organisational differences can create a challenge to this, so too can clashes in organisational cultures and values (Miller, 2016). Transforming attitudes and values is therefore crucial to creating meaningful interprofessional relationships between clinicians to provide effective person-centred care (Stucky et al., 2022). As discussed in Chapter 5, interprofessional education (IPE) provides such a platform by building upon the premise that affective domain development can be influenced by students from different disciplines working and learning together about their own and other's professions (Stephens & Ormandy, 2018), with a growing evidence base demonstrating the impact of IPE on attitudes and professional knowledge and skills (Reeves et al., 2013).

Seminal work by Epstein (1977) explored learning in the affective domain, developing a three-staged process (compliance, identification, and internalisation) which purported to measure how values, attitudes, and behaviour are influenced by communication. Whilst Epstein's (1977) work has limitations, it has provided a useful framework for other scholars to establish new conceptual models to measure affective domain development (Stephens & Ormandy, 2018). Whilst IPE is involved in pre-registered student learning, other models have been developed which situate themselves in clinical practice to facilitate IPE and learning amongst qualified practitioners to allow them to work more effectively in a multidisciplinary team, providing integrated care. An advanced care model such as the Patient-Centered Medical Home (Stout et al., 2017) observed the value of preparing the workforce to work effectively as a high-functioning team and highlighted the need for effective leadership. The Professionals Accelerating Clinical and Educational Redesign (PACER) was a model designed to develop practice-based learning and teamwork through IPE with the aim of building trusting professional relationships and transforming practice (Eiff et al., 2020).

A further concept which adds a different dimension to transforming values and culture, is that of interprofessional socialisation (IPS), which describes the process whereby individuals develop professional and interprofessional identities through shared interprofessional values and behaviours, thus enabling better integrated working (Khalili et al., 2019). The IPS framework (IPSF) developed by Khalili et al. (2013) presents a three-stage process (breaking down barriers, interprofessional role learning, dual identity development) which in many ways is a model which complements existing IPE programs.

In transforming values and culture in healthcare, one of the most influential factors to be considered is leadership (West et al., 2015). Effective leadership should establish a vision and commitment to safety (Bellandi et al., 2021) whilst ensuring a positive work environment and high-quality care provision (Wei et al., 2018). Stucky et al. (2022) assert that leaders in nursing utilise a framework of relational coordination to assist interprofessional practitioners to work more effectively to create what Gittell (2020) describes as a culture of inclusivity, shared goals, shared knowledge, and mutual respect.

As stated in Chapter 5, integrated practice aims to provide *person-centred care*, tailored to the needs of the individual. However, to deliver person-centred care which is based on the needs, beliefs, and values of the individual within the context of their life, family, resources, and agency, transformation at different levels of operation from organisation to individual is required. Health and social care can therefore be visualised to operate across three levels: the macro level (policy or sector level), the meso level (organisational or professional level), and the micro level (clinical or interventional level).

Table 21.1 gives a summary of the contextual factors which need consideration to enable collaboration.

Macro-level integrated working involves interventions and advocacy on a large scale, affecting entire communities, states, or even countries. It helps patients, clients, service users, and residents by intervening in large systems that may seem beyond the reach of individuals (Curry & Ham, 2010). Macro-level integration improves efficiency, quality, and user satisfaction (Suter et al., 2009) with values, principles, and standards in care being derived from the professional and ethical codes for health and social care professionals (Meulenbergs et al., 2004). Within the context of the UK,

TABLE 21.1   Contextual Factors

Operational Level	Considerations
Macro level	Policy Coordination of services Funding Professional regulation, professional education and development
Meso level	Organisational structure Information systems
Micro level	Day-to-day clinical interactions between practitioners and service users Relationship building/developing mutual trust Power sharing Knowledge sharing

the Health and Care Bill (UK Parliament, 2022) proposes to bring in integrated care partnerships (ICPs) and integrated care boards (ICBs) from April 2022. ICPs will establish alliances between organisations, stakeholders, local authorities, and the NHS, becoming a forum to develop integrated care strategies to improve health outcomes for the local population. ICBs will then become the commissioners of healthcare services for the ICP's local area.

Transforming culture and values though integrated working at a meso level is described as the collaborative process whereby the different sectors of the NHS work together with local authorities and the third sector to tackle the needs of the population, which ideally includes the wider determinants of health (Ham, 2018). However, integrated care should not be seen as a sole intervention but more as a facilitator which embodies a set of principles and policies which aim to improve services, health outcomes, and patient experience (Hughes et al., 2020). Meso-level integrated working addresses group issues and is a valuable tool for creating small-scale institutional, social, and cultural change.

Micro-level integrated working includes the day-to-day activities of the professionals and disciplines who work within a team to provide person-centred care (Curry & Ham, 2010), with professional behaviour, decision-making, and values being guided by professional codes (Meulenbergs et al., 2004). In a UK context, examples of transforming culture and values through integrated care at a micro level includes trials of early versions of integrated care models which focused on preventing hospitalisation for individuals with long-term conditions, often with a disease-specific focus (World Health Organization (WHO), 2016). Since then, three major national pilot programmes were developed for integrated care in the UK: the *Integrated Care Pilots* (Department of Health, 2008), the *Integrated Care and Support Pioneers* (NHS England, 2014) and *New Care Model 'Vanguards'* (NHS England, 2016).

GOVERNANCE

When examining integrated practice within health and social care, attention must be given to the overarching governance, which can be described as the rules governing the roles, remits, and responsibilities of care providers and policymakers around service users (WHO, 2015). Governance is the process by which accountability for the quality of care is maintained and monitored, underpinned by the principles of transparency, accountability, participation, integrity, and capability. The need for strong governance is highlighted by the WHO (WHO, 2015) who observed that meso-level organisations should strengthen health system governance to establish a framework for decision-making and policy implementation (Nicholson et al., 2018). Furthermore, there is a need for health and social care professions and disciplines to develop collaborative interdisciplinary learning, to establish an environment which promotes parity of esteem, and to move forward the agenda of interdisciplinary working.

CONCLUSION AND RECOMMENDATIONS

This chapter explored how values and culture can be transformed by integrated practice, drawing on ideas around person-centred care and IPE. Transforming

---

CASE STUDY

In 2021, a feasibility study was developed to implement and evaluate an IPE student training placement scheme across three care homes across Greater Manchester. Fifteen undergraduate students in their second and final year of study were recruited to undertake their placement in one of the three participating care homes. Students came from a variety of disciplines, including nursing, physiotherapy, social work, podiatry, and sports rehabilitation programmes. Some students attended as part of their natural placement cycle, whilst others self-selected to join as part of a 'bespoke' learning opportunity. The study took place over 6 weeks, with students working the same shift patterns to optimise learning from one another. To further enable interprofessional development and reflection, students, care home staff, residents, academics, and practice education facilitators took part in weekly multidisciplinary team meetings. In the meeting, residents set goals that they would like to work towards with the help of the students across the 6 weeks. The students then engaged in a cycle of action and reflection to address these goals as a collaborative team.

The principle aim of the study was to promote IPE and thereby improve standards of care in care homes. On a macro level, the study had a marked value on the current and future students' professional education and development, transforming culture and values through shared identity perspectives, and challenging care environments to become person-centred. A broader issue which emerged from findings was the change in student attitudes around the perception of care homes as innovative environments for education, training, and career development.

On a meso level, the study highlighted the need for shared governance, as care home staff were encouraged by students to change practice and implement innovative care and support through greater autonomy and collective energy among the team. It should also be recognised that decisions at the meso level, from the owners of the care homes, can have a significant impact on the ability to implement change when profit-centred values limit innovation in favour of a more task-orientated focus.

On a micro level, students sometimes found it difficult to navigate hierarchical power dynamics embedded in care home practice, often voicing concerns of 'overstepping the mark' or 'knowing their place'. This was particularly apparent in homes where the wider body of staff were not involved in the study and, in such cases, students found contradictions arose when the culture was not nurturing interprofessional practice in the everyday. The weekly meetings with the residents were recognised to be a new and rewarding addition to practice that harnessed expertise not ordinarily available in the setting and ensured the values, needs, and experiences of the residents guided clinical decision-making. Values of effective communication were also developed that allowed the staff to learn about and implement new practices, whilst giving students the opportunity to strengthen their own professional identity by learning about the cultures and values of other groups.

culture and values will not happen overnight; fostering innovation and cultivating collaborative practice is a challenging process and change is dependent on the culture and context in which it is implemented. It is also important to consider that there is no singular integrated model that can be applied to all health and social care settings, and that different learning programmes and approaches to IPE ensure diverse groups can benefit in meaningful and appropriate ways. While integrated working offers a unique opportunity to prepare and strengthen the future workforce, it should not be pictured as the only solution to systemic and ongoing issues within health and social care, since a strong infrastructure needs to be in place for such innovation to continue to grow and flourish. The case study described in this chapter demonstrates the positive impacts of IPE for staff, students, and residents in a care home environment. Indeed, IPE could provide pre-registration students and qualified clinicians alike a way to enhance collaborative practice and teamworking when facilitated by effective leadership and strong governance.

References

Bellandi, T., Romani-Vidal, A., Sousa, P., & Tanzini, M. (2021). Adverse event investigation and risk assessment. In L. Donaldson, W. Ricciardi, S. Sheridan, & R. Tartaglia. (Eds.), *Textbook of patient safety and clinical risk management* (pp. 129–142). Springer.

Chitty, K. K., & Black, B. P. (2007). *Professional nursing: concepts and challenges* (5th ed.). St. Louis: Saunders/Elsevier.

Curry, N., & Ham, C. (2010). *Clinical and service integration: The route to improve outcomes*. London: King's Fund.

Department of Health. (2008). *Integrated Care Pilots: an introductory guide*. London: Department of Health.

du Toit, D. (1995). A sociological analysis of the extent and influence of professional socialization on the development of a nursing identity among nursing students at two universities in Brisbane, Australia. *Journal of Advanced Nursing, 21*(1), 164–171. https://doi.org/10.1046/j.1365-2648.1995.21010164.x

Eiff, M. P., Fuqua-Miller, M., Valenzuela, S., Saseen, J. J., Zierler, B., Carraccio, C., McDonald, F. S., Green, L., & Carney, P. A. (2020). A model for accelerating educational and clinical transformation in primary care by building interprofessional faculty teams: findings from PACER. *Journal of Interprofessional Education & Practice, 19*, 100336. https://doi.org/10.1016/j.xjep.2020.100336

Epstein, R. (1977). Evaluating the effective domain of student learning. *NLN Publications*, 67–80.

Gittell, J. H. (2020). *Transforming relationships for high performance: The power of relational coordination*. Stanford: Stanford University Press.

Ham, C. (2018). *Making sense of integrated care systems, integrated care partnerships and accountable care organisations in the NHS in England*. London: The King's Fund.

Hughes, G., Shaw, S. E., & Greenhalgh, T. (2020). Rethinking integrated care: a systematic hermeneutic review of the literature on integrated care strategies and concepts. *Milbank Quarterly, 98*(2), 446–492. https://doi.org/10.1111/1468-0009.12459

Khalili, H., Orchard, C., Laschinger, H. K. S., & Farah, R. (2013). An interprofessional socialization framework for developing an interprofessional identity among health professions students. *Journal of Interprofessional Care, 27*(6), 448–453. https://doi.org/10.3109/13561820.2013.804042

Khalili, H., Thistlethwaite, J., El-Awaisi, A., Pfeifle, A., Gilbert, J., Lising, D., MacMillan, K., Maxwell, B., Grymonpre, R., Rodrigues, F., Snyman, S., & Xyrichis, A. (2019). *Guidance on global interprofessional education and collaborative practice research: Discussion paper*. https://interprofessionalresearch.global/wp-content/uploads/2019/10/Guidance-on-Global-Interprofessional-Education-and-Collaborative-Practice-Research_Discussion-Paper_FINAL-WEB.pdf

Meulenbergs, T., Verpeet, E., Schotsmans, P., & Gastmans, C. (2004). Professional codes in a changing nursing context: literature review. *Journal of Advanced Nursing, 46*(3), 331–336.

Miller, R. (2016). Crossing the cultural and value divide between health and social care. *International Journal of Integrated Care, 16*(4), 10. https://doi.org/10.5334/ijic.2534

NHS England. (2014). *Integrated care and support pioneer programme*. London: NHS England.

NHS England. (2016). *New Care Models: Vanguards—developing a blueprint for the future of NHS and care services*. London: NHS England.

NHS England. (2020). *We Are The NHS: People Plan 2020/21 – action for us all*. London: NHS England.

Nicholson, C., Hepworth, J., Burridge, L., Marley, J., & Jackson, C. (2018). Translating the elements of health governance for integrated care from theory to practice: a case study approach. *International Journal of Integrated Care, 18*(1), 11. https://doi.org/10.5334/ijic.3106

Reeves, S., Perrier, L., Goldman, J., Freeth, D., & Zwarenstein, M. (2013). Interprofessional education: Effects on professional practice and healthcare outcomes. *(update). Cochrane Database of Systematic Reviews, 2013*(3), CD002213. https://doi.org/10.1002/14651858.cd002213.pub3

Stephens, M., & Ormandy, P. (2018). Extending conceptual understanding: how interprofessional education influences affective domain development. *Journal of Interprofessional Care, 32*(3), 348–357. https://doi.org/10.1080/13561820.2018.1425291

Stout, S., Zallman, L., Arsenault, L., Sayah, A., & Hacker, K. (2017). Developing high-functioning teams: factors associated with operating as a "real team" and implications for patient-centered medical home development. *Inquiry, 54* 0046958017707296 https://doi.org/10.1177/0046958017707296.

Stucky, C. H., Wymer, J. A., & House, S. (2022). Nurse leaders: transforming interprofessional relationships to bridge healthcare quality and safety. *Nurse Leader, 20*(4), 375–380. https://doi.org/10.1016/j.mnl.2021.12.003

Suter, E., Oelke, N. D., Adair, C. E., & Armitage, G. D. (2009). Ten key principles for successful health systems integration. *Healthcare Quarterly*, *13*, 16–23. https://doi.org/10.12927/hcq.2009.21092

UK Parliament. (2022). *Health and Care Bill (HL Bill 71)*. https://publications.parliament.uk/pa/bills/lbill/58-02/071/5802071_en_1.html

Wei, H., Sewell, K. A., Woody, G., & Rose, M. A. (2018). The state of the science of nurse work environments in the United States: a systematic review. *International Journal of Nursing Sciences*, *5*(3), 287–300. https://doi.org/10.1016/j.ijnss.2018.04.010

West, M., Armit, K., Loewenthal, L., Eckart, R., West, T., & Lee, A. (2015). *Leadership and leadership development in health care: the evidence base*. London: Faculty of Medical Leadership and Management, King's Fund. https://www.kingsfund.org.uk/sites/default/files/field/field_publication_file/leadershipleadership-development-health-care-feb-2015.pdf

World Health Organization. (2015). *WHO global strategy on people-centred and integrated health services: Interim Report*. Geneva: WHO Press.

World Health Organization. (2016). *Strengthening health system governance: Better policies, stronger performance*. Maidenhead: McGraw-Hill.

Further Reading

Book

Boykin, A., Schoenhofer, S., & Valentine, K. (2013). *Health care system transformation for nursing and health care leaders: Implementing a culture of caring*. New York: Springer.

A practical guide for practitioners who wish to change their health and social care systems based on caring values and the promotion of intra- and interprofessional dialogue among stakeholders.

Book Chapter

Miller, R., & Andrade, M. D. (2021). Values and culture for integrated care: different ways of seeing, being, knowing and doing. In V. Amelung, V. Stein, E. Suter, N. Goodwin, E. Nolte, & R. Balicer. (Eds.), *Handbook integrated care* (pp. 131–146). Springer.

This chapter considers what is meant by 'culture' and 'values' and how they have been connected in relation to integration. Two key approaches, teamwork and interprofessional learning, are discussed and reflected upon. Culture and values are explored through the framework of relative-relational inquiry with a final exploration of the importance of reflection to integrated practice.

Articles

André, B., Sjøvold, E., Rannestad, T., & Ringdal, G. I. (2014). The impact of work culture on quality of care in nursing homes—a review study. *Scandinavian Journal of Caring Sciences*, *28*(3), 449–457. https://doi.org/10.1111/scs.12086

The aim of this review was to identify which factors characterise the relationship between work culture and quality of care in nursing homes.

Baker, L., Egan-Lee, E., Martimianakis, M. A., & Reeves, S. (2011). Relationships of power: implications for interprofessional education. *Journal of Interprofessional Care*, *25*(2), 98–104. https://doi.org/10.3109/13561820.2010.505350

Witz's model of professional closure (1992) was used in this large evaluation of IPE to explore the perspectives and the experiences of participants and the power relations between them.

Grealish, L., Henderson, A., Quero, F., Phillips, R., & Surawski, M. (2015). The significance of 'facilitator as a change agent'—organisational learning culture in aged care home settings. *Journal of Clinical Nursing*, *24*(7-8), 961–969. https://doi.org/10.1111/jocn.12656

The aim of this study was to explore the impact of an educational programme focused on social behaviours and relationships on organisational learning culture in the residential aged care context.

Hall, P. (2005). Interprofessional teamwork: professional cultures as barriers. *Journal of Interprofessional Care*, *19*, 188–196. https://doi.org/10.1080/13561820500081745

The aim of this paper is to provide insight into the educational, systemic, and personal factors which contribute to the culture of the professions that can help guide the development of innovative educational methodologies to improve interprofessional collaborative practice.

22

Supporting Integrated Teams in Maintaining Quality—A Case Study of the Role of The Quality Matrons

Shirley Fisher and Dr Kirsty Marshall

KEY CONCEPTS

- Quality assurance
- Workforce
- Nursing services
- Leaders

INTRODUCTION

This chapter seeks to highlight how quality assurance (QA) forms not just an essential part of healthcare management, but also a vital part of ensuring safe, effective, and quality care as services transition to integrated delivery. The chapter will also highlight how the use of dedicated roles can support wider neighbourhood teams to take control of QA and facilitate a positive quality culture.

The chapter will explore the introduction of a community Quality Matron role within an NHS integrated care organisation (ICO) and critique how this role was used to support, improve, and ensure quality. The chapter will explore QA within community services including defining QA within a community nursing context, identifying some of the barriers and challenges in assuring quality, and finally reflect on how the movement to neighbourhood working provides opportunities for development of robust team-level QA and leadership.

The case study within the chapter is taken from an NHS ICO in the northwest of the UK and explores how the Quality Matron role was used to transform management of quality during the transition to neighbourhood working.

QUALITY CARE AND QUALITY ASSURANCE

QA can be described as a proactive approach to achieving quality (NHS-GGC, 2021), and quality has been described as a combination of patient experience, safety, and clinical effectiveness. Quality, therefore, is recognised as a

key marker of operational performance (Charles, 2022; Menezes, 2015; NHS England, 2021). Bowers (2014) highlights a significant challenge in that quality care has been interpreted differently by different professional and other groups, making it harder to quantify the exact nature of quality. Harvey and Green (1993) described quality as a 'a slippery concept'; quality is a dynamic concept rather than a stationary definition and different circumstances require different definitions and approaches (Van Kemenade & van der Vlegel-Brouwer, 2019). Taking account of the vague descriptions and variance in interpretation of what quality is, it is not surprising that there are conflicting priorities in defining how it can be measured (Bowers, 2014). However, as integrated care becomes the dominate paradigm of health and social care systems, quality needs to be more visible at every level. In particular, complex teams with both virtual and physical integrated practices need to be able to assess their performance to drive forward improvements in practice and assure the public that new systems are robustly monitored. It was within this context that the community Quality Matron role was developed from the commencement of the role.

Context of Community Nursing and Quality Assurance in the UK

In the UK, community nursing teams have undergone significant change over the last 20 years and subsequent government policies have led to community teams changing organisations, structures, and functions (Department of Health (DH), 2009; NHS England, 2000, 2014, 2019). Community nursing has been managed by primary care trusts, the private sector, mental health organisations, and acute trusts and has been self-managing, which has impacted on a wider sense of belonging for teams. As the UK moves to a more integrated care model through the introduction of integrated care systems (Health and Care

CASE STUDY **Quality Matron**

In 2019, the Rochdale ICO took the decision to raise the profile of QA within adult community services. To achieve this, a new role was introduced: the Quality Matron. The aim of this role was to drive the quality agenda and ensure that QA was embedded within the emergent integrated teams. The vision for this new role was to develop quality as a golden thread in every frontline community team to ensure safe and effective delivery of care.

Prior to the introduction of the Quality Matron role, pre-pandemic QA in the service was managed through two defined routes. Firstly, outcomes were reported to meet commissioned contractual performance indicators with emphasis on the impact of integrated services, waiting times for treatment, and generalised service-wide activity collected primarily from the electronic patient record data system. Secondly, reports were submitted to the divisional and trust boards using data extracted in various reports from trust data systems linked to operational performance, finance, incident, audit and risk management, workforce, and patient experience with limited breakdown linked specifically to individual community teams.

Whilst both sets of reports provided key information, the directorate management realised that while this provided assurance through robust data, there was little involvement of frontline team leaders in quality checking and the process did not inspire or engage those delivering services. To bring about a more inclusive approach to QA, a new role was developed to support the transformation of QA to a culture where teams had ownership. This was seen as important in the transition to neighbourhood working where there would be multiple professional group teams from different organisational backgrounds.

A feature of the Quality Matron role would be that, rather than the Matron acting as a monitor or a QA guru, they would adopt a coaching and facilitatory approach with the goal of empowering and engaging teams. To support the teams, three tools were developed:

- A quality and performance dashboard for each team/service also collated into an overall directorate dashboard,
- A monthly QA audit completed through a peer review process,
- A monthly directorate quality report.

These tools were the first step and aimed to make QA visible within teams. Visibility aimed to promote ownership and accountability by providing greater understanding of risk and safety at a team level. Each team was provided with training and support in the management of the data and identifying areas for improvement and early warning triggers of issues that may be developing and poor performance.

Over a 3 year period, the Quality Matron has developed the community QA approach including supporting guidance that allowed clinical teams to understand the value of data and how it is used by the organisation and external agencies. Improved processes have enabled team leaders to have direct access to where data is collated within the trust. Teams level reviewing and exception reporting against their own team data and the production of a visual diagrammatic guide to support ease of access. This has led to improved reporting and early intervention against poor performance.

Within the Trust, the role of the Quality Matron is expected to grow as the neighbourhood model becomes more embedded and the health and social care team align systems and processes. The Quality Matron will play a key role in bringing together the quality agendas of the different teams and will act as a systems convener, translating quality across different professional groups and supporting an integrated quality approach.

Act, 2022), community services will again be required to transform how they deliver care, with emphasis on integrating services to improve patient and carer outcomes (Charles, 2022). In the climate of ongoing transformation, QA is increasingly seen as an important element in maintaining safe and effective nursing care which provides focus on improving the safety and value of services to deliver the highest-quality health outcomes to people.

Whilst there has been a shift of care from hospital to the community in the UK with national policy focusing on reducing secondary care pressures (NHS England, 2019), it is recognised that community services have not had the same national profile, influence, or leadership as other parts of the NHS (Charles, 2019; O'Dowd & Dorning, 2017). A report by Grant Thornton UK (2021) has argued that the low profile has resulted in community services not receiving the same level of scrutiny regarding quality data and targets when compared with secondary care services. De Silva (2015) and Foot et al. (2014) state that an unintended consequence of the lack of quality data could lead to frontline teams having lack of ownership of the quality agenda.

A second issue was that commissioned contract reporting had a focus on community, managed through senior manager and commissioner discussions which detracted from individual team QA and ownership by team leads, resulting in a separation of quality rather than making quality everyone's business.

O'Dowd and Dorning (2017) explain in their briefing report that, due to the complex and multiprofessional nature of community services, the introduction of quality metrics was often poorly understood and weakly accepted. In the case study, the Quality Matron linked the QA and quality improvement process to empower team leaders to recognise the importance of a QA process, take ownership of nursing quality metrics and quality indicators, and drive improvement through data-informed decisions. As the teams move through the radical changes brought about by integration, this approach can be adapted to be adopted by multiprofessional teams to provide assurance that quality standards are being met and accountability structures are embedded (Maben et al., 2012).

Alongside the introduction of integrated care systems in the UK, the COVID-19 global pandemic has had a significant impact on community teams. There have been many examples of innovative and creative changes in practice to rise to the challenges of the pandemic, and several have been cited within this book. However, the pandemic also presented a challenge for fledgling co-joined and co-located health and social teams as many of these teams were necessarily separated through mandated isolation requirements to reduce virus spread (Department of Health & Social Care, 2020). As services entered the recovery phase of the pandemic, the focus turned to how future services would be planned, delivered, and experienced. The pandemic also highlighted cracks in the system as services strained to manage the demand for services in a fragmented system. Post-pandemic, there is an increasing realisation that not only does there need to be greater interconnectivity in services but there is also a need for governance frameworks to be adopted at a strategic level to support a whole-system governance agenda (Mitchell et al., 2020).

QUALITY ASSURANCE AND LEADERSHIP

As systems become more integrated, community nurses increasingly require high-level skills in quality management processes to provide assurance of meeting quality and performance standards (Foot et al., 2014; NHS England, 2020). There are strong links between leadership and QA, and leaders within teams have a vital role in embedding QA, as this supports them in 'knowing their business' and understanding how their team is functioning. Ensuring

quality is even more important with the increasing move to integrated health and care services, which blur boundaries and introduce greater complexity in ensuring quality (Care Quality Commission (CQC), 2022). Integrated care presents several opportunities and challenges as services work closer together and transcend traditional boundaries. Therefore, to ensure teams at a frontline level continue to operate in a safe and effective way, it is essential that QA plays a vital and continued role in maintaining patient safety, experience, and outcomes (CQC, 2022). Increasing team leadership was reflected in the Quality Matron not taking the 'expert' position but rather seeking to build quality into the leadership of teams, enabling the teams to engage and influence the agenda rather than being a passive recipient.

Background to the Matron Role in the UK

The role of the matron has been established in the UK for two decades. Around the early 2000s there was a significant and sustained public outcry about the spread of microorganisms such as methicillin-resistant *Staphylococcus aureus*. The public perception was shaped by the media response that these ongoing issues were due to a reduction in standards and quality in NHS hospital care and 'dirty hospitals' (Boyce et al., 2009). In 2001, modern matrons were introduced by the Department of Health with a view that the 'matron' role would be accepted as a role of authority and high standards as modelled by the traditional matrons of bygone years. The 'modern matron' was initially limited to acute/secondary care settings with the specific purpose to improve the delivery of good quality care (DH, 2001). Community matrons were introduced a few years later but with a primary focus to help improve the quality of life of patients living with long-term conditions (DH, 2004).

Later in the 2000s, following a series of NHS failures (most notably the Mid Staffordshire hospital scandal, documented in the Francis report) (Francis, 2013), the 'modern matron' role was reintroduced with a remit to instil confidence back into the general public. However, it is important to note that the modern matron role was significantly different from the traditional autocratic matron role seen pre-1960s (Rivett, 2006).

Development of the Quality Matron

The introduction of the Quality Matron, while linking to the principle and framework for matrons, had a specific quality mission. One of the unique elements of this role was that it held potential for integrated care development. This is because the Quality Matron was developed as a boundary-spanning role, and the matron is required to engage widely and promote greater collaboration.

Boundary spanners can facilitate information flow across people and groups, which is important in health and social care with their cliques, professional siloes, and tribes (Long et al., 2013). One of the first practical steps that the community matron took was to analysis the gaps in information flow to and from the teams. A gap was identified where quality information was not visible by teams/service areas. To empower teams/service leads to own their own quality data, team dashboards were created, reflecting national policy levers to support integration at a service level of performance and management accountability (Reed et al., 2021). Quality metrics are key components of performance dashboards. Quality metrics and data were available across a range of service targets but needed to be sought out and pulled together, often reported at different meetings in a variety of formats, based on secondary care targets with community data being often limited to patient feedback or clinical contacts (Scobie & Spencer, 2018), which initiated the creation of a dashboard for each team/service area.

Through the development of dashboards, team leaders became familiar with quality and performance standards linked to their teams and services, and a clear shift was seen to ownership and eagerness to challenge when extracted data was visualised in report format and was incorrect or below the expected standard. Team leads are now held to account regarding monthly quality measures. Support for team leads has been provided through a series of 'how to' guides giving simple diagrammatic instructions on how to access trust digital systems to check their teams' linked data. Team leaders across adult community services are predominantly clinicians and most have limited knowledge of information technology (IT) systems and accessing databases or spreadsheets; the 'how to' guides have supported their ability to access these systems.

The Quality Matron and Supporting Peoples' Experience of Services

The NHS Constitution (Department of Health & Social Care, 2021) pledges patient feedback will be used as a cornerstone to improve services. To collate data across a high number of community teams, access to a variety of experience collection methods has been introduced. Many NHS services use the nationally recognised tool, the Friends and Family Test, launched initially in 2013 and updated in 2019, which proposes a quick and simple mechanism for people to complete in order to provide feedback regarding their experience.

Whilst the tool is seemingly easy to complete and designed to be as low a burden as possible (CQC, 2021), when compared to acute and secondary care services, community services have low response rates. For example,

in services like district nursing, patients may remain on the caseloads for many years due to their long-term conditions and they will not be asked to respond to a survey that regularly. The community matron again has a role here in supporting teams to explore other ways of collecting data, that staff see the value in experience data, and moving to a more co-produced approach to patient involvement in QA. As services change and develop under an integrated model, the Quality Matron can act as an advisor and guide to support the involvement and feedback from those who use the service.

CHALLENGES AND BARRIERS TO QUALITY

In reporting framed around secondary care, Drennan et al. (2018) found a wide variety of quality indicators mostly focussed on organisational processes developed in isolation of services or those who use services. Data collection can be problematic due to inadequate information technology, acute sector software, lack of connectivity, and compatibility with other systems (Drennan et al., 2018), and challenges can be further exacerbated as team leads/services leads have not traditionally been directly involved in provision of QA. As Jukes (2021) suggests, service teams are unable to measure and share the quality of service provision, and even at a strategic level, attempts to develop integrated governance frameworks has been met with difficulty and identified as a barrier to moving integrated working forward.

Repeated structural reorganisations, no matter how sensible the rationale for them may be, take time, cause disruption, divert focus and energy, and can delay the path to integration (Reed et al., 2021). They also make assessing change over time difficult (Reed et al., 2021). Data on the performance and outcomes of community health services or social care are limited (Reed et al., 2021), and reports demonstrating performance and quality for community services are vague and limited to basic data, with a lack of information and poor clinical data often cited as a barrier to improvement (De Silva, 2015).

Challenges with data collection exist across integrated services and the vision of how this will function in today's world, where we have gaps in the documentation of community activity and an absence of a shared health and care electronic record, suggests it will be difficult to ensure that integrated data is produced (Grant Thornton UK, 2021). IT systems managed by business intelligence services across organisations extract data which can often be incorrect, inconsistent, or has not been subjected to quality-checking processes, and issues with inputting by community staff completing data whilst out and about in their daily duties can be challenging when digital connectivity is poor (Grant Thornton UK, 2021).

QUALITY ASSURANCE IN CHANGING COMMUNITY SERVICES

Provision of evidence-based QA across adult community services within Rochdale is a complex endeavour due to the variance of teams and their structures, which include community nursing, allied health professional therapy, and clinical scientist-led teams. The majority of care is delivered within patient's homes with staff working independently.

Modern thinking suggests a less directive and bottom-up approach which encourages change in the heart of the team (Gifford, 2012), including priorities for team development of quality dashboards using a traffic light system for each team, which includes key indicators linked to patient safety and harm free-care (e.g., pressure ulcers and medication errors) (Randell et al., 2020), allowing for the quick identification of any hotspots in isolated teams or a helicopter view across the service. Competency of staff working in the community is of vital importance as they are lone working practitioners without supervision where incompetence can be difficult to identify (Keegal, 2013).

CONCLUSION

The impact of implemented QA measures provides a snapshot of how each community team is performing against a set of agreed-upon measures. These measures can be updated or changed in response to trust values, aims, and objectives, and should be pertinent to community settings and professionals within the team (e.g., nursing/multiprofessional/therapy/clinical scientist).

The Quality Matron role is a clear bridge between senior management, the directorate, and the frontline, bringing together the aspects of quality and evidence that community services are meeting and exceeding expected standards.

To implement any quality improvement, there needs to be a clear understanding of what quality means to the frontline staff and team leaders, including understanding of exception reporting, teams being able to analyse their own performance data with confidence to support quality improvement projects being undertaken by anyone at any level, and with support from quality improvement specialists. Often the outcomes can be fantastic as stand-alone projects, with a wider remit for organisation-wide shared learning and ultimately a catalyst for wider service change. In contrast, QA includes the consistent approach to being able to demonstrate quality at the forefront of care delivery for all staff in the team, so each member understands why quality measures are in place and are monitored, why service risks are identified and escalated, why they have to maintain their own level of training and clinical competence, what incidents and complaints have occurred, and how to respond to lessons learned, with the goal of being proud to share their data with the organisation, senior managers, and external sources. Once this has been achieved, the Quality Matron role will be fully embedded.

QA will be a key factor in the growth of integrated care and will be essential when adopting new ways of working which will attract people to take risks. Therefore, considering supportive and facilitative roles such as the Quality Matron could support practitioners while they make sense of the new integrated system and enable them to take control of their neighbourhood team's quality agenda.

References

Bowers, B. (2014). Quality indicators in community care. *Primary Health Care, 24*(2), 32–34. https://doi.org/10.7748/phc2014.02.24.2.32.e843

Boyce, T., Murray, E., & Holmes, A. (2009). What are the drivers of the UK media coverage of meticillin-resistant *Staphylococcus aureus*, the inter-relationships and relative influences. *Journal of Hospital Infection, 73*(4), 400–407. https://doi.org/10.1016/j.jhin.2009.05.022

Care Quality Commission. (2022, October 21). *Systems: challenges and opportunities.* https://www.cqc.org.uk/publication/state-care-202122/systems

Charles, A. (2019, January 14). *Community health services explained.* https://www.kingsfund.org.uk/publications/community-health-services-explained

Charles, A (2022). *Integrated care systems explained: making sense of systems, places and neighbourhoods.* Retrived from https://www.kingsfund.org.uk/publications/integrated-care-systems-explained

Department of Health. (2001). *Implementing the NHS Plan: Modern matrons - strengthening the role of ward sisters and introducing senior sisters (Health Service Circular 2001/010).* London: Department of Health.

Department of Health. (2004). *The NHS Improvement Plan: putting people at the heart of public services.* London: Stationery Office.

Department of Health. (2009). *Transforming community services: enabling new patterns of provision.* London: Stationery Office.

Department of Health and Social Care. (2020, August 25). *Overview of adult social care guidance on coronavirus (COVID-19).* https://www.gov.uk/guidance/overview-of-adult-social-care-guidance-on-coronavirus-covid-19

Department of Health & Social Care. (2021, January 1). *Guidance: The NHS Constitution for England.* https://www.gov.uk/government/publications/the-nhs-constitution-for-england/the-nhs-constitution-for-england

De Silva, D. (2015). *What's getting in the way? Barriers to improvement in the NHS*. London: The Health Foundation.

Drennan, V., Ross, F., Calestani, M., Saunders, M., & West, P. (2018). Learning from an early pilot of the Dutch Buurtzorg model of district nursing in England. *Primary Health Care*, 28(6).

Foot, C., Sonola, L., Bennett, L., Fitzsimons, B., Raleigh, V., & Gregory, S. (2014). *Managing quality in community health care services*. London: King's Fund.

Francis, R. (2013). *Report of the Mid Staffordshire NHS Foundation Trust Public Inquiry: Executive summary*. London: Stationery Office.

Gifford, J. (2012). *What makes change successful in the NHS? A review of change programmes in NHS South of England*. Newbury: NHS South of England.

Grant Thornton UK. (2021). *Improving data quality for costing community and mental health services*. London: Healthcare Costing for Value Institute.

Harvey, L., & Green, D. (1993). Defining quality. *Assessment & Evaluation in Higher Education*, *18*(1), 9–34. https://doi.org/10.1080/0260293930180102

Health and Care Act. (2022). London: Stationery Office.

Jukes, M. (2021). *How to develop a successful quality assurance framework*. Evaluagent. https://www.evaluagent.com/knowledge-hub/how-to-develop-a-successful-qa-framework/

Keegal, T. (2013). Poor performance: managing the first informal stages. *Primary Health Care*, *23*(4), 31–38. https://doi.org/10.7748/phc2013.05.23.4.31.e784

Long, J. C., Cunningham, F. C., & Braithwaite, J. (2013). Bridges, brokers and boundary spanners in collaborative networks: a systematic review. *BMC Health Services Research*, *13*(1), 1–13. https://doi.org/10.1186/1472-6963-13-158

Maben, J., Morrow, E., Ball, J., Glenn, R., & Griffiths, P. (2012). *High quality care metrics for nursing*. London: National Nursing Research Unit, King's College London.

Menezes, J. (2015). Are community matrons truly invisible. *British Journal of Community Nursing*, *20*(11), 525. https://doi.org/10.12968/bjcn.2015.20.11.525

Mitchell, C., Tazzyman, A., Howard, S. J., & Hodgson, D. (2020). More that unites us than divides us? A qualitative study of integration of community health and social care services. *BMC Family Practice*, *21*, 96. https://doi.org/10.1186/s12875-020-01168-z

NHS England. (2000). *The NHS plan. A plan for investment. A plan for reform*. London: Stationery Office.

NHS England. (2014). *Five year forward view*. http://www.england.nhs.uk/wp-content/uploads/2014/10/5yfvweb.pdf

NHS England. (2019). *The NHS long term plan*. http://www.longtermplan.nhs.uk/wp-content/uploads/2019/01/nhs-long-term-plan.pdf

NHS England. (2020). *Integrating care: next steps to build strong and effective integrated care systems across England*. https://www.england.nhs.uk/wp-content/uploads/2021/01/integrating-care-next-steps-to-building-strong-and-effective-integrated-care-systems.pdf

NHS England (2021). *The matron's handbook*. London: NHS England.

NHS-GGC. (2021). *Quality Assurance and Audit*. https://www.nhsggc.scot/staff-recruitment/staff-resources/research-and-innovation/research-governance-nhsggc/quality-assurance-and-audit/

O'Dowd, N., & Dorning, H. (2017). *Community services: What do we know about quality?* The Health Foundation. Nuffield Trust.

Randell, R., Alvarado, N., McVey, L., Ruddle, R. A., Doherty, P., Gale, C., Mamas, M., & Dowding, D. (2020). Requirements for a quality dashboard: lessons from National Clinical Audits. *AMIA Annual Symposium Proceedings*, *2019*, 735–744.

Reed, S., Oung, C., Davies, J., Dayan, M., & Scobie, S. (2021). *Integrating health and social care: a comparison of policy and progress across the four countries of the UK Research report*. London: Nuffield Trust.

Rivett, G. (2006). *NHS History 1948-1967*. https://www.nuffieldtrust.org.uk/health-and-social-care-explained/the-history-of-the-nhs

Scobie, S., & Spencer, J. (2018, August 29). *Making sense of the community services data set*. https://www.nuffieldtrust.org.uk/news-item/making-sense-of-the-community-services-data-set

Van Kemenade, E., & van der Vlegel-Brouwer, W. (2019). Integrated care: a definition from the perspective of the four quality paradigms. *Journal of Integrated Care*, *27*(4), 357–367. https://doi.org/10.1108/JICA-06-2019-0029

23

Transforming the Workforce

Dr Naomi Sharples

KEY CONCEPTS

- Global health and social care workforce
- Workforce planning
- Workforce development

INTRODUCTION

The world of workforce planning (WFP) and transformation in health and care is a world that may have been relatively distant for many service providers. In the UK, with the introduction of integrated care systems (ICSs) delivered across neighbourhoods, locality and specialist providers should lead to effective multidisciplinary team working across systems and services. However, this requires transforming the workforce, making workforce delivery a crucial aspect of people's lives (NHS England, 2021).

Countries around the globe face significant and interrelated health and social care workforce challenges. The impact of global financial problems, pandemics, war and conflict, advances in science and innovations, and political changes all affect the ability to meet the workforce needs of a population (Garattini et al., 2021; World Health Organization (WHO), 2018). In the UK, changes to European worker regulations have seen a significant fall in the workforce from across Europe and in turn has increased the workforce from African and South Asian countries, with significant impact on WFP within these areas strengthening the call for globally shared planning, education, skills, and knowledge. This global theatre directly impacts on local service delivery (Dayan et al., 2021).

BACKGROUND

In the UK, we have come a long way in understanding WFP and development needs. The future integrated care model in the UK will, however, require careful consideration to ensure that the NHS has a workforce fit for the future (Addicott et al., 2015). Faced by greater demands on data, finances, professional skills and scope, workforce supply, and population changes, even the best workforce transformation models find themselves tested.

As part of developing a social care system more fit for purpose and with improvements in financial resources, focus on a more diverse workforce will be required as the ICSs develop and as health and care strive to become more balanced and equitable (NHS England, 2021).

In the process of focussing on workforce transformation, we must consider the environment we find ourselves in, including the impact of the global COVID-19 pandemic; the demand for skilled workforces in other industries such as technology, manufacturing, and hospitality; population changes from increased inequity and longevity; reduced birth rates impacting on supply and demand; the rise in comorbidity and complexity; and the ever-increasing financial challenges.

Transforming the workforce requires a range of foci, service design, WFP to meet the service requirements, and workforce development opportunities for staff to meet the needs of the population they serve (Fig. 23.1).

This chapter will focus on global WFP and development through to local implementation, and the fundamental elements of workforce transformation.

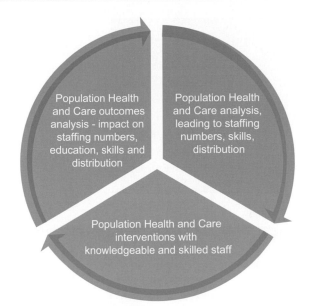

Fig. 23.1 Population health and care.

WORKFORCE PLANNING—GLOBAL TO LOCAL

WFP has been previously described as a 'dark art', where poor data on the current workforce met a concoction of service redesign imperatives, workforce supply issues, over- or undersupply of a profession, a 'retirement bubble', historic under resourcing of placements/assessors, misaligned educational planning, and the ever-increasing demand on services.

Whilst this example may still feel somewhat true for some, we are moving to an ever more improved approach to WFP.

WFP is the process by which any organisation achieves the workforce required to fulfil the organisation's purpose. All WFP (Fig. 23.2), whether at a global, national, regional, or local/service level, goes through a process of analysis, intervention and evaluation.

The model shows the interrelated nature of population health demands, staff skills and numbers, service demands, financial constraints, and the future requirements of a country/region. The levers available come in the form of staff benefits, wages, and terms and conditions of employment, while other levers include service design, numbers of education places/graduates, migration and immigration management, and leadership at all levels and in all areas, including analysis, planning, implementation, and evaluation.

The levers available to influence change and impact the WFP process and outcome at different levels impact the whole system. As discussed, a political change such as withdrawal from the European Union has impacted the workforce supply pipeline, necessitating a 'change of supplier'. In 2022, almost half (48%) of the 48,436 new registrants on the Nursing and Midwifery Council (NMC) had trained internationally. Of those international joiners, 66% had trained in India or the Philippines (NMC, 2022). This shows the impact of a UK system that 'runs hot', with only ever enough nurses and doctors if all is going to plan. Nursing remains on the shortage occupation list by the UK government (GOV.UK, 2020). When service demand outstrips workforce supply for whatever reason, the UK becomes ever more reliant on out-of-country supply, thus impacting on WFP in countries like Nigeria, Ghana, and India (Bond et al., 2020).

As an example, the Ghanaian Health Ministry now needs to factor into their plans not only the nursing workforce numbers and commissions for Ghana, but also the nursing workforce who will leave Ghana to work in the UK. This in turn requires the nurse education providers in Ghana to increase the numbers of student nurses and to shift their focus to diploma and degree education rather than certificate-level education to meet the needs of the UK workforce and their own needs for nurses to work in settings that require increased skills from independent practitioners. Through open negotiations and joint working with the UK, Ghana will be able to carefully plan, manage, and monitor the international demand. The WHO is focused on transparent, supportive, and ethical ways to meet workforce demands around the world, and particularly ways that protect middle-income and developing countries from the demands of wealthier countries.

As we experience more Ghanaian nurses joining the UK workforce, working across a range of health and social care settings, we understand that it is because of global strategic interventions that impact on local service delivery—global to local, strategic planning to localised implementation.

Workforce Supply

As captured by Professor Mason Haire in 1967 (Gibson, 2021), the 'churn' of an organisation's workforce supply gives a framework for considering the four crucial aspects (Fig. 23.3).

To understand workforce supply, we can look at it through a structured lens—from macro, meso, and micro economic and demographic environment levels—to help inform our constructs of the challenges we face and to appreciate the multifaceted drivers involved.

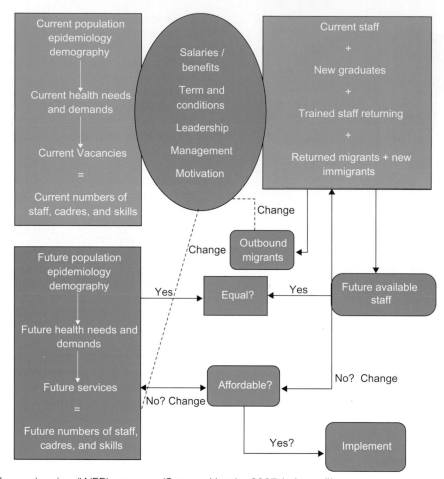

Fig. 23.2 Workforce planning (WFP) process. (Source: Hornby 2007 (adapted)).

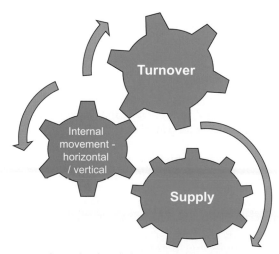

Fig. 23.3 Organisational churn.

Macro-Economic Environment—Whole Population-Level Supply Including International Supply

This data would involve looking at the global health workforce supply, national trends and population data on employment and education, numbers of people leaving school or college, level of education, education programme choices, routes to employment, employment choices, and opportunities which may compete with health and social care (WHO, 2015).

Meso—Regional Population Level Supply

This data focuses more specifically on regions, workforce movement (e.g., from rural to urban), and challenges faced by employers in attracting and keeping employees. Again, it is important to understand the education level of the potential workforce, their education programme options and choices, and their route to employment.

Where there is a 'brain drain' from smaller and more rural communities, it is also essential to understand where people chose to work. Significant shifts can occur within regions with interventions, such as free college bus services taking students from one city to another, the closure of a local college campus or educational programmes, the quality of further education (FE) providers, the availability of placements, and involvement of employers.

Micro-Economic Environment

As the focus on the workforce supply becomes more local to the provider, shifts in population age, demographics, movement, education offers, and employment opportunities are magnified. Does the college in town deliver health and care education at level 2 and 3? Are there plans to bring new companies into the town which may pose competition for health and care providers? Does the local higher education provider offer programmes that meet the needs of the health and care employers in the integrated care system (ICS)? For example, in the northwest of England, as in many regions, there is a pull from the towns to the larger cities. For one large town, this was becoming a recruitment/supply problem, with potential employees tempted by the bright lights of two major cities within 20 miles.

To tackle the need for new entrants to the workforce, the main healthcare provider now works in partnership with the local college and university, delivering a programme offering students in healthcare programmes 'cadetship' placements in the two acute hospitals, plus enhanced learning opportunities with the local higher-education institutions. This enhances students' exposure to healthcare, careers, and health education. In addition, and in partnership with the college and the trust, the local university offers automatic interviews to the cadets to provide a motivating incentive and accelerate entry into nursing programmes for those who choose to learn locally.

The students are supported in their learning in their local community, looking after local people, and developing the experience of serving their own community.

The macro, meso, and micro perspectives can also be used at an organisational level (e.g., local authority), service level (e.g., adult social care), or department level (e.g., a single care home). Analysing the current workforce environment is vital to help target specific interventions.

Benchmark and Baseline

The Hornby model (Hornby, 2007) divides our thinking into 'current' and 'future' paradigms with critical decision-making points. Some challenges that many countries face are understanding the numbers of health and care workers in the system, where they are deployed, who employs them across the public and private sector, how many are registered through the professional regulators, if the registers are

up to date, and if the workforce information is accessible or if it relies on several formats (from simple spreadsheets to online monitoring systems). Can it ever be 'right'?

If you don't know where you are starting from, you will never know where you're going or how you got where you are. When people come to WFP, it may feel like a well-established approach to managing human resources; however, WFP as an organisational tool emerged in the 1960s as part of a mechanistic managerial approach to calculating the human resource need for organisations. As societies go through significant changes such as financial crises, managerial cultural changes, and population pressures, the focus on WFP ebbs and flows.

Having reviewed the wider context of supply and recognising that macro, meso, and micro issues impact directly on workforce supply and as such require scrutiny, benchmarking the current numbers of health and care workforce professionals and support personnel with the services is vital. Service managers will work with their human resource colleagues to fully analyse the numbers of vacancies held in each job area, the retirement trajectory, attrition/retention statistics, and career promotions (internal movement).

Once the benchmark is understood, alignment to the organisational baseline (i.e., the business of the service) must follow. Public and third-sector providers are in the business of health and care delivery, ill-health prevention, and health promotion, in one form or another. In the implementation of ICS organisations, 'baseline' may alter due to changes in focus on population health, developments in collaborative service delivery, or development in the range of primary care services. To understand the service baseline, the organisation could apply the strategic alignment model (Fig. 23.4) to help guide them, as illustrated by Gibson (2021).

Workforce Demand

Looking at the workforce demand can be approached in several ways, including profession-to-population ratios, current service staffing model extrapolations, and staffing according to budget allocations, each with clear resulting limitations. Workforce planners are now embracing a more sophisticated, multifactorial needs-based approach to WFP (Fig. 23.5) which entails addressing the workforce gap, design, demand, supply, and development (Gibson, 2021).

Workforce Gap

The difference between 'supply' and 'demand' creates a gap, which is exemplified by the gap that is being created in many professions with the 'retirement bubble'. Whilst workforce intelligence in the UK was aware of the bubble well in advance, it would take a huge number of WFP and education interventions to start to address the gap in people and skills that have ensued (Gibson, 2021).

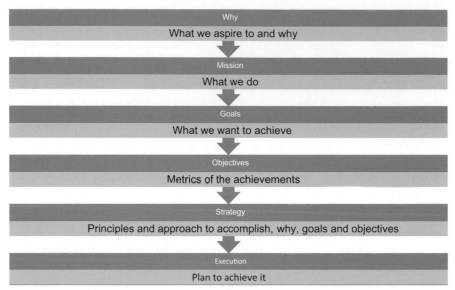

Fig. 23.4 Strategic alignment model—Agile Workforce Planning. (Gibson, 2021).

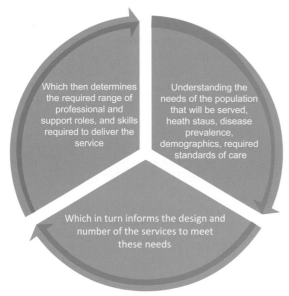

Fig. 23.5 Workforce planning.

Workforce gaps are dynamic and complex, and as such need purposeful attention. Planners need to focus on staff skills and capabilities—are there new roles that could be developed, or roles/scopes of professions extended? Is there flexibility in staffing numbers available according to demand? Are health and care staff released from administration tasks so they can focus on their work more efficiently and effectively? Is the span of support staff, operational staff, and staff who manage and lead effective,

in the right place, deployed at the right time, and within budget? Gaps will also be considered on a variety of time trajectories, including immediate need, 1–3 years, 3–5 years, and more than 5 years.

Gaps in the workforce can be reduced by a variety of interventions in the supply line, including:

- **Alignment activities** to new entrants to the workforce through in-reach activities into colleges of FE, improved academic advice and guidance, strategic curriculum alignment with health and social care career pathways from level 2 through to level 4, and placement provision and live projects planned between employers and education providers. The FE sector is an integral part of the supply line and far too often ignored. Where employers work closely with FE, the benefits extend much further than drawing people into the workplace. FE programmes forge links into communities and into families. Through widening participation, people aspire to greater achievements and attainments.
- **Case example:** A very large NHS Foundation Trust in Greater Manchester has seen its work with a local college bear fruit. Working with their partner university, a satellite school of nursing has been established within the college. This new building and novel delivery model allow the FE health and social care students to see students in the first year of their nursing degree on campus. The first years will not only act as role models, but they will also add to the health education and health promotion dynamic within the college. This community-focused education intervention aims to further

cement the 'living locally, locally educated, locally committed' workforce.

- **International recruitment** as described earlier, using ethical and mutually supportive approaches to international recruitment can satisfy the imbalance of over- and under supply.
  - **Case example:** A regional specialist service, not used to staff recruitment issues until recently, developed an international strategy to work closely with India to offer 3-year rotational roles. The health professionals are supported to move to the UK service for a 3-year deployment. The UK service benefits from qualified staff, new perspectives, and a reduced 'gap' in workforce, and India benefits from staff returning with new skills and different work experience that could impact positively on in-country service delivery.
- **Return to Practice:** Encouraging people back into health and social care roles has always been a useful tool in closing the workforce gap. However, it has not always been very successful, where returners are left unsupported, where cultural and organisational expectations have not been made clear, or where inflexible working practices cause returners to leave for the very same work-life balance reasons that they left for in the first place (Coates & MacFadyen, 2021). This valuable approach needs to be supported by robust education and training support, mentoring, flexible working arrangements, and supportive and skilled leadership.
  - **Case example:** A southern England learning disability trust is keen to attract returners to nursing and to occupational therapy. They offer a clear and structured education and training package with links to the local university. They clearly outline the return-to-practice requirements for both professions and then outline the trust benefits:
    - Commitment to flexible working where this is possible
    - 27 days of annual leave per year plus bank holidays, increasing to 29 days after 5 years and 33 days after 10 years' service
    - Individual personal development plans and a commitment to ongoing training
    - Generous NHS pension scheme
    - Good maternity, paternity, and adoption benefits
    - Health service discounts and online benefits
    - Incremental pay progression
    - Free confidential employee assistance programme 24/7
    - Access to staff networks
    - Health and well being opportunities
    - Cycle to Work Scheme and reduced public transport rates
    - Structured learning and development opportunities

Interestingly, the list of benefits has probably not changed significantly over the past 5 years. Now, with the development of neighbourhood- and place-based services, employers need to think more creatively about what would encourage people back to a profession they had previously left.

Returners find the pressure of work challenging, the development in technology sometimes daunting, and the huge changes in the health and care landscape quite confusing. Addressing these concerns would be quite helpful. This links back to the incentives and terms and conditions illustrated in the bullet points above.

WORKFORCE DEVELOPMENT

Realising the Transformation

Transforming the workforce takes many different routes, from strategic WFP through to workforce training and education. The following case examples illustrate training and education examples in one small part of a huge health and social care workforce in the northwest of England and across the wider workforce.

CASE STUDY   Greater Manchester Cancer Academy

Greater Manchester (GM) has a cancer strategy aimed at improving the lives of people in the region. The strategy is designed to reduce the risk of cancer and improve early diagnosis, treatment, and prognosis with and after cancer, and focuses on developing the cancer workforce and cancer research to further improve the evidence-based approach.

As part of the GM strategy, the Cancer Academy was established to support the development of cancer education across the GM footprint. Supported by innovation funds from Health Education England, the Academy commissioned a review of the urology workforce across GM. The findings indicated:

1. The value of consultant and senior clinicians in providing focus in the delivery of practice-based learning
2. Teaching, training, education, and placement opportunities need to be focused on the practitioner's workplace, drawing on a range of experiences including mentoring, shadowing, workplace supervision, and departmental training
3. Training needs to be relevant to context and workload and focus on band-5 nurses and virtual and accessible learning support
4. A structured approach to succession planning and career development supported by experienced clinicians in post, supported research and development training, clear career pathways, and supporting learning packages.

Building on the findings, the Cancer Academy developed the Urology Training Framework, a range of formal and informal learning programmes and opportunities mapped to each urology role, to support those working in urology in developing the skills required across community, secondary, and specialist urology services.

Case example. Following on from the urology framework, a pilot project to support the urology workforce in their access to training and development ensued.

The Cancer Academy Professional Development Platform project was driven by the need to be able to:

1. Apply a Urology Learning Framework (ULF) for non-medical professionals working in urology to facilitate formal and informal continuing practice development (CPD)
2. Provide the clinicians with a 'one stop' facility which would house their CPD, provide career guidance and direction, support appraisal targets, revalidation evidence, link to external education platforms, and provide reports to clinical and human resource managers to give definitive evidence of required updating and development
3. House the framework and contingent features in an accessible, digital, dynamic form to promote a one-system methodology to improve engagement and align the clinicians' development closer to their clinical practice lives.

This framework, range of learning offers, and career pathway will help to support one specific area of the cancer workforce, transforming the education offer to meet the changing needs of the clinicians, their work, and their alignment to the ICS. On a wider national basis, oncology is moving forwards in developing a career and education framework. This framework would sit across Hornby's WFP model, incorporating current needs and future WFP, impacting on clinicians' motivation, leadership, conditions, and support, all to enhance the experience of people who have cancer, who had cancer, or who care for people with cancer.

The work in GM sits within the national cancer career and education framework of the Aspirant Cancer Career and Education Development programme (ACCEnD).

Case example: The ACCEnD programme is a cancer career and education development programme developed to support nurses and allied professionals who want to move into oncology, and those within cancer services to increase their knowledge, skills, and capability. The focus is to increase and improve the supply of the professional cancer healthcare workforce. It also provides clear career advancement routes with associated education and training pathways mapped to roles and specialities. This is a model which could be adopted by a wide range of other areas of service provision.

MULTIDISCIPLINARY TEAM

Primary care is seeing significant changes through the implementation of ICSs; to design multidisciplinary teams (MDTs) for the new primary care settings, Health Education England (HEE) have undertaken a piece of work to support WFP, design, and sustainability. The MDT tool kit (HEE, 2021) offers a range of resources to support primary care MDTs in designing new patient pathways whilst understanding the need for the 'right people, in the right place, with the right knowledge and skills, delivering the right evidence-based care'.

Drawing upon a wide evidence base, the HEE tool kit is applicable not only to primary care but to a wider range of MDTs across the health and care spectrum. During the Year of the Health and Care Worker, project teams from around the globe have been introduced to the tool to adapt and apply to their own country's needs.

CONCLUSION

The aim of this chapter was to introduce the reader to the realm of workforce transformation, to how the work applies at global and local levels, and how the global health workforce is someone's local workforce. Political, social, economic, education, technological, and regulatory influences converge to create a challenging and dynamic workforce environment within which work takes place to transform from the once static and somewhat predictable landscape.

References

Addicott, R., Maguire, D., Honeyman, M., & Jabbal, J. (2015). *Workforce planning in the NHS*. London: King's Fund.

Bond, S., Merriman, C., & Walthall, H. (2020). The experiences of international nurses and midwives transitioning to work in the UK: a qualitative synthesis of the literature from 2010 to 2019. *International Journal of Nursing Studies*, 110, 103693. https://doi.org/10.1016/j.ijnurstu.2020.103693

Coates, M., & Macfadyen, A. (2021). Student experiences of a return to practice programme: a qualitative study. *British Journal of Nursing*, 30(15), 900–908. https://doi.org/10.12968/bjon.2021.30.15.900

Dayan, M., McCarey, M., Hervey, T., Fahy, N., Greer, S. L., Jarman, H., Stewart, E., & Bristow, D. (2021). *Going it alone: Health and brexit in the UK*. London: Nuffield Trust.

Garattini, L., Badinella Martini, M., & Nobili, A. (2021). Integrated care in Europe: time to get it together? *Applied Health Economics and Health Policy*, 20(2), 145–147. https://doi.org/10.1007/s40258-021-00680-2

Gibson, A. (2021). *Agile workforce planning: How to align people with organizational strategy for improved performance*. London: Kogan Page.

GOV.UK. (2020). Corporate report. *Review of the shortage occupation list: 2020*. https://www.gov.uk/government/publications/review-of-the-shortage-occupation-list-2020

Health Education England. (2021). *Multidisciplinary team (MDT) toolkit*. https://www.hee.nhs.uk/our-work/workforce-transformation/multidisciplinary-team-mdt-toolkit

Hornby, P. (2007, December 13–14). *Exploring the use of the World Health Organization human resources for health projection model* [Conference presentation]. HRH Workforce Planning Workshop, Washington DC.

NHS England. (2021). *Building strong integrated care systems everywhere: guidance on the ICS people function*. https://www.england.nhs.uk/wp-content/uploads/2021/06/B0662_Building-strong-integrated-care-systems-everywhere-guidance-on-the-ICS-people-function-August-2021.pdf

Nursing and Midwifery Council. (2022). *The NMC register 1 April 2021 – 31 March 2022*. London: NMC.

World Health Organization. (2015). *Health workforce 2030: towards a global strategy on human resources for health*. https://apps.who.int/iris/bitstream/handle/10665/330092/9789241508629-eng.pdf

World Health Organization. (2018). *Declaration on Primary Health Care*. https://www.who.int/primary-health/conference-phc/declaration

Further Reading

Aspirant Cancer Career and Education Development programme | Health Education England. https://www.hee.nhs.uk/our-work/cancer-diagnostics/aspirant-cancer-career-education-development-programme

Multidisciplinary Team (MDT) Toolkit | Health Education England (hee.nhs.uk)

World Health Organization. (2010). *Models and tools for health workforce planning and projections (2010)*. Geneva: WHO Press.

World Health Organization. (2016). *Global strategy on human resources for health: Workforce 2030*. Geneva: WHO Press.

PART V

Practising Integration

24

Co-production in Practice

Jamie Potts, Sushma Majithia, James Brooks, Erin O'Neill,
Joseph Crammond, Dr Hayley Bamber, Samantha Pywell, and Katie Cairns*

KEY CONCEPTS

- The authors
- How the chapter was developed
- The case context and the role of quality advisors
- What good co-production looks like
- What bad co-production looks like
- What professionals can do to move forward the co-production agenda with service users

INTRODUCTION

The co-production group felt that the introduction to this chapter should provide some information about the authors through using the one-page profile format which is used within their care setting.

Author

Dr Hayley Bamber

What's Important to Me?

My family and friends
My work as a lecturer teaching occupational therapy students
My health and wellbeing
My study to improve co-production in practice

What Do People Like and Admire About Me?

- My determination
- My kindness
- My thoughtfulness
- My leadership and management skills

How to Best Work With Me

- Listen to my views and opinions
- Don't talk over me
- Actively get involved in discussions

- Bring your skills and talents
- Treat me as equal

Author

Sushma Majithia

What's Important to Me?

- My family, friends, and work colleagues
- My quality advisor work
- My health and wellbeing

What Do People Like and Admire About Me?

- I am a kind and helpful person
- I am bubbly, I like to see people happy, and I am a loving and kind person
- Hardworking and always support my team

How to Best Work With Me

- Please tell me clearly and in simple words what work I am supposed to do, as this will help me to understand well
- Please listen to me as I take time to explain
- At times I might feel shy to express myself, so please motivate me
- I try to plan my work and my day, so please let me know what I need to do in advance
- Please do not judge me straight away, I prefer to be told of any mistakes I have done in a polite and positive manner

Author

Jamie Potts

What's Important to Me?

- My family and friends
- My job as a quality advisor
- Going to new places
- I like doing my own thing

---

*Some authors opted to demonstrate the one-page profile

What Do People Like and Admire About Me?

- I am polite
- I am kind
- I like helping people
- People like my smile

How to Best Work With Me

- Talk to me
- Do not do things I have not agreed to
- I like having a laugh and banter

Author

Sam Pywell

What's Important to Me?

- My family, friends, and work colleagues
- Pulling my weight
- Innovation
- Sleep

What Do People Like and Admire About Me?

- Innovation and creativity
- Risk taking
- Commitment
- Finisher

How to Best Work With Me

- Feed me at 11:30 and 2:45 or I get angry
- Talk with me, not at me
- Let me recharge on my terms (don't force me to be in social situations)
- Don't expect me to function well in meetings that go past 1 hour—I need breaks

HOW THIS CHAPTER WAS DEVELOPED

It was important that this chapter was co-produced and actively included the voices of service users to truly reflect on what is working well, what is not working as well, and what professionals can do moving forward to foster effective co-production relationships with the people they work with. The case context below outlines the role that the authors hold within their organisation, but their dual roles as service user and quality advisor were seen as unique viewpoints for this chapter's construction. Academic authors supported discussions with the group to enable exploration of the chapter's structure and content. These discussions were recorded via Microsoft Teams and auto-transcribed to ensure that, as far as possible, the authors' exact words were presented for authenticity. They then worked to build the group's vision and write up the chapter. It is essential to note at this point that all service user authors reviewed the book chapter and were part of the editing process.

Case Context

Authors Erin, James, Jamie, Joe, and Sushma are all employed as *Quality Advisors* by a national social care charity, from whom they also receive support. The charity is underpinned by the principles of respect, choice, and dignity and aims to take a person-centred approach and support adults with a learning disability, physical disability, autism, mental health condition, or a combination of care needs to live as independently as possible within the community. The organisation supports over 3500 people nationwide and models of support include supported living, registered care homes, community outreach, supported employment, extra care, and respite services.

The Role of the Quality Advisors Within the Charity

All the authors were keen to explore their current roles and explain what they do and how they help people to support setting the scene for the subsequent discussions:

'Our job role as Quality Advisors is we go around doing audits at different services. We ask the people that we support how they're doing, if they've got a good life, better life, if they're happy with their support.'

(Sushma)

'Basically, I'm a quality advisor and I love my role. We get to go and visit people and people's houses and ask them about their lives and ask them what they've been doing, whether they're happy with their support, whether they need to change anything, and if they need anything changing, I request it to their manager.'

(Jamie)

'We use our experience of living in supported living, so you go and see other houses, speak to the other people who we support, see the level of support they need. What could be improved.'

(Joe)

'And we also help people like have a voice and to be able to say what they feel without being judged by people and we take it in our stride too, give people our experiences so that they can learn from us and then to be able to achieve what they want to achieve.'

(Erin)

'We just started doing this voice group in the south region, to get the people we support together and work together. If all goes well, to start in other regions as well, hopefully even Scotland. But we also do things like working with policies, so making things easier so people can understand them a lot clearer. If a policy is 10 pages long, might be a bit boring to read in the end. So we try to cut it down, make it understandable. A bit more appealing.'

(Joe)

'We also do easy-reads and we are involved with different policies and also with voluntary work as well.'

(Sushma)

This section is going to explore what professionals will do to support engagement in co-production. One of the key elements identified by all authors was listening and being heard.

WHAT GOOD CO-PRODUCTION LOOKS LIKE

Within this section, the authors explore previous experiences from both their job role and the support they receive from health and social care services to identify what they find positive in relation to partnership working, co-production, and involvement in service provision.

Working together was a prominent discussion and the authors outline their perceptions of the benefits and the integral components required to ensure working in partnership is successful. The importance of not working in isolation and how this can support the ability to meet proposed aims and enhance the generation of ideas was empathised.

'It makes the job easier to do. It's not just us working alone to do it.'

(Joe)

'Working together means we're working as a team, not on our own, think of ideas together as a group.'

(Jamie)

Additionally, the authors also highlighted how working in partnership could provide a source of assurance and confidence in their own abilities:

'Working together is an excellent way to work because everyone has their input and if any of us forget to say one thing, the other person can say it for us. If that makes sense.'

(Jamie)

'So like if I have an idea and like my support workers put in input, then it really helps. Because then it helps me feel more confident in what I'm doing in my work.'

(Erin)

'Having a side person there so you feel confident. You don't feel shy or scared, nothing like that. Then it's really good to work with a team.'

(Sushma)

Opportunities for equal input from all of those involved and support from others were seen as positive features within the authors' experiences of working in partnership with colleagues and health professionals (Bamber, 2020). It was stressed that the service user is integral to co-production's success:

'Nothing about me, without me, like sort of thing. Because it's obviously you know, my life and stuff. I should make decisions about the stuff I wanna do or stuff that I don't wanna do, or even if there's you know, certain aspects of my life that I'm still unsure about … it should still be done with me.'

(James)

The authors believe that when they are given choices and involved in decision-making, they feel that they have control, empowerment, and independence. The authors felt that this was good co-production. Jamie recalled a time he had been involved with his care and support and making a crucial decision about living independently and how having the opportunity to make this decision and choice about his life supported him to feel more in control:

'When I first moved in my flat, cause I felt in control of my life. Based on that I can live on my own and make decisions because when I live on my own, I follow my own rules.'

(Jamie)

Sushma mirrored this opinion when she described how being able to make decisions around changing her support provision through removing previously imposed restrictions resulted in increased independence:

'I wasn't allowed to go on the buses. I wasn't allowed to hold the knife. But since I've been with [care provider] for like 9 years, I can do everything, I can speak up. So that has changed, and I think that I've done the right thing.'

(Sushma)

Another illustration of how choice can result in effective co-production with decisions being made which are best for them and thus better outcomes was noted:

'I picked my own support workers. I am a service user so they should really respect that, so I need someone as you say in that relation, we can do those things.'

(Sushma)

Input from the other people involved, such as health and social care professionals and the insights and skills they could provide, also appeared to be highly regarded and valued by the authors and there was recognition as to how working in partnership could support joint problem solving and provide a supportive environment:

'There's always like someone there to discuss and help you and stuff which is good.'

(James)

'I think working together is really important because if you like sort of need a like a helping hand or if you're stuck on anything.'

(Sushma)

Authors were also keen to recognise the need for everyone's skills to be used so that people feel involved, supported, and secure (Davies et al., 2014; Roberts et al., 2012). Erin illustrated this in her description of the support that the disability nurses provide:

'I find that disability nurses are brilliant because then they can come and visit and give you like the easy read of what a procedure is or what treatment you're gonna get because a lot of people disabili-

ties might not understand the concept, you know, like a cervical smear test or what does it mean by such and such? Whereas if you have a disability nurse that can give you an easy read of it then it's less scary and like, probably reassuring them as well that they're in a safe environment, nothing bad can happen to them.'

(Erin)

Authors stressed that good co-production requires not only usage of skills and equal involvement, but it also needs to be accessible and flexible to ensure that needs are met:

'On our way round, you know what I mean? Not on their way around, you know, it should not be like that, it should be flexible, working around us.'

(Sushma)

With a key emphasis on valuing the input of all those involved and partnership working as a mutually supportive process that can aid the generation of ideas, meet shared aims, increase independence and raise confidence, one author indicated that for collaboration to be beneficial, then it is essential that people's values are respected and that agreed boundaries are in place:

'And we understand everyone's values and them, and we understand like boundaries. Like before we do meetings, we always let people know what rules there are. It means that I can collaborate with my work colleagues, also my carers, and still like what we're doing.'

(Erin)

In addition to valuing others, developing and continuing to work on building a rapport between people was identified as being a positive contributor to good co-production:

'I think if we get along as a team, makes it a lot easier to do the work.'

(Joe)

'As long as we're working as a team and then you know like what Joe said, it's more easier, which is very important because if you don't have that support then how are you meant to do your job properly? Because you know, like, sometimes it must be difficult for someone to try and say what they feel, but feel that they can't.'

(Erin)

Sushma further described 'one-page profiles' as a useful tool for both service users and professionals in which to establish rapport and to better understand each other:

'So it's got everything in there for that person. I mean, it's not just for the people that we support, it's for everybody, so we know what your likes are, what your dislikes are and it shows the person who we talking to as well. You know it's really good to work with a team you know.'

(Sushma)

Authors explored how the recognition of their strengths and achievements was critical to co-production's success. Authors discussed examples where they were encouraged to share strengths and how this massively impacted on their confidence, recovery, and wellbeing. Erin shared an experience of a time when a social worker supported her and gave her the confidence to read a poem she had written for her dad's funeral:

'He gave me advice and he was like, just do what you, just do what you can because your dad will be so proud of you and he will want you to achieve this. And so then I stood up, did the poem and everyone cheered and clapped.'

(Erin)

Joe highlighted how one professional had recognised his long-term interest in photography and encouraged and supported him to pursue further opportunities and use his talent. Jamie also recalled how being involved in making a video for the organisation improved feelings of confidence and feeling valued and listened to:

'I felt really confident of doing it so you. I felt like people understood what I had to say … felt that I'm wanted and listened to.'

(Jamie)

Authors were keen to share their views on what good co-production looked like and felt that there were clear examples of where this was happening as illustrated in some of their examples. To surmise, authors felt the key

aspects of good co-production were not working in isolation, teamwork, equality, skill usage, choice, flexibility, relationships, and recognition of strengths and achievements. Whilst these positive discussions clearly highlight the strengths of co-production, the authors also shared experiences of when co-production did not work as well and aim to highlight what some of the pitfalls may be for professionals and organisations looking to co-produce with their service users.

WHAT BAD CO-PRODUCTION LOOKS LIKE

The main cause of bad co-production was identified as *communication* (Bamber, 2020; Marshall & Bamber, 2021).

'lack of communication, not involving other people when they should'

(Jamie)

This is not new information but is important. Historically we know that poor communication has been the root cause of many incidents and challenges within health and social care (Francis, 2013) and hence is likely to be a cause of bad co-production and missed service user opportunities (Turnnas et al., 2015). The challenge for the quality advisors is that this can impact their feeling of being equal and involved as illustrated by James:

'It's kind of like we just like submit the report, but I did sort of like try to … sort of follow up. But like I didn't hear anything back. And I was like, that's a that's a bit odd. Like I was emailing her and phone and her and stuff. And then I found out from my line manager and stuff that what had happened. I was like, I would have rather prefer to hear it from, you know. Obviously, the manager then to hear it from you.'

(James)

This action of lack of effective communication by staff toward service users, and impact, was raised by Erin:

'When someone wants a social worker and they'll say, Oh yeah, you will get back to you, but then no one gets back to you and then you think what, what's actually happening and like what Joseph said quite rightly, you know, like it must be like a very difficult, lonely time for.'

(Erin)

As well as a lack of communication, there are several behaviours which can lead to individuals not being heard, such as turn-taking (Hall et al., 2021), which can lead to disgruntlement and disengagement:

'so only sometimes when people are talking at the same time. Everyone don't have a chance to say what they wanna say'

(Jamie)

'I'm not involved in the interviews anymore'

(Jamie)

A further behaviour which impacts on relationship building is the approach of the staff in their communication and how this leaves service users feeling (Weinstein, 2010):

'Because sometimes being strict can really upset someone if they don't understand what's happening.'

(Erin)

'They feel intimidated, so to speak.'

(Joe)

Erin expressed that the consequences of poor communication and ineffective co-production can be significant:

'They might feel lonely, they might feel suicidal, they might drink to try and block off the pain that they feel, or they might just cut contact with people in the field.'

(Erin)

James explores one of the challenging cases he worked with where the approach of the staff was significantly impacting on the wellbeing of the service user. He identified that miscommunication can lead to poor techniques for attempting to manage behaviour which can be perceived as sanctions by service users, which can be extremely detrimental (McDonnell, 2011):

'Not sanction her all the time, because there were really doing it for, like, stupid things like she would open a window and stuff, and that was her saying that you wanted to leave, but obviously the staff didn't realise

that, so there was sanctioned for that and then, you know, should go outside and they were sanctioned for that because she wasn't supposed to leave her room.'

(James)

These issues with communication can have a knock-on effect and impact on individuals feeling as though they are not truly being heard (Blanchard & Ridge, 2013):

'When I go into meetings with people and we hear like, oh, this person didn't get a voice, this person didn't, you know, get a voice and then. Somebody out there needs to listen to them and to make sure that they're safe and well.'

(Erin)

Critical to co-production is the authenticity of being listened to and not just involved as a token gesture (Bamber, 2020):

'in some ways I'm not listened to all the time'

(Jamie)

Some communication issues stem from a lack of understanding of roles (like the quality advisor role) that can positively impact work within the integrated care system (Abudi & Abudi, 2015). This was highlighted by authors as a common issue on the cause of bad co-production:

'… in a way, I don't think they do feel that people can make services better now which they should do because obviously I come from a supportive thing. We have knowledge of which part is bad support is, you know, like we can share that knowledge with them, but think they're just we're looked into sometimes.'

(James)

Lack of choices and ownership grows bad co-production (Bamber, 2020); for example, a lack of co-production of an individual's care plan:

'you know when someone says to you right your support work at NHS says to you right you need to get into bed at 10:00 o'clock. But then it's your choice. I mean they can't say to you they can't be strict'

(Sushma)

'we didn't get much choices of food'

(James)

Organisational processes can be a barrier to effective co-production and lead to frustration (Marshall & Bamber, 2021):

'for example, if you made a complaint and spoke to the support work. That support work has spoken to the service leader. Then the service leader spoken to somebody in the complete teams and they took ... a while ... I'm going back and it's just not been, Not sorted out and I'm thinking that is it. Is it because of lack of communication or is that lack of this? But I think that it should be done better.'

(Sushma)

The authors noted that challenges remain when engaging service users in service development (Hulatt & Lowes, 2013). Although there have been significant benefits to the introduction of quality advisors, the barriers which the authors have faced clearly illustrate a need for more effective co-production:

'Like I'd never got to see my support plans, OK plans because we're all locked in a like a Cabinet thing.'

(James)

'They should really give us a better chance because they know who we are, what job roles we do. So I think the services should give us a chance.'

(Sushma)

Despite the challenges which authors have faced, they remain excited and determined to make changes that truly support co-production with service users. They provided several suggestions which will be explored in the following section.

WHAT PROFESSIONALS CAN DO TO MOVE FORWARD THE CO-PRODUCTION AGENDA WITH SERVICE USERS

The co-production group were keen from the outset to ensure that there were practical ideas presented to support professionals with engaging service users in

co-production. Several key aspects of the discussion included how to promote co-production (so people know what it is), what service users need (to feel able to engage in co-production), and practical actions (which could assist the co-production relationship).

Promote Co-production

All authors noted that the definition of co-production is not easy to understand (Osborne et al., 2016):

'Just seems long and complicated'

(Joe)

'I have heard of it. I am not entirely sure on what, what it is or what it means ... People working together for the same outcome sort of thing.'

(James)

Discussions then progressed to how co-production can be better understood and promoted:

'I think it's like for me, it's been like partnered with all by different organisations.'

(James)

'Coming along together, having different ideas.'

(Sushma)

'Maybe an open day ... a day where they can discuss ... and have like professionals there like ... Occupational therapy services like social work, doctors, nurses, nutritionists'

(Erin)

'Like websites and publicity on TV.'

(Joe)

An important aspect of the discussion was ensuring that the right people were able to engage in co-production (Bamber, 2020):

'Activities accessible.'

(James)

The group progressed their ideas to consider how co-production involving the service user on a more regular basis can led to them having a greater knowledge of what is going on and a sense of involvement in their own care (Tembo et al., 2021):

'That should have regular meetings … So, we can be involved with more instead of having like maybe six months times. I think it should, a meeting should be maybe two weeks. So, we know what's going on and we should be involved with the meetings. Yes, definitely. So, we can have our voices heard have our sayings.'

(Sushma)

Sushma was keen to explore how the role of the quality advisors can support co-production and assist in ensuring that service users have someone relatable to talk to when they feel unable to engage with professionals:

'So, I was talking to, and she was Asian and and I said, look, don't be scared. You can talk to me if you want to. You don't have to talk to your support workers. You don't have to talk to your family. You don't have to talk to your doctors who can talk to me, and you don't. You know what she did? Talk to me … And that was amazing.'

(Sushma)

All the authors were able to recall instances where they were able to support people in a unique way due to their intimate knowledge of their struggles. This asserts the viewpoint that the involvement of service users in co-production activities can have a significant positive impact on outcomes (NCVO, 2019):

'At an elderly people's home and there was this woman, and she was getting sad. She said, "Ohh" and "need help" and I was like, "OK," she was like "I'm getting sanctioned all the time from the staff and I don't know why." And then she said, "oh, this continues I'm gonna do something like really bad." I was like, "OK, so what would you like instead?" She said "I wanna get out of here and live closer to my relatives." I was like, so I put all that in the report and then I sent it to the manager of the care home … Couple of weeks went past and that and then I heard that she moved to her own place, got her own shower and that.'

(James)

'This lady, wasn't allowed to have a front door key, so I said why not? And the staff said no, she keeps losing. Then I guess everybody loses their front door keys or their bus pass. So, you know she wants that and so can you. Please make sure that she does. So, after about maybe a month time I had a phone call from the manager saying that she's just got the front door key. So, it's really good for that lady as well and it's good for me that I did my job properly you know.'

(Sushma)

Authors clearly recognise the benefits of being both service users and quality advisors and how this can position them to support co-production activities. They were also adamant in the fact that co-production without service users is not co-production at all (Social Care Institute for Excellence (SCIE), 2015). Authors also extended their discussion to consider what service users need to be able to engage fully in co-production.

WHAT PEOPLE NEED

The authors articulated that there needs to be consideration of what service users need to support them with engaging in co-production (SCIE, 2013). There was recognition that people can feel worried about engaging:

'Having a side person there so you feel confident? You don't. You don't feel shy or scared? Nothing like that. Then it's really good to work with a team like a teamwork.'

(Sushma)

In addition to support, Sushma considered the engagement of service users who are historically more difficult to engage, expressing the belief that more should be done to give people the opportunity to co-produce:

'There's easy ways of of doing this, but then some people don't have the access able to do it, so we need to, we need to put in place, we need to tell them, right? Do you have it or not? Get it. You know, why haven't you got it? You know? So, we need to look at that first. That do they have a tablet? Are they allowed to use it? If not, then get your next of kin or get your support worker to help you.'

(Sushma)

It was clear from all the authors that having a say in who supports them is critical to successful outcomes (Social Care Wales, 2021):

'Yeah, because like I used to have someone that because I like doing loads of stuff like going to temples. I like going to different bus routes, I like sightseeing, I like taking photographs. And the person who supported me didn't even like doing that. So, then that's not fair. You know what I mean? So, I can't have someone doing their choices. I need someone that because I get supported because I'm a service user so they should really respect that, so I need someone as you say in that relation, we can do those things.'

(Sushma)

Authors strongly recommend considering individual need when commencing co-production activities and extended this concept to think of practical ways in which professionals can foster the reciprocal relationships which are critical for successful co-production and better service user outcomes (SCIE, 2013).

Practical Things

Authors suggested that there are some interpersonal things that professionals could do which would support service users with feeling more confident in the relationship and more willing to engage:

'Maybe having a good demeanour by themselves.'

(Erin)

'In a nice way not in a horrible way.'

(Jamie)

'being polite … like trying to build a good conversation'

(Erin)

'Being friendly, don't be all strict and mean.'

(Joe)

In addition to being personable with service users, the authors felt more was needed (Hughes & Youngson, 2009)—professionals need to have a sound knowledge of the issues service users are facing prior to meeting with them:

'Support people like in the right way. So, I have Williams syndrome and not very many people understand what Williams Syndrome is.'

(Erin)

As well as having knowledge, professionals need to share the knowledge they have to build a trusting relationship with the people they work with (Barnes & Cotterell, 2012):

'let you know what's happening rather than being stuck in a loop.'

(Erin)

'Everything we should know, everything. What's written about us? What's said about us? … And we are entitled to.'

(Sushma)

'Just basically telling me what they wrote in my notes. And whether they have any … concerns about me … giving … feedback'

(Jamie)

James and Joe summed up how this relationship could work:

'They give us knowledge; we give them knowledge like it goes back to them and then they bring it back to us and then we develop.'

(James)

'They can ask for feedback from you … and give you feedback'

(Joe)

Authors strongly felt that involving individuals in their own care will have positive outcomes for their health and wellbeing (Barnes & Cotterell, 2012):

'Everyone needs to be involved.'

(James)

'Do you think that being involved in your own care has meant you have had more periods of being well?'

(Hayley)

'Yes. Definitely … if we are involved with this, you know, it makes us happy. We know, like, you know, for example with me, I mean, I like everything on the sport, you know.'

(Sushma)

Another key consideration identified was how professionals can effectively communicate with service users to reduce tension and foster positive relationships:

'By speaking to them, whether they're able to. Ask people. Ask them if they want to get involved, not just leave them. If you just leave them no one will do it.'

(Jamie)

'If you talk to someone face to face, it's a better sort of this almost you can get more out of the individual if you're talking to them face to face. I think rather than on a computer screen.'

(James)

Authors considered how this communication could be extended to people who have challenges with communication:

'Speak to them and communication. Get the person to write a message or that. Theres all different ways verbal or non-verbal'

(Jamie)

'I mean, like you could, you could write, I don't know. Say they called Billy like Billy wants to go at the church or something like that. And then you ask him, he's like, no, I don't wanna do that. Like, well, why the staff writing anything that like you do wanna do that then?'

(James)

Overall, authors stressed that the key to effective communication is honesty and listening (Trofs & Ampe, 2022):

'Just by being honest with the people that you're working with.'

(Erin)

'Just by listening to the person and what they've got to say and following their aspirations and what they wanna do, not what the care staff want to do.'

(Jamie)

Jamie summed up what professionals need to keep in mind when working with service users:

'It's all about the service user, not the staff.'

(Jamie)

CONCLUSION

This chapter aimed to provide some insight into co-production from the service user's perspective and offer some useful suggestions on what could support professionals to develop more effective and successful relationships, which can impact on overall service user wellbeing. Authors wanted to stress that co-production is challenging and getting it right is hard, but working together is the only way for success:

'You know it's not always roses and flowers … and it's not always a walk in the park … and there are going to be some days when it is gonna be upsetting, but as long as we have each other and we work together and do the best we can then we're doing a pretty good job. Aren't we?'

(Erin)

References

Abudi, G., & Abudi, Y. (2015). *Best practices for managing BPI projects: Six steps to success*. London: J Ross Publishing.

Bamber, H. (2020). *Managers' and clinical leads' perspectives of a co-production model for community mental health service improvement in the NHS: a case study* [Professional Doctorate thesis, University of Salford].

Barnes, M., & Cotterell, P. (2012). *Critical perspectives on user involvement*. London: Policy Press.

Blanchard, K., & Ridge, G. (2013). *Improve your career performance*. London: Pearson Education.

Davies, J., Sampson, M., Beesley, F., Smith, D., & Baldwin, V. (2014). An evaluation of knowledge and understanding framework personality disorder awareness training: can a co-production model be effective in a local NHS mental health Trust? *Personality and Mental Health*, *8*(2), 161–168. https://doi.org/10.1002/pmh.1257

Francis, R. (2013). Report of the Mid Staffordshire NHS Foundation Trust Public Enquiry: *Executive Summary*. London: Stationery Office.

Hall, C., Tanja, D., Kirsi, J., & Koprowska, J. (2021). *Interprofessional collaboration and service user participation: Analysing meetings in social welfare*. London: Policy Press.

Hughes, J., & Youngson, S. (2009). *Personal development and clinical psychology*. London: Wiley.

Hulatt, I., & Lowes, L. (2013). *Involving service users in health and social care Research*. London: Taylor and Francis.

Marshall, K., & Bamber, H. (2022). Using co-production in the implementation of community integrated care: a scoping review. *Primary Health Care*, *32*(6). https://doi.org/10.7748/phc.2022.e1753

McDonnell, A. A. (2011). *Managing aggressive behaviour in care settings: Understanding and applying low arousal approaches*. London: Wiley.

NVCO Know How. (2019). *Co-production and service user involvement*. https://knowhow.ncvo.org.uk/organisation/collaboration/coproduction-and-service-user-involvement

Osborne, S. P., Radnor, Z., & Strokosch, K. (2016). Co-production and the co-creation of value in public services: a suitable case for treatment. *Public Management Review*, *18*(5), 639–653. https://doi.org/10.1080/14719037.2015.1111927

Roberts, A., Greenhill, B., Talbot, A., & Cuzak, M. (2012). 'Standing up for human rights': a group's journey beyond consultation towards co-production. *British Journal of Learning Disabilities*, *40*(4), 292–301. https://doi.org/10.1111/j.1468-3156.2011.00711.x

Social Care Institute for Excellence. (2013). *Co-production in social care: what it is and how to do it*. London: SCIE.

Social Care Institute for Excellence. (2015). *Co-production in social care: what it is and how to do it*. London: SCIE.

Social Care Wales. (2021, September 25). Understanding an outcomes approach in social care. https://socialcare.wales/service-improvement/understanding-an-outcomes-approach

Tembo, D., Hickey, G., Montenegro, C., Chandler, D., Nelson, E., Porter, K., Dikomitis, L., Chambers, M., Chimbari, M., Mumba, N , Beresford, P., Fkiikina, P. O., Musesengwa, R., Staniszewska, S., Coldham, T., & Rennard, U. (2021). Effective engagement and involvement with community stakeholders in co-production of global health research. *British Medical Journal*, *372*, n178.

Trofs, J., & Ampe, P. (2022). *Person to person: Change your life and fix your world*. London: BookBaby.

Tuurnas, S., Stenvall, M., Rannisto, J., Harisalo, R., & Hakari, M. (2015). Coordinating co-production in complex network settings. *European Journal of Social Work*, *18*(3), 370–382. https://doi.org/10.1080/13691457.2014.930730

Weinstein, J. (2010). *Mental health, service user involvement and recovery*. London: Jessica Kingsley Publishing.

25

Supporting Family Carers Within an Integrated Care Context

Dr Julie Alexandra Lawrence

'Across the UK, millions of people provide unpaid support for an ill, older or disabled family member, or friend. They are unpaid carers but for many they are just a wife, husband, child, parent, friend or good neighbour'

(Carers UK, 2021)

KEY CONCEPTS

- 13.6 million family carers in the UK caring through the pandemic
- Family carers want to see more integration between health and social care
- Family carers play a significant role in supporting the NHS and social care
- Family carers are entitled to legal recognition
- Promotion of wellbeing is paramount

INTRODUCTION

In this chapter, a family carer/carer is described as 'a family member or friend who provides care to someone known to them without pay' (Grant, 2018). Family carers are a 'shadow workforce that provides crucial day-to-day support to family members with complex health conditions' (Wong-Cornall et al., 2017).

The chapter will address the key concepts presented and illustrate how the relevant case study (supporting a spouse with Alzheimer's disease) relies upon co-ordinated services through an integrated care system (ICS) to benefit those in need of support. In other words, it is important that the right information and services are provided at the right time and in the right place.

During Carers Week (8–14 June 2020), new figures were released to illustrate how many people now undertake the role of family carer. There are an estimated 4.5 million people in the UK who have become carers because of the COVID-19 pandemic. This is in addition to the 9.1 million who were already caring before the outbreak, bringing the total to 13.6 million. The majority of additional carers are women (2.7 million); men account for 1.8 million.

Greater integration of health and social care services is something that family carers want to see more of. Many carers' lives are often made much harder when 'holistic' (health and social care) services are not joined up. In addition, frustrations can manifest due to important data not being shared effectively and efficiently between services. Unpaid carers were not initially included in the White Paper (Carers UK, 2021). Subsequently, the current government (Conservative) has redressed this omission and includes carers in public consultations, decisions about prevention and treatment of illness, and commissioning of health services.

Carers play an essential role in supporting the NHS and social care systems. Diversity and inclusion are also important in ensuring that voices are heard from community members about their 'lived experiences'. Without this support, our health and care systems would have not been able to cope with the increased demand they have seen. Not only do carers need to be recognised for the important support they provide, but the proposals for integration as outlined in the White Paper (Department of Health & Social Care, 2021) can only work if unpaid carers are visible, recognised, and counted as part of the NHS (Carers UK, 2021). A recent report published by The King's Fund (2021) illustrates these points:

'Integrated care is an ideal opportunity for us all to get involved and to have a say in our health services. By integrating services across communities we will, hopefully, get rid of the delays and gaps in care'

(Thorstensen-Woll et al., 2021)

LEGAL RECOGNITION OF FAMILY CARERS

Many carers carry out complex and difficult tasks without recognised training, and often with little support. The informal status of family carers has led to ambiguity about their role and capabilities. It is, in part, this uncertainty that has led family carers and those they care for to experience fewer opportunities than healthcare providers to contribute to decisions about care and treatment, co-ordination of services, and provision of self-management support (Wong-Cornall et al., 2017).

NHS legislation currently does not need to regard carers' own wellbeing explicitly, nor does it have to identify carers. This is not the case for social care, which treats carers equally in legislation (Care Act, 2014: section 3) alongside people who use services. Closer integration between health and social care means that one system recognises carers legally as an equal part, the other does not. For effective integration across the system to be achieved, both the NHS and social care need to have a statutory duty to have regard for carers and to promote their wellbeing. Fig. 25.1 outlines how the lack of systematic identification and support for carers across the NHS has significant risks for the carers:

It is also important to recognise the limitations of what legislation can achieve. It is not possible to legislate for collaboration and co-ordination of local services. This requires changes to the behaviours, attitudes, and relationships of staff and leaders right across the health and

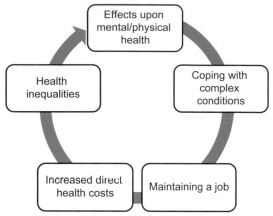

Fig. 25.1 Lack of systematic identification and support for carers across the NHS. (Carers UK, 2021).

care system, including within the national bodies. This makes the government's implementation plan very important, especially as the legislation leaves so much to local (and national) discretion (McKenna, 2021).

Ethical Dilemmas

Individuals respond to caring in different ways, and so 'help' needs to be flexible in approach. It is not a case of 'one size fits all' but rather a more person-centred approach towards those such as Chandra and Hari whose

---

CASE STUDY   Chandra's Story—The Effects of Alzheimer's Disease on Family Dynamics

Dementia is a syndrome (progressive 'brain failure') affecting higher functions of the brain (Rahman & Howard, 2018). Dementia is not a disease in itself but can be caused by one of several different diseases that affect the brain. It involves a decline in people's thinking skills. This can affect our memory, ability to reason and solve problems, ability to communicate, and other types of thinking. People living with dementia have difficulty carrying out daily activities like preparing food, paying bills, or going to the supermarket. At the time of writing, dementia affects around 850,000 people in the UK, of which Alzheimer's disease (AD) is the most common cause (62%). Scientists believe that, for most people, AD is caused by a combination of genetic, lifestyle, and environmental factors that affect the brain over time (Rahman & Howard, 2018). Typical early symptoms of AD may include those outlined in Fig. 25.2.

Chandra (70 years) and Hari (75 years) are a married couple of Indian (Hindu) descent. They have lived in a terraced house in England for the past 45 years. English is their second language. They have three adult children (two boys, one girl), all of whom were born in England and live within a 30-mile radius of them. Hari was showing signs of early-onset AD before the age of 65 years. He became very forgetful and disorientated around his familiar environment. In addition, his ability to reason with his children about his care needs became difficult and resulted in regular arguments with his two sons in particular. More recently, he has become doubly incontinent. Chandra has supported Hari constantly as the AD developed. However, she has felt overwhelmed and exhausted by his endless demands and became fearful about his outbursts of 'rage' due to his frustrations associated with his AD. She is in contact with her children and a community nurse about Hari's incontinence, resulting in additional care needs. During the last home visit, the community nurse suggested that a short period of residential respite care would benefit Hari and not least, Chandra. In addition, during his respite stay, Hari's health and social care needs could

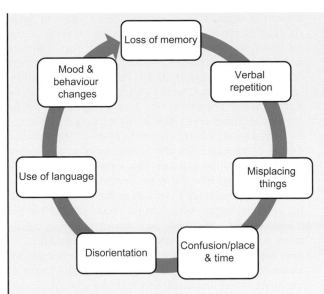

Fig. 25.2 Alzheimer's disease develops over time, but the speed of change varies between people. (Alzheimer's Research UK, 2021).

be reassessed to establish the levels of support needed from the integrated care team. The community nurse also offered to advocate (and co-ordinate translation) on behalf of Chandra, due to her limited understanding of English.

Discussion: Reflections Upon the Case Study

Initially, the solution to the scenario (respite care) sounds ideal. However, what also needs to be taken into consideration is the impact of caring for someone over a long period of time. Rahman and Howard (2018) argue that caring can affect psychological and physical health, the negative health consequences of looking after a family member. Caring for a family member can change family relationships. Changes in behaviour and personality can cause family carers to treat their loved one in a different, more childlike way. In this scenario, Chandra has maintained her relationships with her children, although her capacity to continue caring is questionable. The expectations and responsibility to continue caring for Hari has increased over time. Chandra is now more dependent upon her two sons and daughter to

'step up to the plate' and support her and Hari on a regular basis. The option of residential respite care is unacceptable to Hari, and due to his cultural values, he expects Chandra, as his wife, to continue caring for him. Another consideration in this scenario is the dynamics between the siblings and their attitude(s) towards their parents. Their father has increasingly dependent needs as the AD progresses. Their mother is becoming isolated and distressed and fears that she is not able to continue caring. She had one friend whom she did confide in, but recently, her friend (female in a similar situation) has withdrawn contact, due to her own family commitments.

The integrated care team members (nursing/social work professionals) have a duty of care (Care Act, 2014: section 3) to assess the holistic needs of both Hari and Chandra. The assessment determines that the local authority will contribute towards the care, through relevant eligibility criteria. An eligible care need is the level of need(s) that Hari and Chandra must have for consideration regarding funding. Any NHS provision such as incontinence pads could be free at the point of delivery. In this scenario, respite care can take several forms, such as day care outside the home, house-sitting arrangements whereby the carer can take a break for a few hours, or regular planned breaks within a residential setting—as suggested by the community nurse.

However, there are several reasons why respite care can be counterproductive. Greenwood et al. (2019) discussed their research findings undertaken with older carers (70+). The researchers emphasised that accessing and using health and social care services were appreciated although they were perceived as creating considerable work. Carers highlighted 'multiple tiring, frustrating, time consuming challenges of accessing and using support' (Greenwood et al., 2019). There were conversations between participants (n=45) about the paucity of useful information, poor communication between professionals and services and, not least, onerous form-filling. There was also a lot of discussion about poor services in terms of the quality of the support and professionals' generally poor understanding of, for example, dementia (AD), which added to their stress (Greenwood et al., 2019).

holistic needs vary over time. Chandra recognised that her own advancing age and ethnicity could hinder access to additional formal support. There were potential language barriers to consider, although translation input had been suggested by the community nurse. Chandra experienced periods of isolation and loneliness, due to

her friend and children being preoccupied with their own concerns. The fact that Chandra had been caring for so long and 'caring' was rooted in her long-term relationship with Hari created an ethical dilemma as to whether she felt motivated (and/or guilty) about seeking additional help.

Her daughter, although sympathetic, had her own mental health needs and therefore asking for her support was difficult, given her reduced capacity to offer help. Both Chandra's sons viewed their father as 'difficult' due to fractious exchanges between them. They held the view that their father's confusion (AD) about the extent and therefore demands of his health and social care needs were not fully appreciated. Consequently, their father's expectations from his family were that everyone should be 'looking after him'. This attitude affected his two sons in such a way they resisted any input which would distract them from their own busy family lives.

Person-Centred Care

Person-centred care moves away from professionals deciding what is best for an individual and places the person at the centre, as an expert of their own experience. The person and their family, where appropriate, become an equal partner in the planning of their care and support, ensuring it meets their needs, goals, and outcomes. Person-centred care relies on several aspects, as illustrated in Fig. 25.3.

Person-centeredness is not a new concept, 'but its exact roots in relation to humanistic psychology continue to attract scrutiny' (Rahman & Howard, 2018). As mentioned in Fig. 25.3, one of the most important aspects of this approach is a person's values and beliefs. In this scenario, Hari expects his immediate family to care for him, regardless of the high levels of care which are required. Chandra does have access to some formal support through the community nurse, but there are limitations about the

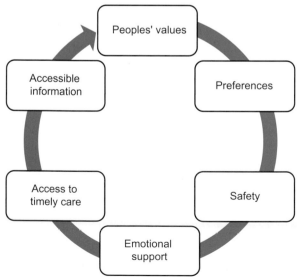

Fig. 25.3 Person's values and beliefs. (Social Care Institute for Excellence, 2021).

amount of support which can be offered linked to financial considerations. In theory, decision-making about his health and care needs should include Hari, although whether this is a realistic option would be dependent upon the progression of AD and its affects upon his reasoning ability. From Chandra's perspective, she could be torn between protecting Hari and trying to ensure he remains included when decisions are being made about his overall needs, which affect both of them. This could be further compounded by the unavailability and reticence of their three adult children. The Alzheimer's Society UK (2021) espouses that there are benefits when a person-centred care approach is applied within family scenarios. For example, someone such as Hari could take part in the things he enjoys and it can be a way of managing behavioural and psychological symptoms of AD. In addition, he may appreciate the opportunity to have conversations and relationships with other people outside the home. At the heart of this approach, and that of a strengths-based approach, is the promotion of a 'can do mind set' (Dix et al., 2019). The emphasis of both practitioners within an integrated care context and family carers such as Chandra is to recognise that everyone has strengths, capabilities, and resources, which are emphasised to promote a hopeful (and realistic) attitude (Dix et al., 2019).

IMPACT ON PEOPLE

Ethnicity and Dementia

In this case study, an important aspect which impacts upon both Chandra and Hari are their cultural needs (i.e., in accordance with Hinduism). A diagnosis of AD could also manifest as a cultural stigma for the family once the news was known in their wider community(s). Any potential service providers, such as those either providing residential respite care or volunteers providing an appropriate 'friendship scheme' at home (Age UK, 2021), would need to consider how to provide culturally appropriate services. Iliffe and Manthorpe (2004) discussed the importance of issues for service providers to consider in such circumstances. These included language, religious belief and observance, cultural practices (including food and personal care practices), and social support and coping mechanisms. The importance, therefore, is to offer an integrated service (via health and social care) rather than to develop segregated or specialised services. This approach can also facilitate a positive person-centred focus with an emphasis upon well-being for both Hari and Chandra, assured that their specific preferences are addressed.

Further, a study of three minority ethnic community groups in Manchester (Temple et al., 2002) suggested that many older people do not have a strong desire for separate services but associate quality with good service delivery rather than different kinds of provision.

The aforementioned friendship scheme was supported by NHS (Coventry) (until 2012) and developed by Age UK (Coventry). Specially trained volunteers visited those individuals identified as having dementia. The referral base came from a variety of health and social work professionals. The visits were once a week for a minimum of 2 hours and cost £20, which could either be spent in the home or accompanying the person to an activity, the point being that the person chooses what they would like to do with the time and activities. The activities could include anything from tea and chat, attending a friendship group or craft activity, and/or going for a lunch/walk. Since 2012, the scheme has been financially supported through the Big Lottery Fund. Thus, it is subjected to both internal and external evaluations in terms of outcomes related to improved social contact, increased activity, and improved wellbeing. This is a good example of how identified needs can be met using personal budgets and/or a direct payment once the assessment and eligibility criteria has been confirmed.

Of course, not everyone with AD can participate within friendship schemes. In some instances, a more formal structured approach (residential care) is necessary, factoring in health and safety issues. However, as mentioned previously, the emphasis and impact is upon autonomy and control—enabling the individual and their carer to have input about additional support required within difficult circumstances.

CONCLUSION

Family carers undertake a significant role when caring for a loved one. There is, to a certain extent, formal legal recognition through the Care Act (2014) about the importance of the caring role. This principle is underpinned by a desire to maintain equilibrium between those who care and those who are cared for through the entitlement to assessments and provision of either formal or informal (voluntary) services. What matters to carers is co-ordinated quality provision which is best suited to their individual circumstances. However, a major concern is the growing numbers (currently 13.6 million) of carers who will continue to need services on behalf of their loved ones and, not least, themselves. It is imperative therefore, that whilst the debates about integrated care and commissioning continue, we do not lose sight of the fact that the current fragmentation between the NHS and social care provision is detrimental to both individuals and their carers who are entitled to live better quality lives.

References

Age UK Coventry & Warwickshire. (2021). https://www.ageuk.org.uk/coventryandwarwickshire/

Alzheimer's Research UK. (2021). https://www.alzheimersresearchuk.org/

Alzheimer's Society UK. (2021). https://www.alzheimers.org.uk/

Care Act 2014. London: Stationery Office.

Carers UK. (2021). http://www.carersuk.org

Department of Health & Social Care. (2021). *Health and Care White Paper, Integration and Innovation: working together to improve health and social care for all.* London: Stationery Office.

Dix, H., Hollinrake, S., & Meade, J. (2019). *Relationship-based social work with adults.* St Albans: Critical Publishing.

Grant, V. (2018). *Working with family carers.* St Albans: Critical Publishing.

Greenwood, N., Pound, C., Brearley, S., & Smith, R. (2019). A qualitative study of older informal carers' experience and perceptions of their caring role. *Maturitas, 124,* 1–7. https://doi.org/10.1016/j.maturitas.2019.03.006

Iliffe, S., & Manthorpe, J. (2004). The debate on ethnicity and dementia: From category fallacy to person-centred care? *Aging & Mental Health, 8*(4), 283–292. https://doi.org/10.1080/1360786041000170965

McKenna, H. (2021, March 9). The health and social care White Paper explained. https://www.kingsfund.org.uk/publications/health-social-care-white-paper-explained

Rahman, S., & Howard, R. (2018). https://www.kingsfund.org.uk/publications/health-social-care-white-paper-explained. London: Jessica Kingsley.

Social Care Institute for Excellence. (2021). https://www.scie.org.uk/

Temple, B., Glenister, C., & Raynes, N. (2002). Prioritising home care needs: Research with older people from three minority community groups. *Health and Social Care in the Community, 10*(3), 179–186. https://doi.org/10.1046/j.1365-2524.2002.00360.x

Thorstensen-Woll, C., Wellings, D., Crump, H., & Graham, C. (2021, July 21). *Understanding integration: How to listen to and learn from people and communities.* https://www.kingsfund.org.uk/publications/understanding-integration-listen-people-communities

Wong-Cornall, C., Parsons, J., Sheridan, N., Kenealy, T., & Peckham, A. (2017). Extending continuity of care to include the contribution of family carers. *International Journal of Integrated Care, 17*(2), 11. https://doi.org/10.5334/ijic.2545

Further Reading

The Carers Trust (2021) raises awareness of unpaid carers in the UK. It gives carers a voice and highlights their work to the public. Campaign work is also a main feature of the Carers Trust:

https://carers.org/help-and-info/introduction

The King's Fund Podcast (November, 2021): The hidden value of unpaid carers (Fatima Khan-Shah):

http://kingsfund.libsyn.com/the-hidden-value-of-unpaid-carers-and-authentic- leadership-fatima-khan-shah

Ethnicity and Dementia

Botsford, J., Clarke, C. L., & Gibb, C. E. (2011). Research and dementia, caring and ethnicity: A review of the literature. *Journal of Research in Nursing*, *16*(5). https://doi.org/10.1177/1744987111414531

Parveen, S., Peltier, C., & Oyebode, J. R. (2017). Perceptions of dementia and use of services in minority ethnic communities. *Health and Social Care in the Community*, *25*(2), 734–742. https://doi.org/10.1111/hsc.12363

26

Integrated Care for LGBTQ+ People

Dr Claire Brown

KEY CONCEPTS

Working definitions of identity descriptors are provided to support shared understandings of lesbian, gay, bisexual, trans, and queer (**LGBTQ+)** identities to promote integrated working. However, it should be acknowledged that gender and sexual identities are individually experienced, and that discourse to describe the complexity of personal identity will necessarily evolve as societal understanding and language develops (Serano, 2016; Stryker & Aizura, 2013).

- **Lesbian**, **gay**, and **bisexual** describe people who are sexually or romantically attracted to people of the same gender as them, or to more than one gender.
- **Trans** (short for transgender) is an umbrella term used to describe a person whose assigned gender differs to that which was ascribed to them by medical staff at birth, based on visual and societally dictated definitions.
- **Cis** (cisgender) describes a person whose experience of their gender aligns with that ascribed to them at birth.
- **Queer** may be used as a self-descriptor denoting a sexual or gender identity that does not sit within traditional definitions constructed within normative ideas of sexuality and gender.
- **Non-binary** is a further umbrella term for people whose gender identity does not align with 'male' or 'female', either all or some of the time.
- **+** aims to capture a range of sexual and gender identities, and to include new identity descriptors as they develop.

(Schilt & Westbrook, 2009; Stonewall, 2017a).

INTRODUCTION

Many people with non-cis-het (cisgender, heterosexual) gender and sexual identities still lack understanding and appreciation within wider society (Hines, 2013), and

specifically within health and social care sectors (Bachman & Gooch, 2018; Brown & Rogers, 2020; Hudson-Sharp, 2018). This lack of understanding has been linked to significant disparities in use of healthcare services (Johnson et al., 2020), higher rates of chronicity (Dragon et al., 2017), and poor outcomes for sexual and reproductive health (Imborek et al., 2017). It has been argued that these poor outcomes result from a complex picture of social and economic inequality (Mink et al., 2014). Core issues in disparity include interlinking factors of employment discrimination, financial and housing insecurity, experience of domestic abuse and sexual violence, and direct discrimination extant across a range of health services. Further, reviews of the literature indicate that the experiences of those at the intersection of multiple sites of discrimination (such as Black, trans, and disabled people) are thus far insufficiently studied. However, there is an indication that those experiencing multiple forms of discrimination will be further subjugated (Brown, 2021b; Lampe & Nowakowski, 2020).

While LGBTQ+ people have received markedly increased media coverage over the past two decades, certain identities have been afforded greater societal acceptance and legal rights (Biblarz & Savci, 2010; Brown, 2021b; Tasker & Lavender-Stott, 2020). The process of increased LGBTQ+ awareness has not necessarily been productive towards including all identities; indeed, it can have the effect of 'othering' some LGBTQ+ identities (Sue, 2010). The experiences of bisexual, pansexual, trans, and non-binary people have historically been relatively neglected within LGBTQ+ family research (Biblarz & Savci, 2010; Brown, 2021b), including research focusing on reproductive choice (Riggs & Bartholameus, 2018; Sterling & Garcia, 2020).

Although the sociopolitical effects of austerity and the COVID-19 pandemic are yet to be fully understood, fertility research implicates a trajectory of increasingly disproportionate disadvantaging of LGBTQ+ people

(Harvey & Inghraham, 2021). It can be argued that family is the most highly regulated context within society, prescribed by specific rules of social legitimacy (Coontz, 2003; Kressier & Bryant, 1996). As such, the way 'outliers' such as LGBTQ+-headed families are treated by professionals within systems of health and social care is both an issue affected by, and productive of, stigma and inclusion (Brown, 2021b; Tyler, 2020; Tyler & Slater, 2018). With the pandemic both exposing cracks (Marmot et al., 2021) and highlighting innovations (Horton et al., 2021) in health and social care systems, a new era of development presents itself. This chapter sets out examples of opportunities for creating LGBTQ+ inclusive models of integrated care that align with a wider agenda addressing the inconsistent inclusion of LGBTQ+ people in UK society (Hines, 2013).

As explained in Chapter 5, attempts to develop integrated systems require exploration of integrated care at macro, meso, and micro levels; therefore, a focus on populations, systems, organisations, professionals, and individuals is essential (Charles, 2022). The first section of this chapter imagines how the successful integration of services could improve care for LGBTQ+ people in a range of domains that are key to their health, wellbeing, and participation in societal life (Brown, 2021b). To do so, a fictional case study will be drawn upon to illustrate how health and social care systems can better work together to ensure understanding joined-up and co-ordinated care (Charles, 2022; World Health Organisation (WHO), 2016). The case study raises several challenges that LGBTQ+ people face when accessing services in a UK context. The ensuing discussion will explore the case study to identify ways to build integrated systems that foster greater inclusivity, equity, and co-production.

The second section of this chapter aims to provide an overview of some of the barriers to good overall health and equality of opportunity that LGBTQ+ people face today. It lays out practical advice for making health and social care systems more inclusive and recognises that co-production is an essential component of integrated care (Marshall & Bamber, 2022). Giving thought to LGBTQ+-inclusive practice is timely considering there is likely to be a raft of service development work associated with embedding the WHO's Core Principles of Integrated Care (WHO, 2016). There is an opportunity to adapt or rebuild systems, procedures, and policies with LGBTQ+ equality in mind.

INTEGRATING SERVICES: IMPROVING CARE FOR LGBTQ+ PEOPLE

At its core, integrated care aims to provide the support that people need across the NHS, local councils, voluntary sector, and other partners in a way that improves health and reduces inequalities (WHO, 2016). When clashes in perspective and communication failures exist within and between individuals, populations, organisations, and systems, service provision ceases to be co-ordinated, continuous, holistic, and governed through shared accountability and whole-systems thinking (Charles, 2022; WHO, 2016). A lack of understanding of the needs of LGBTQ+ people can influence negative outcomes in mental and physical health (Jaspal et al., 2018; LGBT Foundation, 2017; Pearce, 2018), reduce LGBTQ+ people's opportunities to become parents, and reduce options for children needing permanent substitute homes (Brown, 2021b; Hicks, 2006; Wood, 2016). Increased co-production and sharing of knowledge and best practice can produce dramatically different results (Marshall & Bamber, 2022).

When considering this scenario through the lens of integrated care, truly integrated services seek out and work with community assets viewing health as more than episodic care and adopting a population health approach (Charles, 2022). This is particularly important within primary care, which for many is the first point of contact. A place-based approach incorporating social prescribing could enable identification of pockets of concentrated or complex disadvantage to enable targeted initiatives for LGBTQ+ inclusion work (Todd et al., 2021). Charlie and Pete's case highlights an area of practice where a more integrated approach can benefit the experience and outcomes for a whole family. As the first point of access, social work and medical staff with knowledge of the breadth of LGBTQ+ people's potential needs and wants in relation to starting a family can help them provide effective information to those in the process of determining their route and methods of starting and raising children (McDonald et al., 2016; Riggs et al., 2020b; White, 2018).

In the case study, an integrated approach enabled the couple to access wider services as well as enabling the GP to consult with relevant peers who have examined the body of research on trans fertility (BSUH, 2021). This encouraged the offering of information on assisted fertility options that enabled Charlie to carry a pregnancy (Human Fertilisation and Embryology Authority, 2022; White, 2018). The treatment options offered align with World Professional Association for Transgender Health (WPATH, 2012) and Care Quality Commission (CQC, 2022). If a miscarriage had resulted, the professionals involved in Charlie's care could enhance their ability to support Charlie and Pete, drawing from co-produced research (Riggs et al., 2020a). In a case of domestic abuse, Galop can provide support to LGBTQ+ people (Galop, 2022). The support offered by psychological services for Charlie's postnatal depression is again best delivered by professionals with

CASE STUDY

Charlie is a 28-year-old non-binary person (pronouns: they/them) married to Pete, a 31-year-old cisgender man. Charlie and Pete had been trying to conceive via intercourse for 2 years but no pregnancy had resulted. The couple were interested in adoption or fostering, and so attended open days held by local authority and independent adoption and fostering agencies. A social worker who had accessed LGBTQ+ inclusion training and resources signposted Charlie and Pete to New Family Social (2022), a national charity that offers information and support to LGBTQ+ people interested in adopting or fostering a child, and Proud 2b Parents (2022), an inclusive organisation for all routes to parenthood for LGBTQ+ people. Charlie and Pete attended a monthly Proud2b Parents social group, which gave them the opportunity to speak to LGBTQ+ adopters, foster carers, and birth parents. The agency also put them in touch with a non-binary person living near them who had given birth and chestfed their baby. Charlie and Pete realised that although they are open to growing their family via adoption or fostering, they wanted to experience having a child by birth too.

Charlie and Pete attended an appointment with their GP to enquire about fertility support. This was the first time in 5 years that Charlie had accessed NHS medical services because Charlie had been misgendered on multiple occasions by their previous GP, receptionist, and nursing staff. Experience of being misgendered was a trigger for onset of anxiety and depression for Charlie. Charlie used private medical services to provide treatment including testosterone (often referred to as T) and top surgery to remove their chest tissue because the wait for the NHS gender identity service was lengthy, and there was no guarantee of support for gender confirmation surgery at the conclusion of an assessment. Charlie did not take up fertility preservation options ahead of starting T.

Charlie's new GP had no prior experience of working with non-binary people, and so following the initial consultation, she advised Charlie and Pete that she would need to increase her knowledge ahead of a follow-up appointment with them. Using good practice set out by Brighton and Sussex University Hospitals NHS Trust (BSUH, 2021), the GP checked Charlie's preference regarding the gender of the staff who would support them. Anne, a gender inclusion midwife was appointed to support Charlie and Pete. Following Care Quality Commission (CQC) guidance (CQC, 2022), Anne spoke to the GP about Charlie and Pete's options for conception, and they jointly discussed these with Charlie and Pete. Charlie decided that they would reduce the T treatment they were taking to increase the chances of a pregnancy by in vitro fertilisation treatment provided by the Human Fertilisation and Embryo Authority (2022). Charlie's GP and midwife noted on their medical records the negative impact that misgendering can have on Charlie's mental health.

A pregnancy resulted and the gender inclusion midwife supported Charlie throughout the pregnancy. Anne enabled the GP, support staff, and Charlie's health visitor to access gender inclusion training. Charlie used pronoun stickers when attending scan appointments. Anne gave Charlie and Pete a tour of the hospital facilities they chose to have their baby in, and shared details of the personalised birth plan they had produced together with the ward sister. This included Charlie's wish for their chest and external pelvic area to be named as such (CQC, 2022). Charlie accessed information about chest-feeding from La Leche League (2022) but decided to bottle feed as they felt that chest-feeding may induce dysphoria that could negatively impact on their mental health. Charlie's health visitor contacted a local parenting group that Charlie wanted to attend to speak to its co-ordinator about gender inclusion and the provision of facilities such as a gender-neutral toilet. Charlie wanted to share their trans identity with group members when they felt ready, so the health visitor did not share details of their trans identity. Charlie experienced postnatal depression, for which they received medication and support from a therapist with knowledge of gender diversity.

knowledge of how to support LGBTQ+ people (BSUH, 2021; Riggs et al., 2019; Royal College of Psychiatrists, 2019). Transnormativity could make Charlie feel excluded from both cis and trans groups as their identity does not fit binary norms (Riggs et al., 2019). Support and signposting to an appropriate counselling service for trans and

non-binary people and their families can be accessed via the Beaumont Society (2018).

An earlier adoption of integrated care systems could have further broadened Charlie and Pete's options. For example, the previous GP could have gained knowledge through networks of T treatments, as this treatment can reduce fertility (Coleman et al., 2011; White, 2018; WPATH, 2012). Indeed, it is essential for GPs and nursing staff to be aware that T does not prohibit natural conception in all cases; trans people taking it have become pregnant (Coleman et al., 2011; MacDonald et al., 2016). Knowledge of trans pregnancy and sexual health is integral to wider health and wellbeing agendas (Lampe & Nowakowski, 2021; Mavuso, 2021). Non-government organisations such as the LGBT Foundation have taken a key role in this endeavour, training thousands of health professionals to feel more confident and knowledgeable treating LGBTQ+ patients (LGBT Foundation, 2018).

The GP's mobilisation of her networks enabled her to give Charlie the information to consider a temporary T reduction to maximise their chances of a pregnancy (Coleman, 2011; MacDonald et al., 2016). Opportunities for peer support helped improve knowledge for all the health and social work staff involved in Charlie and Pete's care. The couple may also wish to consider a surrogate, which is a method of having a genetically related child that some trans people have utilised. There are increasing examples of how primary care can act as a support for LGBTQ+ people preparing for and during pregnancy (BSUH, 2021; Coleman et al., 2011; Human Fertilisation and Embryology Authority, 2022). Forging new partnerships and working with a range of experts from within the community have demonstrated that trans masculine and non-binary people can engage their bodies to become pregnant and chest-feed (MacDonald et al., 2016; Riggs et al., 2020b). The examples included within this research benefit from co-produced knowledge that enhances the credibility and practice applicability of the findings (Marshall & Bamber, 2022). Liaising with wider groups helped increase knowledge and expand the range of options offered to Charlie and Pete. GPs should be given the time and opportunity for liaising with colleagues who can support their vital role in providing equitable gatekeeping for LGBTQ+ people into other services.

In the UK, the NHS funds support for fertility treatment. However, this is known to be a postcode lottery for cis-het people, with support for LGBTQ+ people lagging even further behind (Harvey & Ingraham, 2021). Where fertility treatment is not funded for LGBTQ+ people, this presents a further barrier to inclusion. This is particularly relevant when considering that LGBTQ+ people in the UK experience discrimination in housing and employment that can impact upon finances (Bachman & Gooch, 2018; LGBT Foundation, 2017).

The research base suggests that inclusion is differential, based on the closeness of fit that an LGBTQ+ person has to established mainstream norms of gender and sexuality (Brown, 2021a; Hicks, 2000, 2006; Wood, 2016). As such, a lesbian, gay, or trans person or family that closely mirrors the central characteristics of a heterosexual cisgender person/family may receive more favourable treatment, while a person whose characteristics do not align with expected cis-het norms may experience pronounced discrimination (Bachman & Gooch, 2018; LGBT Foundation, 2017; Stonewall, 2017b). Indeed, there is an amassing body of research suggesting that specific detriment exists for non-binary people (Matsuno & Budge, 2017). Recent research highlights the prevalence of hetero-cis-normativity in relation to various forms of parenting (Worthen & Herbolsheimer, 2022).

A challenge faced when moving to a whole-systems approach is the management of information sharing across agencies (Kodner, 2009). When sharing medical notes with other agencies such as local authorities and independent adoption and fostering agencies, medical staff should be aware of and committed to including context where relevant. Likewise, those reading reports should be open to considering the wider context and reasons for medical issues. For example, a period of poor mental and physical health such as that described earlier could have been triggered by the stress of a perceived loss. Charlie and Pete had hoped to have a birth child and although no physical loss was incurred, they had to accept that they would not become birth parents. A process similar to another grief and loss can be experienced by some people (Brown, 2021b).

Any incidence of misgendering or gender-based discrimination can likewise trigger stress responses that have the potential to impair physical and mental health (Brown, 2021b). An acknowledgement of this could firstly limit the associated stress response, and secondly could elicit a different response when sharing medical information with an adoption panel. Kodner and Spreeuwenberg (2002) explain that when services fail to integrate, all aspects of care can be affected, people get lost in systems and services can fail to deliver an equitable service, and quality of care declines.

LEGISLATION AND POLICY'S CURRENT PROTECTIONS

Taking a UK example, The Gender Recognition Act 2004 aimed to set out additional rights for trans people. The Equality Act 2010 should provide an overarching framework that meets the needs of LGBTQ+ people when accessing health and social care services, as it affords protection based on protected characteristics of sexual orientation, sex, and gender assignment. However, limitations of the application and contemporary remit of both acts have been questioned by recent research showing that LGBTQ+ people experience frequent and significant discrimination in public and social life (Bachman & Gooch, 2018; LGBT Foundation, 2017; Stonewall, 2017b).

Protections supposedly afforded by legislation and policy have indeed failed to protect the rights of LGBTQ+ individuals across a range of health and social care practice areas. The '*Transgender Equality*' report emphasised how trans people have been failed in a range of domains from media representation to hate crime, prison and probation, education, and health and social care (House of Commons Women and Equalities Committee, 2016). Trans people experience disproportionately high rates of mental illness, unemployment, homelessness, and domestic abuse (Bachman & Gooch, 2018; LGBT Foundation, 2017). As such, it can be surmised that the protections these acts should overarchingly provide are insufficient to ensure equitable treatment of LGBTQ+ within health and social services.

NON-BINARY (IN)VISIBILITY

While it can be argued that strides have been made in expanding the possibilities for non-binary gender expression for non-binary people in the West in recent years, there is still much work to be done. Instances of good practice are emerging, like the UK civil service bringing in a non-binary identity option (Monro & Van der Ros, 2017) and the increased visibility of non-binary people in clinical settings (Motmans et al., 2019). However, health monitoring systems do not uniformly include non-binary identities; thus, where suitable options are not provided, non-binary identities are erased (Jaspal et al., 2018). Visibility of non-binary people remains a prominent issue (Taylor et al., 2018). A recent UK study found that 76% of non-binary people avoided expressing their gender identity because they were afraid of negative reactions to it (Government Equalities Office, 2018).

It has been argued that current legislation purporting to govern equality for all only extends protections to those with normative expressions of gender and sexuality (Hunter, 2018). In this way, UK health and social care's policy and legislative context may only serve to mask structural inequalities, perpetuating a neoliberal idea of diversity that itself represents a shallow, depoliticised classification of difference. Indeed, it seems that attempts to deepen and broaden equality protections for gender and sexual diversity are stalled before meaningful change is proposed. For example, reforms were put on hold following a 3-year consultation period hoped to culminate in updates to legal frameworks in England, Wales, and Scotland (Hines, 2020). Reasons cited include concerns about implications for wider gendered policy and service delivery, as well as access to women's spaces. The act of stalling reform in the name of harm reduction can, however, be readily disputed with findings showing that LGBTQ+ people experience multiple disadvantages that lead to poor health and social care outcomes (Bachman & Gooch, 2018; LGBT Foundation, 2017).

There may be marked differences between the way in which LGBTQ+ and intersectional experiences of disability and mental illness are understood and supported by the medical and social models (Shakespeare, 2017). A social model of understanding problems related to being LGBTQ+, disabled, or mentally ill would hold that the problems are not inherent to the person, rather that they are created by a society that fails to appreciate gender and sexual diversity (Davis, 2017). A lack of co-ordination and communication between various health and social care systems can perpetuate both health and social care problems. LGBTQ+ people can be enabled rather than prevented from taking full part in the family life they desire by social care staff and systems that consciously seek to remove barriers for them. The responsibility of deconstructing decades of normative ideas relating to gender and sexual orientation should not fall on individual staff; rather, a co-ordinated approach to tackling inequalities is needed. This can be done in a manner that is inclusive of diverse gender and sexual identities by increasing communication between and understanding of the different roles that different agencies have in Charlie and Pete's lives.

IMPACT ON PEOPLE: SUPPORTING BEST PRACTICE

The case study and supporting evidence included within this chapter makes a strong case for a greater integration of health and social care services. Embedding principles of integrated care within health and social service organisations could be the key to addressing huge disparities in a wide range of health and social outcomes for LGBTQ+ people (WHO, 2016). Ensuring that LGBTQ+ people are supported and included by increasing service integration could improve mental and physical health and family and social life.

Fig. 26.1 demonstrates a systems-level example of how integrated care aligns with and can support LBGTQ+-inclusive practice.

In relation to the case study, best practice can be achieved by providing joined-up care and holistic support for the physical and mental health needs and family wishes that Charlie and Pete have. Where systems work together to ensure understanding and joined-up care, Charlie and Pete enjoyed better physical and mental health (Charles, 2022). Charlie's ability to undergo the assessment and matching processes to adopt a child could also be supported by clear and open communication about the facts of their medical history. The inclusion of contextualising

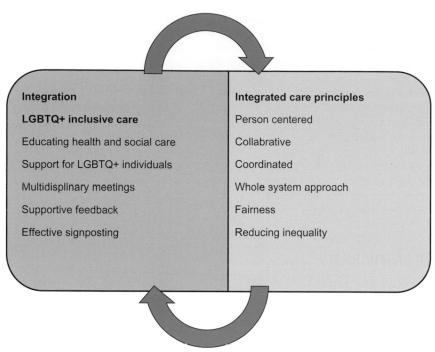

Integration	Integrated care principles
LGBTQ+ inclusive care	Person centered
Educating health and social care	Collabrative
Support for LGBTQ+ individuals	Coordinated
Multidisplinary meetings	Whole system approach
Supportive feedback	Fairness
Effective signposting	Reducing inequality

Fig. 26.1 Alignment of inclusive care and integrated care.

information regarding the impact that heterosexism and cisgenderism (the unfavourable treatment of those who diverge from expected sexual or gender norms) can have upon LGBTQ+ people's overall health and mental and emotional wellbeing could help adoption social workers understand the reasons behind a deterioration in health (Riggs et al., 2019). Indeed, a wider reconsideration of the way we respond to and produce gender and sexual norms within families could benefit a range of families. An understanding of the ways in which people are socialised into norms of masculinity and femininity can help us better support individuals and families (Roy & Allen, 2022).

More equitable care provision could have secondary positive impacts upon domains as divergent as finance and economics too (Bachman & Gooch, 2018; LGBT Foundation, 2017). Within the case study, Charlie and Pete could be more financially secure and have more available income to support a family if they did not have to self-fund gender-affirming medical treatments. Importantly, the needs of birth children and children needing homes via adoption could be better met by an integrated care system that supported their parent/carer. Although the implementation of co-ordinated care requires a change of cultural norms and established thinking, it is argued that joined-up care is essential to the physical and mental wellbeing of LGBTQ+ people and their families. Although it is beyond the scope of this chapter to detail best practice in relation to the range of health and social care services provided in the UK, it is highlighted that co-producing knowledge with trans and non-binary youth is an essential aspect of whole-family support for LGBTQ+ people (Carlile, 2020).

Where bias and prejudice exist in the system, we must challenge it. However, it must be acknowledged that not all bias is overt or conscious (Brown, 2021b). Professionals need to continuously examine their potential unconscious biases and motivators. This process can be supported by co-ordinated peer communication and support. In this way, care provision can be seen as a holistic and equitable process, supported by joined-up, preventative working. Integrated care provision can enable comprehensive, continuous, and long-term support for LGBTQ+ people. Professionals can work together to provide respectful and empowering care interactions that include those who are diverse in gender or sexuality. In doing so, it is imperative to continue developing the evidence base to improve care, drawing from co-produced knowledge (Marshall & Bamber, 2022). Shared accountability and whole-systems thinking is needed to enable LGBTQ+ people to challenge practice that fails to include them and encourages services to consider ethical dilemmas to promote health and social justice (Charles, 2022; WHO, 2016).

CONCLUSION

Health and social care staff and systems can work together to build a shared knowledge and understanding of LGBTQ+ people, as well as a co-ordinated approach to assessing and responding to their specific needs. Addressing tensions in the medical and social models' different approaches to LGBTQ+ people will be essential to the project of developing LGBTQ+-inclusive services that embody the Core Principles of Integrated Care (WHO, 2016). Furthermore, the role of co-production in inclusive research, policy, and practice is fore-fronted, as it is clear that experts by experience can provide important direction to health and social care organisations. There is an opportunity to rebuild systems, procedures, and policies using contemporary knowledge of LGBTQ+ peoples' lives to contribute to a more inclusive form of integrated care. It is hoped that in doing so, the public sector can embody an integrated care approach that includes and empowers LGBTQ+ voices and perspectives to inform ethical, respectful, and equitable practice.

References

Bachman, C. L., & Gooch, B. (2018). *LGBT in Britain: Trans report*. London: Stonewall.

Beaumount Society. (2018). https://www.beaumontsociety.org.uk/

Biblarz, T. J., & Savci, E. (2010). Lesbian, gay, bisexual, and transgender families. *Journal of Marriage and Family, 72*(3), 480–497. https://doi.org/10.1111/j.1741-3737.2010.00714.x

Brighton and Sussex University Hospitals NHS Trust (2021). *Support for trans and non binary people during pregnancy, birth and the postnatal period*. https://www.bsuh.nhs.uk/documents/support-for-trans-and-non-binary-people-during-pregnancy-birth-and-the-postnatal-period/

Brown, C. (2021a). Exploring trans people's experiences of adoption and fostering in the United Kingdom: a qualitative study. *International Journal of Transgender Health, 22*(1), 89–100. https://doi.org/10.1080/26895269.2020.1867396

Brown, C. (2021b). *EnGendering inclusive practice: exploring trans people's experiences of adoption and fostering in England and Wales* [PhD thesis, University of Sheffield].

Brown, C., & Rogers, M. (2020). Removing gender barriers: promoting inclusion for trans and non-binary carers in fostering and adoption. *Child & Family Social Work, 25*(3), 594–601. https://doi.org/10.1111/cfs.12731

Care Quality Commission. (2022, May 12). *Adult trans care pathway: what CQC expects from GP practices.* https://www.cqc.org.uk/guidance-providers/gps/adult-trans-care-pathway-what-cqc-expects-gp-practices-0

Carlile, A. (2020). The experiences of transgender and non-binary children and young people and their parents in healthcare settings in England, UK: interviews with members of a family support group. *International Journal of Transgender Health, 21*(1), 16–32. https://doi.org/10.1080/15532739.2019.1693472

Charles, A. (2022, August 19). *Integrated care systems explained: making sense of systems, places and neighbourhoods.* https://www.kingsfund.org.uk/publications/integrated-care-systems-explained

Coleman, E., Bockting, W., Botzer, M., Cohen-Kettenis, P., DeCuypere, G., Feldman, J., Fraser, L., Green, J., Knudson, G., Meyer, W. J., Monstrey, S., Adler, R. K., Brown, G. R., Devor, A. H., Ehrbar, R., Ettner, R., Eyler, E., Garofalo, R., Karasic, D. H. ... Zucker, K. (2011). Standards of care for the health of transsexual, transgender, and gender-nonconforming people, version 7. *International Journal of Transgenderism, 13*(4) 165–232. https://doi.org/10.1080/15532739.2011.700873

Coontz, S. (2003). Diversity and communication values in the family. *Journal of Family Communication, 3*(4), 187–192. https://doi.org/10.1207/S15327698JFC0304_2

Davis, C. (2017). Practice with transgender people. In G. P. Mallon (Ed.), *Social work practice with lesbian, gay, bisexual and transgender people* (pp. 42–65). Routledge.

Dragon, C. N., Guerino, P., Ewald, E., & Laffan, A. M. (2017). Transgender medicare beneficiaries and chronic conditions: exploring fee-for-service claims data. *LGBT Health, 4*(6), 404–411. https://doi.org/10.1089/lgbt.2016.0208

Equality Act. (2010). London: Stationery Office.

Galop. (2022). https://galop.org.uk/

Gender Recognition Act. (2004). London: Stationery Office.

Government Equalities Office. (2018). *National LGBT survey: Summary report*. London: Stationery Office.

Harvey, P., & Ingraham, N. (2021). LGBTQ+ family expansion in the age of COVID-19: a brief report. *Annals of LGBTQ Public and Population Health, 2*(2), 1–9. https://doi.org/10.1891/LGBTQ-2020-0046

Hicks, S. (2000). "Good lesbian, bad lesbian...": regulating heterosexuality in fostering and adoption assessments. *Child & Family Social Work, 5*(2), 157–168. https://doi.org/10.1046/j.1365-2206.2000.00153.x

Hicks, S. (2006). Maternal men—perverts and deviants? Making sense of gay men as foster carers and adopters. *Journal of GLBT Family Studies, 2*(1), 93–114. https://doi.org/10.1300/J461v02n01_05

Hines, S. (2013). *Gender diversity, recognition and citizenship: Towards a politics of difference*. London: Palgrave Macmillan.

Hines, S. (2020). Sex wars and (trans) gender panics: identity and body politics in contemporary UK feminism. *The Sociological Review Monographs, 68*(4), 699–717. https://doi.org/10.1177/0038026120934684

Horton, T., Hardie, T., Mahadeva, S., & Warburton, W. (2021). *Securing a positive health care technology legacy from COVID-19*. London: Health Foundation.

House of Commons Women and Equalities Committee. (2016). *Transgender equality: First report of session 2015–16*. London: House of Commons.

Hudson-Sharp, N. (2018). *Transgender awareness in child and family social work education*. London: Department for Education, National Institute of Economic and Social Research.

Human Fertilisation and Embryology Authority. (2022). *Information for trans and non-binary people seeking fertility treatment*. https://www.hfea.gov.uk/treatments/fertility-preservation/information-for-trans-and-non-binary-people-seeking-fertility-treatment/

Hunter, C. (2018). *The Equality Act 2010 and Empty Diversity: neoliberal legislation and inequality in the lives of trans and sexgender nonconforming people* [PhD thesis, London Metropolitan University].

Imborek, K. L., Graf, E. M., & McCune, K. (2017). Preventive health for transgender men and women. *Seminars in Reproductive Medicine, 35*(5), 426–433. https://doi.org/10.1055/s-0037-1604457

Jaspal, R., Nambiar, K. Z., Delpech, V., & Tariq, S. (2018). HIV and trans and non-binary people in the UK. *BMJ, 94*(5), 318–319. https://doi.org/10.1136/sextrans-2018-053570

Johnson, A. H., Hill, I., Beach-Ferrara, J., Rogers, B. A., & Bradford, A. (2020). Common barriers to healthcare for transgender people in the U.S. Southeast. *International Journal of Transgenderism, 21*(1), 70–78. https://doi.org/10.1080/15532739.2019.1700203

Kodner, D. L. (2009). All together now: a conceptual exploration of integrated care. *Healthcare Quarterly, 13*, 6–15. https://doi.org/10.12927/hcq.2009.21091

Kodner, D. L., & Spreeuwenberg, C. (2002). Integrated care: meaning, logic, applications, and implications – a discussion paper. *International Journal of Integrated Care, 2*(4), e12. https://doi.org/10.5334/ijic.67

Kressier, D. K., & Bryant, C. D. (1996). Adoption as deviance: socially constructed parent-child kinship as a stigmatized and legally burdened relationship. *Deviant Behavior, 17*(4), 391–415. https://doi.org/10.1080/01639625.1996.9968037

La Leche League G.B. (2022). *Support for transgender & non-binary parents*. https://www.laleche.org.uk/support-transgender-non-binary-parents/

Lampe, N. M., & Nowakowski, A. C. H. (2020). New horizons in trans and non-binary health care: Bridging identity affirmation with chronicity management in sexual and reproductive services. *International Journal of Transgender Health, 22*(1-2), 141–153. https://doi.org/10.1080/26895269.2020.1829244

LGBT Foundation. (2017). *Transforming Outcomes: A review of the needs and assets of the trans community*. Manchester: LGBT Foundation.

LGBT Foundation. (2018). *Pride in practice: Excellence in lesbian, gay, bisexual and trans healthcare*. Manchester: LGBT Foundation.

MacDonald, T., Noel-Weiss, J., West, D., Walks, M., Biener, M., Kibbe, A., & Myler, E. (2016). Transmasculine individuals' experiences with lactation, chestfeeding, and gender identity: a qualitative study. *BMC Pregnancy Childbirth, 16*, 106. https://doi.org/10.1186/s12884-016-0907-y

Marmot, M., Allen, J., Goldblatt, P., Herd, E., & Morrison, J. (2021). *Build Back Fairer: The COVID-19 Marmot Review*. London: The Health Foundation.

Marshall, K., & Bamber, H. (2022). Using co-production in the implementation of community integrated care: a scoping review. *Primary Health Care, 33*(1). https://doi.org/10.7748/phc.2022.e1753

Matsuno, E., & Budge, S. L. (2017). Non-binary/genderqueer identities: a critical review of the literature. *Current Sexual Health Reports, 9*(3), 116–120. https://doi.org/10.1007/s11930-017-0111-8

Mavuso, J. M.-J. J. (2021). Understanding the violation of directive anti-abortion counselling [and cisnormativity]: obstruction to access or reproductive violence? *Agenda, 35*(3), 69–81. https://doi.org/10.1080/10130950.2021.1949692

Mink, M. D., Lindley, L. L., & Weinstein, A. A. (2014). Stress, stigma, and sexual minority status: the intersectional ecology model of LGBTQ health. *Journal of Gay & Lesbian Social Services, 26*(4), 502–521. https://doi.org/10.1080/10538720.2014.953660

Monro, S., & Van der Ros, J. (2017). Trans and gender variant citizenship and the state in Norway. *Critical Social Policy, 38*(1), 57–78. https://doi.org/10.1177/0261018317733084

Motmans, J., Nieder, T. O., & Bouman, W. P. (2019). Transforming the paradigm of nonbinary transgender health: a field in transition. *International Journal of Transgenderism, 20*(2-3), 119–125. https://doi.org/10.1080/15532739.2019.1640514

New Family Social. (2022). *Who we are*. https://newfamilysocial.org.uk/nfs-who-we-are

Pearce, R. (2018). *Understanding trans health: Discourse, power and possibility*. Bristol: Policy Press.

Proud 2B Parents. (2022). *About us*. https://www.proud2bparents.co.uk/about

Riggs, D., & Bartholomaeus, C. (2018). Fertility preservation decision making amongst Australian transgender and non-binary adults. *Reproductive Health, 15*(1), 181–191. https://doi.org/10.1186/s12978-018-0627-z

Riggs, D. W., Pearce, R., Pfeffer, C. A., Hines, S., White, F., & Ruspini, E. (2019). Transnormativity in the psy disciplines: constructing pathology in the Diagnostic and Statistical Manual of Mental Disorders and Standards of Care. *American Psychologist, 74*(8), 912–924. https://doi.org/10.1037/amp0000545

Riggs, D. W., Pearce, R., Pfeffer, C., Hines, S., White, F. R., & Ruspini, E. (2020a). Men, trans/masculine, and non-binary people's experiences of pregnancy loss: an international qualitative study. *BMC Pregnancy and Childbirth, 20*(1), 482. https://doi.org/10.1186/s12884-020-03166-6

Riggs, D. W., Pfeffer, C., Pearce, R., Hines, S., & White, F. R. (2020b). Men, trans/masculine, and non-binary people negotiating conception: normative resistance and inventive pragmatism. *International Journal of Transgender Health, 22*(1-2), 6–17. https://doi.org/10.1080/15532739.2020.1808554

Roy, K. M., & Allen, S. H. (2022). Men, families, and the reconceptualization of masculinities. *Journal of Family Theory & Review, 14*(1), 28–43. https://doi.org/10.1111/jftr.1244116

Royal College of Psychiatrists. (2019). *Supporting transgender and gender-diverse people*. London: Royal College of Psychiatrists.

Schilt, K., & Westbrook, L. (2009). Doing gender, doing heteronormativity: 'gender normals', transgender people, and the social maintenance of heterosexuality. *Gender and Society*, 23(4), 440–464. https://doi.org/10.1177/0891243209340034

Serano, J. (2016). *Whipping girl: A transsexual woman on sexism and the scapegoating of femininity* (2nd ed.). Seal Press. Berkeley: CA: Seal Press.

Shakespeare, T. (2017). The social model of disability In L. J. Davis (Ed.), *The disability studies reader* (5th ed., pp. 195–203). Routledge.

Sterling, J., & Garcia, M. M. (2020). Fertility preservation options for transgender individuals. *Journal of Translational Andrology and Urology*, 9(2), 215–226. https://doi.org/10.21037/tau.2019.09.28

Stonewall. (2017a). *Glossary of terms*. https://www.stonewall.org.uk/help-advice/faqs-and-glossary/glossary-terms

Stonewall. (2017b). *LGBT in Britain: Hate crime and discrimination*. London: Stonewall.

Stryker, S., & Aizura, A. Z. (2013). *The transgender studies reader 2*. New York: Routledge.

Sue, D. W. (2010). *Microaggressions in everyday life: Race, gender, and sexual orientation*. Hoboken: John Wiley & Sons.

Tasker, F., & Lavender-Stott, E. S. (2020). LGBTQ parenting post-heterosexual relationship dissolution In A. E. Goldberg & K. R. Allen (Eds.), *LGBTQ-parent families: Innovations in research and implications for practice* (2nd ed., pp. 3–24). Springer.

Taylor, J., Zalewska, A., Gates, J. J., & Millon, G. (2018). An exploration of the lived experiences of non-binary individuals who have presented at a gender identity clinic in the United Kingdom. *International Journal of Transgenderism*, 20(2-3), 195–293. https://doi.org/10.1080/15532739.2018.1445056

Todd, K., Eastwood, J. G., Fotheringham, P., Salinas-Perez, J. A., & Salvador-Carulla, L. (2021). Using geospatial analysis to inform development of a place-based integrated care initiative: the Healthy Homes and Neighbourhoods experience. *International Journal of Integrated Care*, 21(2), 23. https://doi.org/10.5334/ijic.5430

Tyler, I. (2020). *Stigma: The machinery of inequality*. London: Zed Books.

Tyler, I., & Slater, T. (2018). Rethinking the sociology of stigma. *The Sociological Review*, 66(4), 721–743. https://doi.org/10.1177/0038026118777425

White, F. R. (2018). *Trans pregnancy: An international exploration of transmasculine practices of reproduction: Law and policy review: United Kingdom*. University of Westminster. London: University of Westminster.

Wood, K. (2016). 'It's all a bit pantomime': an exploratory study of gay and lesbian adopters and foster-carers in England and Wales. *British Journal of Social Work*, 46(6), 1708–1723. https://doi.org/10.1093/bjsw/bcv115

World Health Organization. (2016). *Integrated care models: an overview*. https://www.euro.who.int/__data/assets/pdf_file/0005/322475/Integrated-care-models-overview.pdf

World Professional Association for Transgender Health. (2012). Standards of care for the health of transsexual, transgender, and gender nonconforming people [7th Version]. https://www.wpath.org/publications/soc

Worthen, M. G. F., & Herbolsheimer, C. (2022). "Mom and dad = cis woman + cis man" and the stigmatization of trans parents: an empirical test of norm-centered stigma theory. *International Journal of Transgender Health*. https://doi.org/10.1080/26895269.2021.2016539

Further Reading

Brown, C. (2021b). *EnGendering inclusive practice: exploring trans people's experiences of adoption and fostering in England and Wales* [PhD thesis, University of Sheffield].

Brown, C., & Rogers, M. (2020). Removing gender barriers: promoting inclusion for trans and non-binary carers in fostering and adoption. *Child & Family Social Work*, 25(3), 594–601. https://doi.org/10.1111/cfs.12731

Hicks, S. (2000). "Good lesbian, bad lesbian...": regulating heterosexuality in fostering and adoption assessments. *Child & Family Social Work*, 5(2), 157–168. https://doi.org/10.1046/j.1365-2206.2000.00153.x

Hicks, S. (2006). Maternal men–perverts and deviants? Making sense of gay men as foster carers and adopters. *Journal of GLBT Family Studies*, 2(1), 93–114. https://doi.org/10.1300/J461v02n01_05

Pearce, R. (2018). *Understanding trans health: Discourse, power and possibility*. Bristol: Policy Press.

Wood, K. (2016). 'It's all a bit pantomime': an exploratory study of gay and lesbian adopters and foster-carers in England and Wales. *British Journal of Social Work*, 46(6), 1708–1723. https://doi.org/10.1093/bjsw/bcv115

27

Integrated Practice in Learning Disability

Dr Ruth Garbutt, Cindy-Leigh Fallows, Lucy Power, Georgia Thorpe, Kim Powell, and Lisa Lewis

KEY CONCEPTS

- Integrated practice in learning disability
- Person-centred practice
- Sharing information and working with others
- Transition from children's services to adult services
- Communication and communication aids
- The importance of respect and dignity

INTRODUCTION

This chapter looks at integrated practice in learning disability. Mencap defines a learning disability as:

'… a reduced intellectual ability and difficulty with everyday activities – for example household tasks, socialising or managing money – which affects someone for their whole life…. People with a learning disability tend to take longer to learn and may need support to develop new skills, understand complicated information and interact with other people.'

(https://www.mencap.org.uk/learning-disability-explained)

Many community learning disability teams in the UK follow an integrated approach. Typically, there could be the following professionals in a community learning disability team: psychiatrists, psychologists, physiotherapists, dietitians, occupational therapists, speech and language therapists, learning disability nurses, behaviour specialists, and social workers. Practice within a learning disability community team encourages all professionals to work together and to work with strong values.

This chapter will outline a fictional case study relevant to a community learning disability team. It will explore how this case study would be approached in an integrated way and some of the issues arising. The University of Salford delivers a unique degree, the BSc (Hons) Integrated Practice (learning disability nursing and social work). The authors of this chapter include academics from this integrated degree, learning disability practitioners who qualified from the integrated degree, parents, and people with learning disabilities. The information in the chapter comes from our own knowledge, understanding, and joint experiences in one specific region and might not be representative of wider experiences.

The key points from the case study that will be discussed are communication, transitions, and sexualised behaviour. This chapter will show the importance of an integrated approach for these three aspects.

FICTIONAL CASE STUDY

Background

Shane is a 16-year-old boy who lives at home with his mum and younger sister. Shane also spends two overnights weekly with his dad. Shane has a diagnosis of autism and severe learning disability. Shane is preverbal and communicates with photographs and visual symbols. Shane has a package with respite and receives one overnight stay, alongside 6 additional hours spread throughout the week.

Why Referred?

Shane has been referred to the learning disabilities nursing team for 'sexualised behaviour'. Shane is 'thrusting', particularly when receiving personal care. Shane's mum also said that Shane is hitting and scratching her at this time, and that this is usually on her face. She also thinks that Shane has anxiety and has recently started to withdraw from her. She has said that she notices every time Shane has a growth spurt or hair growth (e.g., moustache), he starts to thrust on her. She said it is 'tricky' to move Shane when he is thrusting on her and she is worried about him hurting his younger sister. She said that Shane is currently getting his pads changed in his bedroom and this can be challenging, due to Shane hitting and scratching his mum's face.

Where Next?

Since the referral to the learning disability nurse team, Shane will now be starting college (post 16) in 2 months. Direct observations are recorded via video camera to aid the assessment. Shane's parents felt that behaviours might not be seen if someone was in the same environment of the scene. This helped professionals to clearly identify a trigger for his behaviour. The learning disability nursing team have finished their assessment and analysis and have hypothesised that Shane's behaviours are due to:

- Sensory needs: Shane was thrusting due to hormonal influx.

- Social interaction: Shane wants to be independent and to communicate back his needs/wants.
- Expressing stress: Shane appears to be stressed due to transitioning into college and expresses stress because he is aware that he is leaving school, but he is not fully sure of where he is going, etc.

A one-page profile and an updated communication passport was made to help Shane have a smoother transition. This included reports from occupational therapy/speech and language therapy and was shared in all environments that Shane visits. An Assessment of Sexual Knowledge (ASK) was completed by the adult learning disability nursing team and shared with the children's learning disability nurse, occupational therapist, speech and language therapist, and all professionals involved. This included some strategies based around Shane's understanding of sexual needs and puberty. Shane transitioned well into college by using social stories and having photographs of the staff. Shane now uses visual symbols to ask when he wants his pad changed or have private time.

COMMUNICATION

A learning disability can affect the way people understand new and complex information which is being communicated to them. Some people may struggle to read and write, and some people may find it difficult to find the right words or verbalise what they want to say, and this can lead to frustration or disengagement from services. With this is mind, it is vital that all practitioners work together to ensure they are communicating in a way which is easily accessible and understood by the person they are working with.

It is noted in the case study that Shane uses photographs and visual symbols to communicate with others; therefore, all practitioners should have access to his communication passport which will describe in detail what visual resources he understands and how best to use them. Bunning (in Atherton & Crickmore, 2011) states:

'The point of a communication passport is to capture the unique, and sometimes subtle or idiosyncratic ways an individual communicates and represents this profile to the people who matter to the individual, for example, carers, teachers, support staff, GP etc.'

The communication passport, therefore, is a good example of a tool that can help to share information with other professionals and, in consequence, provide better care for an individual. This passport-style document is

usually created by a speech and language therapist who will carry out an in-depth assessment of the individual's communication methods.

Talking Mats can also be used as a communication tool, which could be especially useful when gaining Shane's wishes and feelings in relation to his care and support needs. Talking Mats is:

'... an interactive resource that uses three sets of picture symbols—topics, options and a visual scale ...'

(Murphy and Cameron, 2002, p. 8).

Talking Mats can be used to gain a better understanding of Shane's feelings around his personal care routine. The more information gathered, the more informed practitioners can be when carrying out their assessments. Easy-read resources can also be used when explaining complex health information such as bodily changes during puberty.

By making sure you can communicate effectively, you are giving the person the best chance to be at the centre of any decisions being made. This gives them greater choice and control over their situation and allows them to use their own voice to determine their support. By showing this level of respect, Shane will feel listened to and understood, empowering him to be able to make his own decisions. From talking to people who have a learning disability, it was acknowledged that showing a little bit of respect goes along way.

It is also important to keep channels of communication open between different fields of practice. Information needs to be shared and accessible to all practitioners through regular team meetings. It may often be the case that the person develops a good relationship with one particular practitioner who can then update the team effectively with what the person has communicated. This is important because when lots of different professionals are working with someone, the person may become overwhelmed or confused with all the different messages they are hearing. It is also acknowledged that not all practitioners have had training on what a learning disability is and how they can best support someone. Therefore, it is vital to take a team approach to the assessment process so that important pieces of information are not lost. It is only by creating a network of professionals around the person with a learning disability that they can easily tap into, that the person feels fully supported, as, for many people with a learning disability or autism, they may feel unsupported or misunderstood, commonly leading to feelings of isolation and helplessness.

TRANSITIONS

It is evident in current practice that there is a struggle for people with learning disabilities when they transition from children's services into adult services (NICE, 2016). Williams (2006) states:

'Transition can be a particularly complicated and stressful experience for a young person with learning disabilities and his or her family.' (p. 47)

The case study describes many challenges for Shane, and this shows how important it is to support a smooth transition for individuals with a diagnosis of a learning disability. This may not always be the case due to there being such a large age gap around the transition. This often requires a variety of different professionals to be involved, to share information, and ensure the individual is supported effectively.

Transitions start when the young person reaches the age of 16 and a full transition can take up to age 25, in accordance with the Children and Families Act (2014). This is because young people with learning disabilities still have an Educational Health Care Plan up until age 25. For example, there is children's social care and adult social care involvement at the same time, and they may work jointly with learning disability nurses, therapists, and other specialists. This may be done in multidisciplinary meetings where all professionals involved with working

with the individual should attend and discuss planning and how to avoid or prevent challenges that may occur for the person.

Health and social care services are often stretched, and therefore resources and funding become problematic. This often leads to longer waiting times for the individual or even missed information. It is crucial that services share information in an integrated way, and this should be done in a timely manner to help reduce waiting times and support the individual appropriately. This may also help to reduce safeguarding risks and prevent neglecting the individual/service user's needs.

Some information on supporting the individual can be shared through person-centred plans, one-page profiles, and care plans. This information should be reviewed and updated regularly, as and when required. People with learning disabilities should be supported to change their needs, dreams, and desires too.

Positive behaviour support plans are often a useful resource that provide evidence-based strategies to help promote independent skills, augment communication methods, and reduce behaviours of concern. This would be beneficial for Shane in the case study because he is preverbal. It might be possible for him to find an alternative way to present his current 'sexualised behaviour' in a safer way. Sharing all this relevant information not only shows respect and equality but also gives a voice to the person being supported by several professionals.

The importance of an integrated approach to transitions cannot be emphasised enough, as Williams (2012) states:

'While the personalised aspect of transition is essential, nevertheless, it's important that planners and managers in all agencies, take on individual information and plan ahead for services and supports ... however person-centred we become at an individual level, nothing will ever really change until there are systemic shifts, more resources, more opportunities and changes in attitude.' (p. 130)

SEXUALISED BEHAVIOUR

A clear issue that arises from the case study is the sexualised behaviour displayed by Shane. This is a key area for an integrated approach. It is important to note that sexualised behaviour might be seen differently depending on the professionals involved and on the service setting:

'What is unacceptable sexual behaviour for some, can be seen as positive by others'

(McCarthy & Thompson, 2010).

Since Shane has autism, a learning disability, and is pre-verbal, his behaviour could indicate numerous things, such as sexual urges, development of puberty, a 'nice feeling', frustration, expressing stress, and worries about changes in his life (e.g., college). However, if not addressed, he might think that his thrusting behaviour is acceptable and then he might then also do this with other people.

The case study states that he has been referred to a learning disability nursing team and that he has undertaken an ASK assessment. The ASK assessment is designed for a broad range of professionals to use. In the case study, the ASK assessment was carried out by the adult learning disability nursing team and shared with the children's learning disability nurse, occupational therapist, speech and language therapist, and all professionals involved.

From the outcome of this assessment, it was recommended that Shane should get some form of sex education that is appropriate for his needs and his level of understanding. An integrated approach to teaching sex education is important. It is very easy for each professional to assume another professional has the responsibility for teaching sex education and, as a result, a person can then end up with no sex education. Quite often, the parents might end up providing sex education to their son or daughter. However, parents often lack the confidence, training, and/or resources to do this effectively. The mother might worry that, by introducing her son to sex education, this might escalate his behaviour. As a professional, it is important to reassure parents that sex education will be less about teaching people to have sex and more about understanding boundaries, what is appropriate, public/private space, and understanding what is and is not abuse.

Good practice in relation to addressing sexualised behaviour with someone with a learning disability would involve using an integrated approach that had consistent communication between all the professions involved (including appropriate communication with the person themselves); having a service response/policy around addressing sexual needs that possibly outlines a process for staff to follow is also important. A holistic, person-centred practice is important, as Thompson (2000) states:

'... the ba sic point is quite a simple one really, namely the importance of treating people with respect—not treating them in a way that you would object to if other people treated you like that'.

Barriers to good practice can include pressure from the family to avoid addressing sexualised behaviour or sex education. There might also be concerns about risk, protection from harm, and wider societal attitudes. Williams (2012) states:

'Recognising people with learning disabilities as emotional and sexual beings is a challenge to many service providers and families.'

(Williams, 2012, p. 112).

It is important that, when addressing sexualised behaviour, all professionals work together to follow a clear, consistent approach and a respectful attitude, and that they plan ahead to offer appropriate information, education, and support.

IMPACT ON PEOPLE

The issues of communication, transitions, and sexualised behaviour identified in this chapter will impact on most people with learning disabilities and their families at some time.

Richardson (2011) states that:

'A range of values underpin the provision of good-quality support for people with learning disabilities.'

Richardson goes on to say that these values include human dignity, self-actualisation, person-centred approaches, working in partnership, and supporting families.

Historically, people with learning disabilities have tended to receive support in segregated services, based on a perception that all people with learning disabilities will fit into a generalised service. Person-centred approaches challenge this idea. Person-centred planning is:

'... a way of discovering what people want, the support they need and how they can get it. It is evidence-based practice that assists people in leading an independent and inclusive life. Person-centred planning is both an empowering philosophy and a set of tools for change, at an individual, a team and an organisational level. It shifts power from professionals to people who use services.'

(Department of Health, 2010)

A person-centred approach is rooted in the belief that people with disabilities are entitled to the same rights, opportunities, and choices as other members of the community (Department of Health, 2001). A person-centred approach puts the person with a learning disability at the centre of their own care and provides people with learning disabilities with choice and control. This, in turn, also helps the wider family to feel supported and valued.

There are numerous pieces of UK legislation and policy that support people with learning disabilities to have independent and dignified lives and exercise their human rights, such as the Human Rights Act (1998), The Equality Act (2010), Valuing People (2001), Valuing People Now (2009), and Putting People First: Personalisation/ Transforming Social Care (2007). These documents back up the need for a person-centred approach and for good integrated working.

This chapter has shown that the best way to support a person with a learning disability in relation to communication, transitions, and sexualised behaviour is for all professionals to work together and to see the person as an individual, with their own needs and wishes. Working within a person-centred approach will have an impact on the quality of life of a person with a learning disability and their family and carers.

CONCLUSION

This chapter has explored integrated practice in relation to people with learning disabilities. By using a case study, we have highlighted the importance of integrated practice in relation to communication, transitions, and sexualised behaviour. We have argued that much of the focus of good practice involves a person-centred approach in which the person with a learning disability is listened to and is empowered to have their own choices. Mencap states that:

'It's important to remember that, with the right support, most people with a learning disability in the UK can lead independent lives.'

(https://www.mencap.org.uk/learning-disability-explained)

Working in an integrated way is not unusual in community learning disability teams in the UK. Ultimately, an integrated approach can have a huge impact on the quality of life, the life chances, and even life expectancy of a person with a learning disability. At present, the life expectancy of people with learning disabilities is at least 15 to 20 years shorter than the general population, with a high proportion (36.9%) of deaths that could have been prevented with effective healthcare. Improving health services for people with learning disabilities, including mainstream hospital services and working in an integrated way, is a high priority for the UK government (Coppus, 2013). The Learning Disabilities Mortality Review Programme (LeDeR), which was established in 2016, was set up to review deaths of people with a learning disability, with the purpose of creating improvements in the quality of

health and social care for people with learning disabilities in England and to advise on best practice. The outcomes of the LeDeR reviews emphasise the importance of an integrated care system to improve services and address health inequalities experienced by people with learning disabilities. The review states that a more joined-up approach results in a better quality of life and reduces health inequalities for all people with learning disabilities.

This chapter has shown that learning disability awareness for all professionals is hugely important. Most professionals will come across a person with a learning disability in their work at some point, and an understanding of learning disability, including communication needs, is vital for the best outcomes for a person with a learning disability. One of the key themes in this chapter is the importance of respect. This includes having underpinning professional values emphasising dignity and respect.

The key message from this chapter is that all professionals who work with people with learning disabilities should work in an integrated way, as this results in better outcomes for people with learning disabilities and their families. Although working in an integrated way is not always easy, this chapter has shown how a community learning disability team, where numerous professionals work together as part of one team, provides a useful model for this to happen.

References

Children and Families Act (2014).

Coppus, A. M. W. (2013). People with intellectual disability: What do we know about adulthood and life expectancy? *Developmental Disabilities Research Reviews*, *18*(1), 6–16. https://doi.org/10.1002/ddrr.1123

Department of Health. (2001). *Valuing People: A new strategy for learning disability in the 21st century*. London: Stationery Office.

Department of Health. (2010). *Personalisation through person-centred planning*. London: Stationery Office.

Human Rights Act (1998).

McCarthy, M., & Thompson, D. (2010). *Sexuality and learning disabilities: A handbook*. West Sussex: Pavilion Publishing.

Murphy, J., & Cameron, L. (2002). *Talking Mats and learning disability: A low tech resource to help people to express their views and feelings*. Stirling: University of Stirling.

National Institute for Health and Care Excellence (NICE). (2016). *Transition from children's to adults' services for young people using health or social care services*. https://www.nice.org.uk/guidance/ng43

Putting People First: Personalisation/ Transforming Social Care (2007).

Richardson, M. (2011). Values-based support. In H. Atherton & D. Crickmore (Eds.), *Learning disabilities: Towards inclusion*. Elsevier.

The Equality Act (2010).

Thompson, N. (2000). *Understanding social work: Preparing for practice*. London: Macmillan.

Valuing People (2001).

Valuing People Now (2009).

Williams, P. (2006). *Social work with people with learning difficulties*. Exeter: Learning Matters.

Williams, V. (2012). *Learning disability policy and practice: Changing lives?* London: Palgrave Macmillan.

Further reading

Books

Atherton, H., & Crickmore, D. (2022). *Learning disabilities: Towards inclusion.* (6th ed.). Edinburgh: Elsevier.

Brown, M. (2002). *Learning disability: A handbook for integrated care*. Fivepin.

Jones, V., & Haydon-Laurelut, M. (2019). *Working with people with learning disabilities: Systemic approaches*. New York: Bloomsbury Academic.

Northway, R., & Hopes, P. (2022). *Learning disability nursing: Developing professional practice*. St. Albans: Critical Publishing.

Swanson, L., Harris, K., & Graham, S. (2013). *Handbook of learning disabilities.* (2nd ed.). New York: Guildford Press.

Williams, V. (2012). *Learning disability policy and practice: Changing lives?* London: Palgrave Macmillan.

Journal articles

Farrington, C., Clare, I. C. H., Holland, A. J., Barrett, M., & Oborn, E. (2015). Knowledge exchange and integrated services: Experiences from an integrated community intellectual (learning) disability service for adults. *Journal of Intellectual Disability Research*, *59*(3), 238–247. https://doi.org/10.1111/jir.12131

Sims, D. (2011). Achieving collaborative competence through interprofessional education: Lessons learnt from joint training in learning disability nursing and social work. *Social Work Education*, *30*(1), 98–112. https://doi.org/10.1080/02615471003748056

Slevin, E., Truesdale-Kennedy, M., McConkey, R., Barr, O., & Taggart, L. (2008). Community learning disability teams: Developments, composition and good practice: a review of the literature. *Journal of Intellectual Disabilities*, *12*(1), 59–79. https://doi.org/10.1177/1744629507083583

28

How to Implement an Integrated Care Approach to Reduce Falls and Fall-Related Injuries in People With Learning Disabilities

Dr Evangelia Petropoulou and Dr Lisa O'Leary

KEY CONCEPTS

- Falls and fall-related injuries in people with learning disabilities: incidence, modifiable and non modifiable risk factors, risk assessment
- Supported-living service providers: recorded and reported fall injury data
- Integrated practice in learning disability, health and social care integration
- Co-production and empowerment
- Social determinants of health

INTRODUCTION

People with learning disabilities now live longer, with the life expectancy of adults with mild learning disabilities approaching that of the general population (Patja et al., 2000). Although increased longevity is considered the fundamental measure of population health and wellbeing, it is still important to tackle the challenge of adding healthy and quality years onto their lives (Williams et al., 2020). This includes reducing the psychological impact that injuries and fall-injuries have on people with learning disabilities (Cahill et al., 2014; Finlayson et al., 2014) along with the consequences on physical activity and independence (Scottish Government, 2013).

Falls and fall-related injuries to older people in the general population have added significant costs to health and social care services. For example, in 2014–2015, more than £2 billion was spent on health and social care services. This was due to the cost of hip fractures of more than 250,000 older adults (over 65 years) living in England (Public Health England, 2017). Fall and fall-related injuries in older people can be particularly costly for community care. For example, a study undertaken in England by Tian et al. (2013) compared the care costs for older people before and after a fall incident. They reported that community care costs increased by 160% after a fall incident compared to social care costs and acute hospital care costs, which increased by 37% and 35%, respectively (Tian et al., 2013).

As in the general population, people with learning disabilities experience high rates of falls and fall-related injuries but at a younger age (Pal et al., 2014). A recent systematic review conducted by Ho et al. (2019) revealed that the mean age for falls amongst people with learning disabilities was much younger (47.6 years) in comparison to the general population, where falls are not identified as an issue until an older age (65 years). Falls and fall-related injuries are considered avoidable causes of frailty and death (NICE, 2013) which could be avoided by improving the quality of the health and social care received by service users.

SUPPORTING FALL REDUCTION

There is considerable heterogeneity in defining falls, with some definitions focusing on the presence of acute medical events, such as syncope and seizures, on contact with furniture or wall, or on behavioural aspects, such as accidental falls (Currie, 2008). The Prevention of Falls Network Europe (ProFANE) group defines a fall as *'an unexpected event in which the participant comes to rest on the ground, floor, or lower level'* (Lamb et al., 2005). This definition relates to falls that occur from all causes and it is widely accepted amongst researchers and practitioners in services for people with learning disabilities, as a high proportion of the service users are unable to offer reliable description of their injuries. In our case study, Duncan was found injured and lying on the floor without being able to explain what happened. This definition may enable people who care for or support Duncan to hypothesise that Duncan has just experienced a fall, so they can continue with monitoring and recording process of the event.

CASE STUDY

Duncan is a 52-year-old Scottish man with a mild learning disability. He has epilepsy, he is overweight, and wears glasses. Duncan lives in a supported-living group home with two other tenants, and he needs extra support in his daily life. Duncan is sedentary, spending most of the day in front of his computer or watching TV. He has only one sister, who lives 50 miles away, but she does not visit him that often.

Duncan was in the toilet when the support worker, Zoe, who was on a sleepover shift heard a thud at the door at 3:00 am. When Zoe went in, Duncan was lying on the floor behind his bathroom door following a fall, and potentially hitting the wall or handrail on the wall. Although conscious, he was not speaking initially, but after a few moments he responded by saying that his back was sore, and his eye was bleeding. The ambulance was called due to eye injury and Duncan was taken into the hospital. On examination, blood pressure was too high when Duncan was in a standing position. Duncan was kept in hospital for a day, as some of the medication that he was taking could make him feel dizzy. Zoe reported the incident immediately. She also stressed the importance of a referral, as Duncan was involved in another fall injury prior to this incident. He tripped over his rollator whilst walking from the kitchen to the living room. Duncan was walking unaided by his rollator. He was not wearing his glasses and the corridor was dark. Duncan had a graze to the left knee, and he complained of a sore right ankle.

Staff have raised concerns in relation to the increase in Duncan's number of falls (more than five) during the last 2 months. Duncan is reluctant to go outside or to engage in any type of physical exercise, as he fears that he will fall again. The support worker (Zoe) referred Duncan to a social worker, occupational therapist, physiotherapist, learning disability nurse, psychologist, and general practitioner (GP) for advice relating to this problem.

A multidisciplinary team meeting was organised to identify how an integrated care package could be developed to prevent another fall-related injury for Duncan. This comprised a support package and reasonable adjustments that could be implemented. Duncan and Zoe were invited to the meeting so that they could both advocate for Duncan's needs and wishes and so that they could contribute to co-producing this package.

It was identified that the GP could review the medication that Duncan was taking to identify if Duncan could take an alternative or lower dose of a specific medication to reduce the risk of dizziness side effects. Environmental safeguards were agreed upon to prevent Duncan experiencing harm from a fall in the future. All professionals agree that the lighting should be kept on in the corridor at night in Duncan's residence to reduce the risk of Duncan tripping in the dark. It was also identified that the occupational therapist should visit the residence and assess the environmental factors that might influence Duncan's risk of future fall. It was organised that the social worker would regularly visit Duncan to identify if there is any reduction in his incidence of falling. The occupational therapist and physiotherapist also agreed to assess Duncan's walking aid to see if he required an alternative to enable his mobility.

Duncan's fear of falling and his reluctance to go outside for exercise was explored by the psychologist. Duncan expressed that he would be willing to try to do exercise if he had more carer support with this and if the risks of him falling were reduced. He said that he used to like going to the local park for walks and to feed the ducks but that he would need two carers to walk on either side with him to protect him from falling. It was identified that Duncan should be supported to do this again following other measures to reduce his risk of falling outside (potentially change medication following review to avoid dizziness, only going for walks if it is bright outside, avoiding certain terrain).

Claire (who is Zoe's line manager and is the learning disability nurse on the team) indicated that resources and staff shortage had previously been a barrier to getting two staff on board to support Duncan with walks. Claire identified that she could provide organisational support in freeing up two support staff to initially go on a short walk every other day in the local park with Duncan. Following other measures such as recruitment of some more staff, this could potentially be increased. Other options of support that were discussed included informing Duncan's sister about the outcome of the meeting and inviting her to a follow-up meeting to see if she would be interested in supporting him on occasional walks. Duncan agreed to this. The physiotherapist also suggested some gentle exercises for Duncan to undertake inside to reduce his sedentary activity until he is comfortable going outside.

A written record of the issues that were discussed and agreed-upon action points was produced and shared amongst the professionals. This enabled professionals to share accountability and responsibility for avoiding incidences of falls and improving Duncan's capacity to engage in any form of physical activity. A date was established for a follow-up meeting to discuss the outcome of the actions in preventing fall related injuries for Duncan.

Data from several studies that have focussed on people with learning disabilities have suggested that the prevalence of falls among adults with learning disabilities (aged 20–80 years) ranges from 12.1% to 70% across different settings. These include studies undertaken in institutional and community settings (Chiba et al., 2009; Cox et al., 2010; Finlayson et al., 2010; Grant et al., 2001; Pal et al., 2014; Petropoulou et al., 2017; Salb et al., 2015; Smulders et al., 2013; Van Hanegem et al., 2014; Wagemans & Cluitmans, 2006). These studies are representative of various countries such as Australia, Canada, Germany, the Netherlands, New Zealand, Sweden, the UK, and the United States. Therefore, falls are common in people with learning disabilities, with 25%–40% experiencing at least one fall per year (Finlayson, 2018). This is similar to high rates of falls (around 30%) in older adults in the general population, but people with learning disabilities are experiencing falls and fall-related injuries at a younger age (Finlayson, 2018).

According to the World Health Organization (2008), a prevention strategy is considered effective when it reduces the risk of falling or the number of individuals who fall—measured as whether a person has any falls (or no falls) within a defined timeframe. For frequent fallers (three or more falls over 12 months) like Duncan in our case study, the risk of having an injury related to the fall is higher, as previous falls has been found to be a risk factor for further falls in adults with learning disabilities (Pal et al., 2014). The factors which contribute to falls are usually multifactorial and are commonly divided into demographic, medical, psychosocial/behavioural, and/or environmental according to many widely used models, such as Cwikel and Fried's model (1992). However, regarding adults with learning disabilities who have elevated levels of physical inactivity, poor physical fitness, and poor dietary habits, the inclusion of physical factors as well within the proposed models is considered as essential.

In this case study, practitioners or anyone else who supports or cares for Duncan should consider all factors that might have contributed to his falls. For example, some potential risk factors might be those listed in Table 28.1.

Indeed, many of these potential contributory factors for Duncan's falls have been found to be risk factors for falls in adults with learning disabilities, such as older age (Cox et al., 2010; Wagemans & Cluitmans, 2006), epilepsy (Finlayson et al., 2010), physical inactivity (Enkelaar et al., 2013), previous history of falls (Pal et al., 2014), and non-use of assistive equipment (Finlayson et al., 2010; Pal et al., 2014). Some of these factors (e.g., older age) are not modifiable, but some others are (e.g., being sedentary or fear of falling); when possible, these modifiable

TABLE 28.1 Potential Risk Factors	
Demographic:	Older age, living conditions, ethnicity
Medical:	Epilepsy, high blood pressure, level of learning disability, body mass index
Psychosocial/ behavioural:	Fear of falling, inactivity
Environmental:	Poor lighting
Physical:	Limited mobility, poor physical fitness

factors should be treated. In that sense, using risk assessment is a vital part of effective support for adults with learning disabilities. Accident-related injury prevention strategies should be based on appropriately collected and evaluated injury and fall-related injury data. It is also important to educate caregivers on these risk factors and strategies for preventing fall-related injuries such as fractures (Pope et al., 2021).

Organisational ethos and environmental support are fundamental to facilitate health promotion for people with learning disabilities (O'Leary et al., 2018; Vlot-van Anrooij et al., 2020). Contextual and environmental factors are also important to address in consideration of risk factors for falls and related injuries in people with learning disabilities. For example, Cahill et al. (2014) identified how a lack of external support to prompt, educate, and warn an individual about a fall can influence the risk of falls and fall-related injuries. Studies have recommended that fall prevention requires adoption of a multilevel approach. This approach would entail individual/carer education and construction of environmental support interventions for fall prevention (Cahill et al., 2014; Pope et al., 2021).

Health and social integration could facilitate this multilevel approach and thus facilitate prevention of fall and fall-related injuries amongst people with learning disabilities. There is a legal drive towards provision of integrated care in specific regions in the UK. For example, in Scotland, key legislation such as the Public Bodies (Joint Working) (Scotland) Act 2014 requires health and social care services to co-ordinate resources and share records and to provide person-centred care for individuals. This legislation requires health and social care services to collectively safeguard, empower, and advocate for the needs and wants of individuals with complex needs such as those with multiple/complex long-term conditions, disabilities, or frailties. This focus on safeguarding and advocating for the needs of potentially vulnerable individuals is also enshrined within other Scottish legislation, such as the Adult Support and Protection Act (2007) and Adults with Incapacity (Scotland Act) (2010).

Empowerment and co-production are central to integration, as health and social care organisations should collectively work with an individual and their families to build a healthcare package that is aligned with the individual's needs and wants. In the case of Duncan, this would require Duncan and Zoe working with the multidisciplinary team to co-produce a strategy to prevent prospective falls or fall-related injuries. This would also require Duncan and Zoe assuming authority and influence over the process of co-producing an accessible and easy-read version of the strategy (Chinn, 2017; Chinn & Pelletier, 2020).

The effective delivery of integrated and co-produced care is shaped by macro-level influences in the form of policy agendas and values and micro-level influences in the form of values and drive of organisation leaders (Chinn & Pelletier, 2020; Connolly et al., 2022). In Duncan's case, it would be vital to have support from Claire and higher management to ensure that integration and co-production is sustained in Duncan's case in relation to the prevention of falls and fall-related injuries.

In addition to the aforementioned, organisations who support adults with learning disabilities to live independently in community, residential, or institutional settings are required to routinely monitor and record all injuries experienced by people with learning disabilities to ensure care standards throughout their services (RIDDOR, 2013). This practice has been found to be particularly helpful in reporting and recording both minor and severe injuries (Petropoulou et al., 2017). Previous studies (Finlayson et al., 2010; Petropoulou et al., 2017) have shown that people

with learning disabilities experience high rates of 'minor' injuries, which can result in individuals losing confidence and developing fear of falling (Tian et al., 2013). Thus, it is important that all information about Duncan's injuries is electronically recorded by all providers who are involved in Duncan's care, so that an integrated approach is adopted to prevent prospective fall incidents and fall-related injuries. Also, it is important that Duncan is involved in co-producing this preventative strategy to ensure that he is fully empowered and involved in this strategy. Indeed, there is some evidence that individuals with learning disabilities (Eldeniz Cetin & Bozac, 2020; Gast et al., 1992; Ozkan, 2013; Spooner et al., 1989) are capable of being trained in and applying procedures for minor injuries, such as first aid for choking, minor burns or wounds, or insect bites. This highlights the need for the workforce to practice within an evidence-based framework, promoting an independent life for people with learning disabilities.

An example of a fall record and monitoring chart is shown in Table 28.2.

By using this kind of injury chart, practitioners and anyone who supports Duncan could identify potential risk factors for his falls based on repeated patterns. These factors may include whether Duncan is more likely to fall indoors than outdoors, what time of day they tend to occur at, if he falls mostly during a particular activity, and whether his injuries are severe or not, among others. It would also be important to design an accessible version of this chart. Duncan's input would also be required in co-designing and co-producing this accessible version, and this may require the chart to be adapted to the needs of an individual with a learning disability. Zoe's input would also be required to advocate for Duncan's need. This would facilitate a person-centred and inclusive approach to risk assessment of falls for Duncan.

TABLE 28.2 Fall Records and Monitoring Chart

Person Injured	Date	Time	Type of Injury	Cause of Injury	Part/s of Body Injured	Place	Hazard/s	Medical Attention	Description (of What Happened)
Duncan	3/3/22	1 pm	Graze	Trip/slip	Left Knee	Hall	Poor lighting/ Not wearing Glasses/ Not using assistive equipment	First-aid staff on site	
Duncan	8/3/22	3 am	Bruise	Falls	Eye Back	Bathroom	Seizure	Hospital	

IMPACT ON PEOPLE

The vast literature documenting the substantial risk of falls and fall-related injuries in people with learning disabilities throughout their lives demonstrates how vital it is for practitioners and carers to have an awareness of the seriousness of the problem, recognise the potential risk factors for falls, and work towards reducing and eliminating these risk factors to support people with learning disabilities to live safely and independently at home. The implementation of a shared electronic database to record and monitor falls and fall-related injuries across health and social care services could enable staff to accurately and promptly assess whether an individual is at risk of falling. This would enable them to respond appropriately by quantifying the risk with a risk assessment tool, followed by relevant preventative strategies. This, of course, requires macro- and micro-level influences to be in place, resulting in a well-trained staff who have the competency to provide accurate and quality data which consequently represent the high-quality service performance.

As described in this chapter, following an effective integrated approach to reduce falls in people with learning disabilities includes co-production so that the person's needs are met. Institutional support is required to ensure that people with learning disabilities and their advocates are empowered to influence and shape risk assessment strategies. Working with families and service users to develop a person-centred approach to reduce falls could provide long-term solutions and benefits, as it maximises the service user's engagement into the agreed-upon support and preventative plans and it also gives them power to make their own decisions.

CONCLUSION

This chapter explored the importance of providing an integrated care approach for people with learning disabilities who experience high rates of falls and fall-related injuries. Risk factors for falls and fall related injuries should be monitored at an early stage for people with learning disabilities, as they have a greater risk of falling at a younger age compared to the general population. In this chapter, an example of an integrated service delivery was discussed, focusing on the additional health needs that people with learning disabilities experience. This chapter highlighted the need for any assessment, intervention, and preventative strategy to be multifactorial. It is vital that health care staff in A&E and other departments collaborate with other services to not only treat people with learning disabilities for fall-related injuries, but also refer people with learning disabilities for management of risk factors. This would empower people with learning disabilities to take greater control of their health by encouraging preventative strategies and regular health checks to take place.

Given the high risk of falls in people with learning disabilities, further research is needed to add knowledge on their aetiology. Therefore, the relationship between fall injuries and intrinsic and extrinsic factors in this population requires further exploration, along with the development and implementation of fall-injury risk assessment tools tailored to this population. The implementation of effective prevention strategies based on a collaborative approach between health and social care sectors—as described in this chapter—could bring benefits not only for service users and their carers, but also for the services, as timely response to any potential falls is promoted.

References

Adult Support and Protection Act (2007).

Adult with Incapacity (Scotland Act) (2010).

Cahill, S., Stancliffe, R. J., Clemson, L., & Durvasula, S. (2014). Reconstructing the fall: individual, behavioural and contextual factors associated with falls in individuals with intellectual disability. *Journal of Intellectual Disability Research*, *58*(4), 321–332. https://doi.org/10.1111/jir.12015

Chiba, Y., Shimada, A., Yoshida, F., Keino, H., Hasegawa, M., Ikari, H., Miyake, S., & Hosokawa, M. (2009). Risk of fall for individuals with intellectual disability. *American Journal on Intellectual & Developmental Disabilities*, *114*((4), 225–236. https://doi.org/10.1352/1944-7558-114.4:225-236

Chinn, D. (2017). Learning how to be (a) patient: Visual analysis of accessible health information leaflets for people with intellectual disabilities. *Disability & Society*, *32*(10), 1485–1509. https://doi.org/10.1080/09687599.2017

Chinn, D., & Pelletier, C. (2020). Deconstructing the co-production ideal: Dilemmas of knowledge and representation in a co-design project with people with intellectual disabilities. *Journal of Intellectual & Developmental Disability*, *45*(4), 326–336. https://doi.org/10.3109/13668250.2020.1795820

Connolly, J., Munro, A., Macgillivra, S., Mulherin, T., Toma, M., Gray, N., & Anderson, J. (2022). The leadership of co-production in health and social care integration in Scotland: A qualitative study. *Journal of Social Policy*, 1–20. https://doi.org/10.1017/S0047279421000799

Cox, C. R., Clemson, L., Stancliffe, R. J., Durvasula, S., & Sherrington, C. (2010). Incidence of and risk factors for falls among adults with an intellectual disability. *Journal of Intellectual Disability Research*, *54*(12), 1045–1057. https://doi.org/10.1111/j.1365-2788.2010.01333.x

Currie, L. (2008). Fall and injury prevention. In R. G. Hughes (Ed.), *Patient safety and quality: An evidence-based handbook for nurses*. Rockville, MD: Agency for Healthcare Research and Quality. https://www.ncbi.nlm.nih.gov/books/NBK2653/.

Cwikel, J., & Fried, A. (1992). The social epidemiology of falls among community-dwelling elderly: Guidelines for prevention. *Disability and Rehabilitation, 14*(3), 113–121. https://doi.org/10.3109/09638289209165846

Eldeniz Cetin, M., & Bozak, B. (2020). The effectiveness of a training package prepared to teach first aid skills to individuals with intellectual and additional disabilities. *International Education. Studies, 13*(3), 27–42.

Enkelaar, L., Smulders, E., van Schrojenstein, H., Weerdesteyn, V., & Geurts, A. (2013). Prospective study on risk factors for falling in elderly persons with mild to moderate intellectual disabilities. *Research in Developmental Disabilities, 34*(11), 3754–3765. https://doi.org/10.1016/j.ridd.2013.07.041

Finlayson, J. (2018). Fall prevention for people with learning disabilities: Key points and recommendations for practitioners and researchers. *Tizard Learning Disability Review, 23*(2), 91–99. https://doi.org/10.1108/TLDR-06-2017-0026

Finlayson, J., Morrison, J., Jackson, A., Mantry, D., & Cooper, S.-A. (2010). Injuries, falls and accidents among adults with intellectual disabilities. Prospective cohort study. *Journal of Intellectual Disability Research, 54*(11), 966–980. https://doi.org/10.1111/j.1365-2788.2010.01319.x

Finlayson, J., Morrison, J., Skelton, D. A., Ballinger, C., Mantry, D., Jackson, A., & Cooper, S.- A. (2014). The circumstances and impact of injuries on adults with learning disabilities. *British Journal of Occupational Therapy, 77*(8), 400–409. https://doi.org/10.4276/030802214X14071472109833

Gast, D. L., Winterling, V., Wolery, M., & Farmer, J. A. (1992). Teaching first-aid skills to students with moderate handicaps in small group instruction. *Education and Treatment of Children, 15*(2), 101–124.

Grant, H. J., Pickett, W., Lam, M., O'Connor, M., & Ouellette-Kuntz, H. (2001). Falls among persons who have developmental disabilities in institutional and group home settings. *Journal on Developmental Disabilities, 8*(1), 57–73.

Ho, P., Bulsara, M., Downs, J., Patman, S., Bulsara, C., & Hill, A.-M. (2019). Incidence and prevalence of falls in adults with intellectual disability living in the community: A systematic review. *JBI Evidence Synthesis, 17*(3), 390–413. https://doi.org/10.11124/jbisrir-2017-003798

Lamb, S. E., Jørstad-Stein, E. C., Hauer, K., & Becker, C. (2005). Development of a common outcome data set for fall injury prevention trials: The Prevention of Falls Network Europe consensus. *Journal of the American Geriatrics Society, 53*(9), 1618–1622. https://doi.org/10.1111/j.1532-5415.2005.53455.x

National Institute for Health and Care Excellence (NICE). (2013). *Assessment and prevention of falls in older people.* Manchester: National Institute for Health and Care Excellence.

O'Leary, L., Taggart, L., & Cousins, W. (2018). Healthy lifestyle behaviours for people with intellectual disabilities: An exploration of organizational barriers and enablers. *Journal of Applied Research in Intellectual Disabilities, 31*(1), 122–135. https://doi.org/10.1111/jar.12396

Ozkan, S. Y. (2013). Comparison of peer and self-video modelling in teaching first aid skills to children with intellectual disabilities. *Education and Training in Autism and Developmental Disabilities, 48*(1), 88–102.

Pal, J., Hale, L., Mirfin-Veitch, B., & Claydon, L. (2014). Injuries and falls among adults with intellectual disability: A prospective New Zealand cohort study. *Journal of Intellectual & Developmental Disability, 39*(1), 35–44. https://doi.org/10.3109/13668250.2013.867929

Patja, K., Iivanainen, M., Vesala, H., Oksanen, H., & Ruoppila, I. (2000). Life expectancy of people with intellectual disability: A 35-year follow-up study. *Journal of Intellectual Disability Research, 44*(5), 591–599. https://doi.org/10.1046/j.1365-2788.2000.00280.x

Petropoulou, E., Finlayson, J., Hay, M., Spencer, W., Park, R., Tannock, H., Galbraith, E., Godwin, J., & Skelton, D. A. (2017). Injuries reported and recorded for adults with intellectual disabilities who live with paid support in Scotland: A comparison with Scottish adults in the general population. *Journal of Applied Research in Intellectual Disabilities, 30*(2), 408–415. https://doi.org/10.1111/jar.12244

Pope, J., Truesdale, M., & Brown, M. (2021). Risk factors for falls among adults with intellectual disabilities: A narrative review. *Journal of Applied Research in Intellectual Disabilities, 34*(1), 274–285. https://doi.org/10.1111/jar.12805

Public Bodies (Joint Working) (Scotland) Act 2014.

Public Health England. (2017). *Falls and fracture consensus statement: supporting commissioning for prevention.* London: Public Health England.

Reporting of Injuries, Diseases and Dangerous Occurrences Regulations (RIDDOR). (2013). *HMSO Statutory Instrument 2013 No. 1471.* London, UK.

Salb, J., Woodward, C., Offenhäußer, J., Becker, C., Sieber, C., & Freiberger, E. (2015). Prevalence and characteristics of falls in adults with intellectual disability living in a residential facility: A longitudinal study [PreFallID]. *Intellectual and Developmental Disabilities, 53*(3), 228–239. https://doi.org/10.1352/1934-9556-53.3.228

Scottish Government. (2013). *The keys to life. Improving quality of life for people with learning disabilities.* Edinburgh: Scottish Government.

Smulders, E., Enkelaar, L., Weerdesteyn, V., Geurts, A. C. H., & van Schrojenstein Lantman-de Valk, H. (2013). Falls in older persons with intellectual disabilities: Fall rate, circumstances and consequences. *Journal of Intellectual Disability Research, 57*(12), 1173–1182. https://doi.org/10.1111/j.1365-2788.2012.01643.x

Spooner, F., Stem, B., & Test, D. W. (1989). Teaching first aid skills to adolescents who are moderately mentally handicapped. *Education and Training in Mental Retardation, 24*(4), 341–351.

Tian, Y., Thompson, J., Buck, D., & Sonola, L. (2013). *Exploring the system-wide costs of falls in older people in Torbay.* London: King's Fund.

Van Hanegem, E., Enkelaar, L., Smulders, E., & Weerdesteyn, V. (2014). Obstacle course training can improve mobility and prevent falls in people with intellectual disabilities. *Journal of Intellectual Disability Research, 58*(5), 485–492. https://doi.org/10.1111/jir.12045

Vlot-van Anrooij, K., Koks-Leensen, M. C. J., van der Cruijsen, A., Jansen, H., van der Velden, K., Leusink, G., Hilgenkamp, T. I. M., & Naaldenberg, J. (2020). How can care settings for people with intellectual disabilities embed health promotion. *Journal of Applied Research in Intellectual Disabilities*, *33*(6), 1489–1499. https://doi.org/10.1111/jar.12776

Wagemans, A. M. A., & Cluitmans, J. J. M. (2006). Falls and fractures: A major health risk for adults with intellectual disabilities in residential settings. *Journal of Policy and Practice in Intellectual Disabilities*, *3*(2), 136–138. https://doi.org/10.1111/j.1741-1130.2006.00066.x

Williams, E; Buck, D, Babaloa G, Maguire, D. (2022). What are health inequalities?. https://www.kingsfund.org.uk/publications/what-are-health-inequalities.

World Health Organization. (2008). *WHO global report on falls prevention in older age*. Geneva: WHO Press.

Further Reading

Finlayson, J. (2016). *Injury and fall prevention for people with learning disabilities: Resource guide for people who care for or support people with learning disabilities*. https://agile.csp.org.uk/system/files/injury-and-fall-prevention-for-people-with-learning-disabilities-resource-guide.pdf

29

Severe Mental Illness and Integrated Care

Rachel Price

KEY CONCEPTS

- People experiencing severe mental illness experience challenges accessing and navigating health care.
- Individuals with a mental illness, especially those diagnosed with chronic and enduring mental health problems, experience a reduction in life expectancy of around 10 to 20 years compared with the general population.
- Over 16.5 million people in England, which amounts to 30% of the population, have been diagnosed with one or more long-term conditions. From this population, over 30% will also go on to develop a mental health problem, which is markedly higher than the prevalence rate in the general population (NCCMH, 2018).
- There has been a historical lack of parity of esteem between mental health service provision and physical health care.
- Stigma is a persistent barrier to people with mental health problems receiving care for physical health problems.
- The integration of mental health services into wider health and social care provision serves to address the disparity in life expectancy for people with chronic and severe mental illness, improves preventative health promotion activity, and serves to minimise the impact of long-term conditions on individuals and populations.

INTRODUCTION

In aiming to provide high-quality, sustainable, and effective integrated care for communities and populations, it is essential that consideration is made to the benefits this model of care can have on specific vulnerable groups. Certain populations have historically faced significant challenge in trying to access and navigate healthcare, and one of those groups that have historically been excluded from traditional care delivery models is those that experience severe mental illness (SMI).

It is widely recognised that, compared with the general population, individuals who experience SMI have poorer physical health outcomes and a reduction in life expectancy of around 10 to 20 years. Only a small proportion of these premature deaths can be attributed to causes such as suicide, homicide, or accident, with many early deaths being more likely to occur through comorbid physical health conditions that could be avoidable.

SMI refers to mental health problems that are debilitating to the extent that the individual experiences significant challenges in maintaining daily function and occupational activity. Conditions such as schizophrenia, psychosis, bipolar disorder, schizotypal delusional disorders, schizoaffective disorder, and other significant mood-related disorders are identified in the 10th edition of the International Classification of Diseases (ICD) as conditions which are classed as SMI.

The reasons behind poor physical health outcomes for people experiencing SMI are linked to this population experiencing a higher prevalence of obesity, asthma, diabetes, chronic obstructive pulmonary disease (COPD), chronic heart disease, heart failure, cancer, chronic kidney disease, and stroke. There are numerous factors that contribute to people experiencing SMI developing these potentially life-limiting conditions. Antipsychotic medication, which is often prescribed to treat the symptoms of the SMI, has the potential to increase the risk of stroke and sudden death and can prompt the onset of metabolic side effects. Known as metabolic syndrome, this complication not only leads to poor adherence to treatment and poorer clinical outcomes but also increases waist circumference, prompts the onset of fasting hyperglycaemia, dyslipidaemia, and elevated blood pressure (Carli et al., 2021).

Lifestyle factors also contribute to the onset of comorbid physical illness and disease for people experiencing SMI. Cardiometabolic risk factors are increased in this population through poor diet, physical inactivity, substance misuse, and smoking. Additionally, people experiencing SMI are more likely to experience unemployment, poverty, deprivation, and financial inequality—all factors that can exacerbate poor mental health and prompt the onset of physical health problems and disease.

The complex nature, symptoms, and prognosis of SMI leads to the individual experiencing significant difficulties in motivation, concentration, energy, and the volition to self-manage physical health problems. Consequently, this may lead to low attendance at medical appointments, poorer adherence to medication and treatment plans, and an increase in adverse health behaviour such as smoking, poor diet, and lack of engagement in physical exercise. It is of little surprise that comorbid physical health conditions are frequently developed within this population and higher rates of hospitalisation and use of health services are prevalent.

Additional consideration needs to be made to people experiencing long-term physical health problems as evidence correlates that people experiencing poor physical health, particularly individuals with multiple physical health comorbidities, are more likely to develop significant and enduring mental health problems (Naylor et al., 2016; Stafford et al., 2018). Even with the knowledge that people with SMI are more likely to experience physical health comorbidities, the mortality rate remains persistently higher than that experienced by the general population. This presents an ongoing challenge for service providers and commissioners across the health and social care sector in trying to reduce this gap.

Accessing healthcare remains challenging for people with SMI and the reasons for this are explored in the following.

STIGMA

The stigmatisation of mental illness is a century-old problem and is far more prolific compared to other health conditions. Mental health stigma continues to be prevalent in modern-day society and creates significant barriers for this population to access healthcare. Stigma in mental illness arises in two main forms: public stigma refers to the endorsement of negative stereotypes by communities and society and self-stigma arises when an individual internalises these negative stereotypes.

People experiencing mental illness have commonly reported that they feel dehumanised and dismissed by healthcare professionals who they may encounter. Key elements of these negative experiences relate to feeling excluded, receiving subtle or overt threats to comply with treatment, being made to wait excessively long for help, not being given information about their care or treatment, being treated in a paternalistic manner, being excluded from treatment because of their mental health diagnosis, or being spoken to in a demeaning or stigmatising way (Knaak et al., 2017).

These issues will impact on the individual experiencing mental health problems in seeking health-improving opportunities and encourages reluctance in seeking help. Treatment and health-improving interventions may often be terminated early because of the lived experience of stigmatisation. Another consideration is that people experiencing mental illness have often cited that physical health symptoms are mistakenly attributed to their mental illness and that they do not feel their health issues are taken seriously. This is referred to as diagnostic overshadowing (Thornicroft, 2011) and, consequently, the individual will avoid or limit contact with physical health services as they feel ignored and excluded.

CASE STUDY 1   Stockport Together

Stockport Together in the northwest of England is a partnership of five health and social care organisations that work collaboratively to meet the health and social care needs of the population in Stockport, Greater Manchester. As a multispecialty provider, this alliance developed Stockport Neighbourhood Care with the aim of delivering integrated care to communities to improve life expectancy and reduce health inequality. Eight neighbourhood teams were developed in the locality with the aim of moving care closer to home, supporting residents of the borough to adopt healthier lifestyles, and reduce the impact of ill health through multidisciplinary service provision.

This development highlighted a significant role for registered mental health nurses and mental health support workers to be co-located within the neighbourhood teams. The mental health professionals support the early identification of residents experiencing mental health problems and provide early assessment and interventions to improve outcomes not only in mental health but with physical health. The benefits of having mental health nurses and mental health support workers co-located with social workers, district nurses, GPs, and other health and social care agencies ensures that care for individuals experiencing mental illness is not fragmented and physical health needs are not overlooked.

When addressing the need for mental health professionals to be included in integrated care teams, an important factor to address is that the multifaceted and complex nature of stigma can be experienced by mental health professionals through affiliated stigma. Professionals working in mental healthcare can experience stigmatisation from other organisations and professions because of associating and working with people experiencing SMI, which can lead to this professional group being undervalued and discredited.

A manifestation of this is how mental health nurses are not viewed by some as 'proper nurses', that their role is often difficult to explain ('all you do is drink tea and chat with patients'), demeaning comments about the choice of profession such as 'don't you have to be a bit mad to work with those kinds of patients' have been made, and professional contributions relating to patient care and management are disregarded. Consequently, this affiliated stigma not only undermines the mental health profession, but it can also have consequences on patient care. If such a negative view is held of the mental health professional, then what views will there be on the needs of those needing mental healthcare?

PARITY OF ESTEEM

In the last decade, there has been an increasing emphasis in the UK in ensuring individuals experiencing mental illness have the same access and opportunity to mental healthcare as physical healthcare. This concept seeks to demonstrate a parity of esteem, where value is placed equally on mental health conditions as they are on physical health conditions.

Enshrined in law since the introduction of the Health and Social Care Act in 2012, it is recognised that mental health must be given equal priority as physical health. However, this aim has not been fully realised, with mental health funding being 13% of the total NHS spending while the burden of disease is significantly higher. To put this in context, 5.5% of the UK's health research budget contributes to mental health; in contrast, cancer research is four times higher at 19.6%. This equates to £1,572 per cancer patient in research funding compared to £9.75 per adult with a mental health problem (MQ Mental Health, 2021).

Parity of esteem can be viewed through a patient perspective by health standards being equal in physical and mental health when accessing services, a provider's perspective where care is delivered with an equal focus on mental and physical health, and from a funding standpoint where service should be commissioned to enable equal resource allocation to mental and physical healthcare. The publication of the NHS *'Five Year Forward View'* (NHS, 2014) included a goal of ensuring equal regard and parity of esteem was achieved by 2020; however, with investment not going far enough to reverse years of chronic underfunding in mental health services, and workforce retention and recruitment being in decline as demand for services increases, the goal of achieving parity of esteem so that people with mental health problems can access the same care and services in comparison to those with physical health problems remains some distance away.

INEQUALITIES IN MEDICAL CARE FOR PEOPLE EXPERIENCING SMI

Mass screening programmes serve to identify people in health populations who are at higher risk of disease and illness so that early intervention can be offered to reduce the impact and the mortality associated with the condition under review. In mammography screening, for example, evidence has demonstrated that women with SMI are less likely than women in the general population to access screening appointments. This may be attributed to people experiencing SMI requiring more support to attend appointments, members of this population not being registered with a GP, or those in long-term care not being eligible or supported to access screening services.

People with SMI are more likely to have periodontal problems than the general population. Higher rates of smoking, higher intake of sugar, poor dental hygiene, cost implications, medication side effects, anorexia and other eating disorders, in addition to anxiety and phobic disorders result in people with SMI being three times more likely to lose teeth than the general population (Kisley, 2016).

Medical and surgical care can also be inequitable for people experiencing SMI. In primary care, people with a diagnosis of schizophrenia are less likely to have a record of cardiovascular disease and diabetes, may have low engagement and adherence to treatment plans, and a lack of clinician's knowledge or confidence in supporting people with SMI may compromise medical care for this population. Postoperative outcomes and longer hospital admissions are less favourable for people with a diagnosis of SMI and this has been correlated with stigma, challenges negotiating complex health systems, and a lack of knowledge about psychiatric medication and the interactions with anaesthesia, in addition to people with SMI feeling uncomfortable or unable to speak openly about their mental illness in a physical health setting (McBride et al., 2021).

The COVID-19 pandemic has raised many issues when it comes to people experiencing SMI. Research has highlighted that this vulnerable group were five times more likely to die from COVID-19 and three times more likely to require hospitalisation. This has been linked to this cohort experiencing preexisting comorbid physical health problems and being at greater risk of experiencing complications from diseases that can impact on immunity (Lee et al., 2020; Nemani et al., 2021; Wang et al., 2020). However, this only partially explains the high mortality rate, and factors such as age, gender, ethnicity, lifestyle, and access to physical health services have also played a part.

The COVID-19 pandemic has led to people who experience SMI facing new challenges in navigating healthcare. Numerous services moved to online appointments and telehealth became the predominant way of accessing care. Consequently, people experiencing SMI, who are already widely recognised as being digitally excluded (Spanakis et al., 2021), potentially experienced even more barriers in accessing healthcare than those in the general population.

The presence of mental health professionals in the integrated care team can ensure care and access to services are inclusive and a priority should be made to not only ensure people with SMI have their physical and mental health needs assessed but that they are supported to navigate healthcare systems and obtain support to maintain this engagement.

THE ROLE OF INTEGRATION IN IMPROVING HEALTH OUTCOMES IN SMI

With evidence widely recognising that some primary care providers and non-mental health specialities experience reluctance or challenges when engaging with individuals experiencing SMI, the integration of mental health services into multispeciality provider services is a priority.

As detailed already, there are significant barriers in place that impact on the health outcomes for individuals with SMI and in commissioning mental health professionals to be part of the integrated team, which would support inclusion for vulnerable members of society whose health outcomes are significantly compromised.

Mental health practitioners have a unique skill set that other health professionals may find difficult to articulate. Often, the mental health practitioner can utilise communication and engagement strategies that may be unfamiliar to healthcare providers who have a greater understanding of the biomedical model to deliver care. Mental health practitioners are often able to engage with individuals that have previously not been able to connect with services or who may, because of the nature of the SMI, be reluctant to seek out help. Advocacy plays a significant role in the delivery of effective mental healthcare and these skills can be easily transferred to working within other healthcare settings. The mental health professional can perform the role of a navigator in such circumstances to support the individual with SMI to negotiate the pathways and potential obstacles that may present when they are attempting to access care.

Another valuable component of the mental health professional is their understanding of biopsychosocial approaches to care and how clinical recovery should be substituted for personal recovery (Damsgaard & Angel, 2021). The nature and prognosis of SMI means that focus should be shifted away from the paradigm of cure and rapid stabilisation to one more focused on supporting recovery that has the potential to lead to quality of life and personal recovery.

Psychoeducation plays a significant role in supporting people experiencing SMI, and the mental health professional can not only address the psychological dimension of health but can also support people experiencing SMI to become more empowered to manage their physical health. In this context there is also a reciprocal benefit to the mental health professional working within an integrated team. Provision of learning and education to non-mental health professional groups about mental illness, symptoms, and management is beneficial in reducing stigma and improving health outcomes, and shared development of treatment and care plans ensures there is a parity of esteem. A collaborative multidisciplinary approach to meeting the needs of an individual with an SMI will also help mental health practitioners develop wider knowledge about physical health problems, thus ensuring a more holistic approach to how care is organised and delivered.

A significant challenge that needs to be highlighted relates to the national shortage of psychiatrists and mental health nurses in the UK. The Royal College of Psychiatrists in October 2021 stated that 1 in 10 consultant psychiatrist posts are unfilled, which means there is 1 consultant psychiatrist per 12,567 people in the UK. The mental health nursing profession is also facing significant challenges with more registered mental health nurses leaving the profession than joining it. Twenty percent of all vacant nursing positions in the NHS are in mental healthcare.

It is evident that, for integration to be effective in addressing the needs of people with SMI and to improve physical health outcomes, mental health staff must be actively engaged in developing and delivering integrated care services, and there also must be a larger overview and evaluation of education, training, recruitment, and retention of these valuable practitioners.

CASE STUDY 2   James*

James* is a 68-year-old gentleman with a longstanding diagnosis of schizophrenia. James was involved in a road traffic accident where he was knocked off his bike and sustained a right leg fracture and a dislocated shoulder. James was admitted to hospital for 3 weeks and a referral was made to the community neighbourhood team for follow-up. The hospital discharge notification cited that James would require follow-up as he had been 'non-compliant' with physiotherapy in the ward and there was a possibility he would need a long-term care placement on discharge.

The referral to the neighbourhood team was discussed in the multidisciplinary referral meeting where a mental health nurse, mental health support worker, and physiotherapist began working with the hospital team to plan discharge. The initial visit by the mental health nurse highlighted that James had longstanding paranoid and delusional ideas about people he was unfamiliar with, and he had lost a significant amount of weight on the ward as he believed the ward staff were poisoning his food. The symptoms of his SMI had resulted in James being perceived as a 'difficult' and 'challenging' patient and, consequently, fewer attempts were made in the hospital setting to engage James with discussions about his care. The lack of engagement in ward-based activity and treatment was due to James' ongoing symptoms from the diagnosed SMI and the mental health nurse was able to explain this to the ward staff and physiotherapist. The physiotherapist and

mental health support worker were able to escort James home for a visit prior to discharge and here it was identified that James had experienced difficulties in maintaining independent living and self-care prior to the accident.

A decision was made by James to go into a community intermediate-care placement for a period of 3 weeks whilst he was supported with mobility, nutrition, and weight gain and had his psychiatric medication reviewed. This period enabled James to work with the physiotherapist, mental health nurse, and mental health support worker to maximise his physical and mental health for him to reach a level of recovery which he had identified would enable him to return to independent living. Having the support available enabled James to develop a therapeutic relationship with the mental health staff and the physiotherapist; they were able to work together to not only improve his mobility and mental and physical health, but James was also able to obtain support with his finances and social activity and was registered with a GP for the first time in 8 years. James was able to resume living independently with ongoing support from the GP and the community mental health team and did not require placement in long-term care. The transition from hospital to home with the support from the integrated care team ensured that James' physical, social, and mental health needs were addressed, and he was given the opportunity to remain independent within his local community.

*In line with adhering to strict guidance on patient confidentiality all names and identifying markers have been anonymised and a pseudonym used as per the standards set out in the Nursing and Midwifery Council (2018).

IMPACT ON PEOPLE

Incorporating mental health professionals into the integrated team has many benefits, including supporting wider health professional groups to understand how to provide care for people experiencing distress and mental illness across the life course, improve the visibility of mental health problems in the population and support this vulnerable group to navigate health improvement opportunities, the ability to demonstrate an understanding of the pathophysiology of illness and disease and provide education about how SMI can impact on physical health assessment and treatment, and to implement evidence-based screening, assessment, and treatment which are consequently underpinned by relationship-based problem-solving and patient empowerment.

The presence of mental health nurses in integrated care teams has the potential to influence care outcomes and have a positive impact on the care economy. As previously

highlighted, people experiencing SMI can find it difficult to engage in healthcare, screening opportunities, and may not be afforded the same health opportunities as the general population. Consequently, physical health conditions develop and progress undetected, requiring more intensive and resource-consuming interventions that weigh a heavier burden on health and social care economies.

CONCLUSION

People experiencing SMI have higher mortality rates than the general population and this inequality can be addressed with better collaboration and the integration of mental health professionals into community healthcare services.

Mental health professionals can transform traditional models of care by engaging in the integration process and demonstrate innovative and evidence-based care that ultimately supports the needs of individuals with SMI to access timely and responsive healthcare.

Commissioners of services have an obligation to recognise the value of mental health specialists in integrated teams and there needs to be funding made available to ensure mental health services are resourced adequately to demonstrate parity of esteem when integrated services are being developed.

Improving the physical health of people experiencing SMI is a priority so that the mortality rates prevalent for this vulnerable group can decrease. Improving care for vulnerable populations through the delivery of integrated care provides a real opportunity for care to be co-ordinated and a greater awareness of the challenges facing people experiencing SMI to be addressed. Collaboration between health and social care providers through a model of integrated working demonstrates that there is an opportunity for inclusion and for people with SMI to remove the historical disconnect between physical healthcare providers and mental health services.

Often, people experiencing SMI will have complex physical and mental health needs. When attempts are made to manage these in isolation, the impact on the individual and their opportunity to regain a sense of recovery is reduced by a fragmented approach in meeting their healthcare needs. Breaking down the barriers and viewing mental health services as a valuable contributor to the integration agenda continues to be challenging as there remain many obstacles to overcome, some of which have been highlighted in this chapter.

WHAT IS NEXT?

Underfunding, parity of esteem, stigma, and health inequality has long been associated with SMI, and the high mortality rates that continue to prevail in this population demonstrate that there is much to be done in ensuring this vulnerable population receive healthcare that is meaningful and improves quality of life.

Integrated care provision is one way that inequalities in health experienced by people living with SMI can be addressed; however, for this to be demonstrated effectively there is an ongoing need for investment in recruitment and retention of experienced mental health professionals. A second challenge is for commissioners of integrated services to ensure mental health services are viewed as equal partners in service development rather than perceived as an added luxury for existing integrated teams. It is essential that parity of esteem for both mental health and physical health is reflected in the organisational structure from the outset.

Integrated care has the potential to work in meeting the unmet needs of people experiencing SMI and reducing excessive mortality; however, much more is needed in terms of investment, inclusion, research, training, advocacy, and challenging the stigma associated with SMI for this model of healthcare to benefit this vulnerable population.

References

Carli, M., Kolachalam, S., Longoni, B., Pintaudi, A., Baldini, M., Aringhieri, S., Fasciani, I., Annibale, P., Maggio, R., & Scarselli, M. (2021). Atypical antipsychotics and metabolic syndrome: From molecular mechanisms to clinical differences. *Pharmaceuticals*, *14*(3), 238. https://doi.org/10.3390/ph14030238

Damsgaard, J. B., & Angel, S. (2021). Living a meaningful life while struggling with mental health: Challenging aspects regarding personal recovery encountered in the mental health system. *International Journal of Environmental Research and Public Health*, *18*(5), 2708. https://doi.org/10.3390/ijerph18052708

Health and Social Care Act (2012).

Kisley, S. (2016). No mental health without oral health. *Canadian Journal of Psychiatry*, *61*(5), 277–282. https://doi.org/10.1177/0706743716632523

Knaak, S., Mantler, E., & Szeto, A. (2017). Mental illness related stigma in healthcare: Barriers to access and care and evidence-based solutions. *Healthcare Management Forum*, *30*(20), 111–116. https://doi.org/10.1177/0840470416679413

Lee, S. W., Yang, J. M., Moon, S. Y., Yoo, I. K., Ha, E. K., Kim, S. Y., Park, U. M., Choi, S., Lee, S.-H., Ahn, Y. M., Kim, J.-M., Koh, H. Y., & Yon, D. K. (2020). Association between mental illness and COVID-19 susceptibility and clinical outcomes in South Korea: A nationwide cohort study. *Lancet Psychiatry*, *7*(12), 1025–1031. https://doi.org/10.1016/s2215-0366(20)30421-1

McBride, K. E., Solomon, M. J., Lambert, T., O'Shannassy, S., Yates, C., Ibester, J., & Glozier, N. (2021). Surgical experience for patients with serious mental illness: A qualitative study. *BMC Psychiatry*, *21*(1), 47. https://doi.org/10.1186/s12888-021-03056-x

MQ Mental Health. (2021). *Strategy document: UK mental health research funding 2014–2017*. London: MQ Mental Health.

National Collaborating Centre for Mental Health [NCCMH]. (2018). *The Improving Access to Psychological Therapies (IAPT) pathway for people with long-term physical health conditions and medically unexplained symptoms. Full implementation guidance*. London: National Collaborating Centre for Mental Health.

Naylor, C., Das, P., Ross, S., Honeyman, M., Thompson, J., & Gilburt, H. (2016). *Bringing together physical and mental health: A new frontier for integrated care*. London: King's Fund.

Nemani, K., Li, C., Olfson, M., Blessing, E. M., Razavian, N., Chen, J., Petkova, E., & Goff, D. C. (2021). Association of psychiatric disorders among patients with COVID-19. *JAMA Psychiatry*, *78*(4), 380–386. https://doi.org/10.1001/jamapsychiatry.2020.4442

NHS England (2014). *Five Year Forward View*. London: Stationery office.

Nursing and Midwifery Council. (2018). The code: Professional standards of practice and behaviour for nurses, midwives and nursing associates. London: NMC.

Spanakis, P., Peckham, E., Mathers, A., Shiers, D., & Gilbody, S. (2021). The digital divide: Amplifying health inequalities for people with severe mental illness in the time of COVID-19. *British Journal of Psychiatry*, *219*(4), 529–553. https://doi.org/10.1192/bjp.2021.56

Stafford, M., Steventon, A., Thorlby, R., Fisher, R., Turton, C., & Deeny, S. (2018). *Understanding the health care needs of people with multiple health conditions*. London: The Health Foundation.

Thornicroft, G. (2011). Physical health disparities and mental illness: The scandal of premature mortality. *British Journal of Psychiatry*, *199*(6), 441–442. https://doi.org/10.1192/bjp.bp.111.092718

Wang, Q. Q., Xu, R., & Volkow, N. D. (2020). Increased risk of COVID-19 infection and mortality in people with mental disorders: Analysis from electronic health records in the United States. *World Psychiatry*, *20*(1), 124–130. https://doi.org/10.1002/wps.20806

30

Integrated Care Within 0–19 Services in the UK

Miriam Collett

KEY CONCEPTS

- **School Nursing:** The role of the school nurse in the UK, how they work with families, schools, and local communities.
- **Health Visiting:** The role of health visitors in the UK, how they work with families, wider services, and local communities.
- **Extended Role:** School nurses or health visitors who have completed additional training to work in the opposite field of practice (e.g., a school nurse who extended their role into health visiting).
- **Healthy Child Programme:** The history of the Healthy Child Programme and the introduction of 0–19 in the 2016 delivery model (updated in 2021).
- **0–19 Services:** The inception and purpose of 0–19 services, including benefits and barriers to a more integrated service.

INTRODUCTION

Setting the Scene for Health Visiting and School Nursing in the UK

Health visitors were first employed in the UK in 1862 in Salford, England. Their role focused on visiting homes in areas of high deprivation, advising mothers on maternal and infant health, basic hygiene, and nutrition (Billingham et al., 1996). School nursing has its beginning in the UK in 1892, when Queen's Nurse Amy Hughes visited schools in London to give advice around nutrition. During her visits, she noted that children were suffering from untreated diseases and ailments, consequently offering advice and treatment (Schwab & Gelfman, 2005). Both professions have their roots in reducing health inequalities and improving the health of those in poverty. Over 100 years later, the two professions retain their public health roots and are now even more aligned, both being registered with the Nursing and Midwifery Council (NMC) as specialist community public health nurses (SCPHNs). The roles complement each other in their provision of universal and targeted healthcare to children; the health visitors leading for 0- to 5-year-olds, and school nurses for 5- to 19-year-olds (Public Health England (PHE), 2021). The roles continue to focus on reducing health inequalities through working with parents, carers, and young people, offering health education and support in a community setting.

The Healthy Child Programme—UK National Policy Development

In 2009, the UK government introduced a new approach to school nursing and health visiting with the launch of The Healthy Child Programme, 0–5 and 5–19 (Department of Health (DH), 2009a, 2009b). The programme outlined a range of universal contacts and activities, such as developmental reviews, screening, and immunisations. These are offered to all families, children, and young people in the UK. It also outlined a series of targeted support offers for children with special education needs, long-term medical conditions, or families with safeguarding concerns. The Healthy Child Programme aimed to ensure that every child gets the best start in life and continues with the work begun over a century ago by health visitors and school nurses in reducing the health inequalities in the UK (DH, 2009a, 2009b).

In 2016, PHE updated The Healthy Child Programme, introducing a vision for health visiting and school nursing to be jointly commissioned under new 0–19 services (PHE, 2016), which was a significant move away from the previously quite separate services. Much of the offer outlined built on the original Healthy Child Programme with a continued focus on giving children the best start in life; however, the shift towards a more modern and integrated universal service was evident (PHE, 2016). Alongside the developments in The Healthy Child Programme, the NHS Long Term Plan was published in 2019, creating a vision for the future of NHS services, including a more integrated approach to community services across the life course.

Earlier chapters in this book have worked through the principles of integrated care and models that have been used in practice. This chapter seeks to take those principles of integrated care and apply them to the integration of health visiting and school nursing services to 0–19 services in a UK context. It will explore some of the benefits and barriers to integrated care in a 0–19 context and propose a solution based on a case study of good practice.[1]

CASE STUDY

This case study is taken from the following study with the lead authors' permission:

Peckover, S., Shearn, K., Wood, D., Frankland, S., & Day, P. (2020). Extending the scope of health visiting and school nursing practice within a 0–19 service. *Journal of Health Visiting*, 8(10), 426–434. https://doi.org/10.12968/johv.2020.8.10.426

In response to the national policy recommendations around moving towards an integrated 0–19 service, a 0–19 team in the north of England explored the possibility of extending the training of six of their SCPHNs into the other field of practice. This was done in conjunction with Sheffield Hallam University who put together a work-based learning portfolio for the students to complete. In addition to the portfolio, practitioners were required to complete 50 days of practice in the new field in order to demonstrate competency and experience. The study included four health visitors extending their practice into school nursing, and two school nurses extending their practice into health visiting. The study sought to explore the views of the students, managers, practice teachers, and mentors around the benefits and challenges of extending SCPHN practice. Some of the driving factors for this approach include reduced school nursing numbers, desire to support families across the age spectrum, and flexibility in the teams to cover sickness and absence for either speciality; these will be explored in greater detail later in this chapter.

One of the challenges around work-based learning was the space for students to focus on their extended practice rather than their current role and caseload. Originally, students were given one day a week in their extended practice; however, this was changed to larger chunks of placement time allowing for a more varied and concentrated learning experience. Organisational factors such as shared online diaries and co-location of health visitors and school nurses were found to support students in learning their extended roles.

One of the main benefits reported by the particpants in the study was the flexibility to support the service wherever the needs were. Being qualified in health visiting and school nursing allowed practitioners to support things such as duty across the whole 0–19 spectrum, to complete primary birth visits, and support school immunisation sessions—tasks that traditionally would have required two separate members of staff. This flexibility enables teams to cover sickness and absence more efficiently.

Students completing the extended training noted that they found the process helpful in refreshing their knowledge of existing practice as well as gaining new knowledge. The training supported staff in reflecting on their practice and become what one student described as a 'more conscientious practitioner'. One of the worries expressed by students during their extended role training was the risk of becoming a 'jack of all trades, master of none' and missing doing the thing they were passionate about when they first applied, be that care of parents, babies, teenagers, etc.

Particpants reported that they felt there was a benefit to service users and families of having one single professional involved in their lives. Parents preferred having one practitioner who supported their child with additional needs through the transition into primary school and continued to support them once in school. This was also significant for families that were involved in child-in-need or child protection processes, where one health professional could support all members of the family. This is a further step towards integration from some current practices where one health professional attends meetings but the children stay allocated to a separate health visitor or school nurse. In addition to a single point of contact, practitioners reported that families and children experience a more timely service when being cared for by a practitioner trained in both health visiting and school nursing. Rather than having to refer to a colleague for support, advice, treatment, and referrals can be completed by the practitioner caring for the family as they arise.

This case study demonstrates that, although there can be some organisational and capacity challenges to extending the practice of health visitors and school nurses, there are positive effects on patient care, service delivery, flexibility, and efficiency, which are values at the very core of integrated care (Marshall, 2021).

---

[1] **Note on language:** The NHS Long Term Plan, 2019 (NHS England, 2019) discusses the expansion of 0–19 services to 0–25 services with an aim of reducing the 'cliff edge' of services experienced by many young people as they reach adulthood (18 years of age). The proposed 0–25 services include a broad range of services and professionals. This chapter is focused on the universal services of health visiting and school nursing, currently advised to be commissioned as a '0–19 Service' as per NHS England Commissioning Guides, 2016 (PHE, 2016).

DISCUSSION

Multiagency Working or Integration?

The Healthy Child Programme originally published in 2009 and all subsequent updates encourages an emphasis on 'integrated services' for families, children, and young people through effective multiagency working. School nurses and health visitors have worked together with other professionals to support families, such as teachers, youth workers, social workers, children's centre staff, and early help staff. This is particularly evident for families where there are safeguarding concerns, or families with children with special educational needs or disabilities (Wheeler, 2017). As discussed in Chapter 5, integrated care, at its core, is about reducing silo working, lack of co-ordination, and fragmentation of care experienced by people when they engage with health and/or social care (Thorstensen-Woll et al., 2021). There is a move towards systems and organisations that not only work well along side each other but merge to hold a new identity with a common shared goal of improving the lives of the people it serves (Shaw et al., 2013). The concept therefore of integrated services delivery being achieved through effective multi-agency working is something of an oxymoron. Despite the language in the Healthy Child Programme (describing services that are integrated), what has been seen in practice is more akin to good interprofessional working as opposed to true integration. Howarth and Morrison (2007) describe five levels of interprofessional working, with communication at one end and integration at the other (Fig. 30.1).

These levels can help practitioners and services imagine the process they will go through as they move towards integration. In 2003, the Laming Inquiry (Laming, 2003) was released with significant criticism around inter-agency communication regarding the safeguarding of children. The Laming Inquiry centred around the sad events of Victoria Climbié's life and death, highlighting the lack of joined-up working and communication across health, social care, and voluntary sectors. Since then, several government changes have taken place around the legislation and guidance regarding safeguarding and communication (Department for Education (DE), 2018). There are now formalised processes for early help, child-in-need, and child protection procedures, ensuring that professionals and families meet regularly with plans that are robust, seeking to support children and their families (DE, 2018). Health visitors and school nurses are well versed in working alongside partner agencies to support children and their families in these arenas, where the role of each professional is defined and although there are rarely joint structures (coalition) in place, there are formalised processes ensuring progress is made. However, what about when the child protection plan ends? What about the other children: those who do not meet the threshold for statutory interventions, those without formal structures for communication and planning in place? Are their needs co-ordinated and communicated? Where on Howarth and Morrison's scale would they place their experiences?

The NHS Long Term Plan, 2019 (NHS England, 2019) proposes big changes for service delivery with the establishment of integrated care systems (ICSs). ICSs are designed to bring together providers such as health, social care, education, and voluntary sectors to form new organisations enabling more integrated care to be delivered to our service users (Department of Health and Social Care (DHSC), 2021). The ICSs are anticipated to devolve care to a local or micro level, described in the literature as 'place' level; the details of how this will be outworked are yet to be seen (DHSC, 2021). However, with a little imagination, a world could be envisioned where information is not only shared between organisations, but jointly owned across organisations, where professionals work with families to support them the best they can, without being precious about roles or organisational preferences and with families feeling carefully held within a system rather than bounced around a system. Could there be a future where professionals from schools, social care, and voluntary groups work in the same service as school nurses and health visitors, working together to improve the health and wellbeing of the local population? Could there be a time where new organisations are formed to the extent that the concerns raised by Lord Laming (2003) around interagency communication are a moot point? This may sound a little optimistic, but it is fully anticipated that a much greater integration will occur of services working to support people across the whole life course. This begs the question—how do we get there?

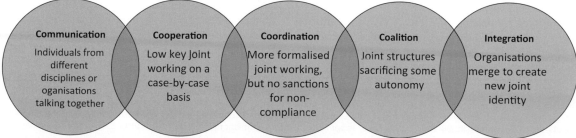

Fig. 30.1 Five levels of interprofessional working. (Howarth & Morrison, 2007).

The macro-level work will be happening behind the scenes: funding streams, national policies, and digital capabilities are all set to change. This chapter is for the people on the ground, at place level—the health visitors and the school nurses. Where do they begin in preparing for and supporting the move away from mere communication towards integration? This chapter suggests that if school nurses and health visitors are to integrate with other services, then they must first look to how they integrate within their service.

Integration Within 0–19

In many areas of the UK, health visiting and school nursing have merged as teams and formed a new title as 0–19 services (PHE, 2016). However, it could be argued that the formation of identity as a 0–19 service is still a work in progress as much of the work is still delivered in an age-bound way (Peckover et al., 2020). This brings into question the purpose of integrating 0–19 services. What are the benefits of an integrated service and are the benefits felt if the work continues with the invisible divide at age 5?

One of the key drivers for integrated care is patient and service user experience. Service users who have multiple practitioners in their lives report that having a more joined-up and co-ordinated service improves their experiences (Marshall, 2021; Shaw et al., 2011). This is particularly relevant in 0–19 when considering families that are in the safeguarding arena, or children with special educational needs or long-term medical conditions. Parents may have, in the past, experienced working with a health visitor for their younger children and working with a school nurse for their school-aged children, and potentially even a second school nurse if they have children in more than one school. The case study demonstrates that by having an integrated service where parents have one practitioner from 0–19 who works with all their children, this can improve communication, a sense of support, and efficient and timely care (Peckover et al., 2020). Poor communication and duplication of work are well evidenced contributing factors to patient errors and high levels of dissatisfaction with services (Coulter et al., 2018).

Children with additional needs often struggle during periods of transition such as starting primary school, moving from primary to high school, and leaving school (Duncan, 2012). Traditionally, health visitors would hand over children to the school nursing team upon starting primary school, bringing a change of practitioner at one of the family's most vulnerable times. Having the same practitioner walk through that transition journey would allow a greater level of support and therefore success in settling into school (Peckover et al., 2020). Having one 0–19 practitioner for a family is arguably a very effective way to improve the experience of families, children, and young people engaging with 0–19 services.

The need to deliver efficient and cost-effective services is a key driver for integrated services (DHSC, 2021). As discussed earlier, with separate health visiting and school nursing services, families could have two or three practitioners meeting with them to discuss the one child they support. This can be overwhelming and confusing for the parent; for the service, there is a significant amount of duplication and time savings to be made in changing this approach. In a truly integrated 0–19 service, one practitioner would be supporting the family, working with the parents or carers and each child, regardless of age. This would also be of benefit from a safeguarding perspective too. One of the many challenges, particularly in cases of childhood neglect, is the risks posed by 'starting again' or looking at a case with 'fresh eyes' (Brandon et al., 2008). New practitioners become involved with the family and give 'the benefit of the doubt' and drift occurs. With one practitioner having oversight of the family as a whole, this has the potential to be reduced, ensuring prompt and appropriate action is taken (DE, 2018).

The approach to care demonstrated in the case study also fits in with the 'Think Family' approach to care. 'Think Family' is in many ways a complementary concept to integrated care as it seeks to support the whole family when a parent or child comes into contact with health services. This represents a move away from working in siloes, where each professional treated their individual patient, towards caring for the family as a whole (McVeigh, 2020).

With such a wealth of positives discussed, not only to children, young people, and their families but also NHS services, why is there not greater integration in health visiting and school nursing services? What are the challenges that face practitioners and service leads?

Challenges

Arguably the biggest barrier to having one 0–19 practitioner is that there currently is no such thing as a 0–19 SCPHN. The titles of SCPHN Health Visitor and SCPHN School Nurse are protected by law and are separate registrations on the NMC register (NMC, 2004). Many of the discussed benefits could only be truly achieved if practitioners are trained and qualified in both health visiting and school nursing. In 2022, the NMC launched the updated SCPHN standards and have maintained the separation of health visiting and school nursing registration, with no 0–19 SCPHN qualification included in the standards (NMC, 2022). The case study demonstrates the answer to this barrier, in the extended training of school nurses and health visitors. In 2006, the NMC (2006) issued an addendum to facilitate SCPHNs registered as a school nurse or health visitor to complete additional training to extend their role into the opposite field of practice. As such they would be qualified to carry out the work of both health visitors and school nurses, although they would only retain NMC registration in their original SCPHN title. This is particularly significant for health visiting, as school nurses who extended their role would be able to complete core health visiting contacts which are required to be completed by a qualified health visitor (PHE, 2021).

Additionally, many practitioners chose to train in either health visiting or school nursing for specific reasons. School nurses need to be skilled in working with teenagers, building a knowledge base around sexual health, substances, and young people's mental health. They also are expected to lead classroom-style teaching sessions, working in a placed-based approach with a whole school population (PHE, 2016; School and Public Health Nurses Association (SAPHNA), 2021). Health visitors must be skilled in care of new-borns and maternal health, working in close proximity with parents or carers and their infants. They are expected to hold specialist knowledge around child development, maternal mental health, breastfeeding, and understanding the impact of attachment and bonding (DH, 2009a, 2009b; Seaman, 2021). Midwives can become health visitors but not school nurses, any registered nurse can train to be either a health visitor or a school nurse (NMC, 2004). Practitioners who have chosen to train as health visitors may not want to work with young people. Equally, practitioners who have chosen to train as school nurses may not want to work with new-borns and new parents. This was highlighted in the case study with some participants commenting that they felt they were becoming a 'jack of all trades, master of none'. What then does this mean for the delivery of good-quality service? If improved patient experience is at the core of integrated care, is the patient experience improved by working with a practitioner who is not comfortable or confident in their work? What is the impact on young people if they have to speak to the same practitioner that their parents or carers speak to? Young people want health services that are accessible and confidential, where they can talk openly without fear of their parents finding out (Lynch et al., 2021; Peckover et al., 2020). This is something that is supported in the new SAPHNA Vision for School Nursing (2021), with accessible and confidential services being a high priority. Nurses who have a preexisting relationship with parents may not present as confidential, potentially preventing a young person accessing support when it is needed. 0–19 staff would need to be careful with boundaries and ensure that confidential services for young people were maintained. The opportunity for extended training presented in the case study does not seek to entirely remove any sense of role preference or speciality for practitioners; however, it does provide some flexibility for both the service and service users.

Difficulties around protecting time off-caseload for practitioners to study their new craft are clearly evidenced in the case study. Numbers of school nurses and health visitors nationally in the UK have been in decline in the last decade, with both the Institute of Health Visiting (iHV) and SAPHNA

calling on the government to reinvest in the roles (iHV, 2020; SAPHNA, 2021). Time will be short for those who wish to extend their role, with safeguarding caseloads having a huge strain on practitioners (Wheeler, 2017). Services that wish to pursue a more integrated service, as demonstrated by the case study, will need to protect the time of their practitioners and ensure adequate access to support is in place. Some of the practitioners in the case study expressed that greater time with university staff and additional learning support resources would have been beneficial, something for SCPHN programme leads to consider when developing programmes (Peckover et al., 2020).

CONCLUSION

The national picture in the UK around service delivery is changing, with much greater investment to be seen in integrating health and social care over the coming years (DHSC, 2021). In 2016, PHE launched a new integrated 0–19 service, joining together health visiting and school nursing services into one service to support parents, carers, children, and young people from birth through to adulthood (PHE, 2016). Health visitors and school nurses need to form a new identity together as one service, putting patient care and experience at the centre of their delivery. There are many challenges to this, including declining numbers, safeguarding caseloads, historical working practices, NMC standards, and preexisting role preferences (NMC, 2004; Peckover et al., 2020; SAPHNA, 2021; Seaman, 2021). In response to these challenges, one 0–19 team in the north of England has invested in extending the training of some of their school nurses and health visitors (Peckover et al., 2020). Despite some challenges around protecting learning time and loss of sense of professional identity, the overarching message is a positive one. Practitioners trained in both health visiting and school nursing were able to flex to the needs of the service and the needs of the client groups. Universities and NHS Trusts need to work together to develop pathways, resources, and approved programmes to support this integration of 0–19 services.

References

Billingham, K., Morrell, J., & Billingham, C. (1996). Reflections on the history of health visiting. *British Journal of Community Health Nursing*, 1(7), 386–392. https://doi.org/10.12968/bjch.1996.1.7.7536

Brandon, M., Belderson, P., Warren, C., Gardner, R., Howe, D., Dodsworth, J., & Black, J. (2008). The preoccupation with thresholds in cases of child death or serious injury through abuse and neglect. *Child Abuse Review*, 17(5), 313–330. https://doi.org/10.1002/car.1043

Department of Education. (2018). Working Together to Safeguard Children A guide to inter-agency working to

safeguard and promote the welfare of children. https://
assets.publishing.service.gov.uk/government/uploads/
system/uploads/attachment_data/file/942454/Working_
together_to_safeguard_children_inter_agency_guidance.pdf

Department of Health. (2009a, October 27). *Healthy child programme: Pregnancy and the first 5 years of life*. https://
www.gov.uk/government/publications/healthy-child-pro-
gramme-pregnancy-and-the-first-5-years-of-life

Department of Health. (2009b). *Healthy child programme: From
5 to 19 years old*. London: Department of Health.

Department of Health & Social Care. (2021, February 11).
*Integration and innovation: Working together to
improve health and social care for all*. https://
www.gov.uk/government/publications/
working-together-to-improve-health-and-social-care-for-all

Duncan, M. (2012). Supporting the transition from primary to
secondary education. *British Journal of School Nursing, 7*(4),
183–187. https://doi.org/10.3390/educsci11090546

Horwath, J., & Morrison, T. (2007). Collaboration, integration
and change in children's services: Critical issues and key
ingredients. *Child Abuse & Neglect, 31*(1), 55–69. https://doi.
org/10.1016/j.chiabu.2006.01.007

Institute of Health Visiting (iHV). (2020). *Health visiting in
England: State of health visiting in England*. https://ihv.org.
uk/wp-content/uploads/2020/02/State-of-Health-Visiting-
survey-FINAL-VERSION-18.2.20.pdf

Laming H. (2003). *The Victoria Climbié Inquiry: Report of an
Inquiry by Lord Laming*. https://www.gov.uk/government/
publications/the-victoria-climbie-inquiry-report-of-an-
inquiry-by-lord-laming

Lynch, L., Moorhead, A., Long, M., & Hawthorne-Steele, I.
(2021). What type of helping relationship do young people
need? Engaging and maintaining young people in mental
health care—A narrative review. *Youth & Society, 53*(8),
1376–1399. https://doi.org/10.1177/0044118X20902786.

Marshall, K. (2021). Development of a framework for preparing organisations and teams for neighbourhood working.
International Journal of Integrated Care, 21(S1), 32. https://
doi.org/10.5334/ijic.ICIC20223

McVeigh, K. (2020). The Think Family Social Work Assessment:
outcomes of a family-focused initiative using The Family
Model. *Advances in Mental Health, 18*(3), 261–275. https://
doi.org/10.1080/18387357.2020.1825969

NHS England (2019). The long term plan. https://www.long-
termplan.nhs.uk/publication/nhs-long-term-plan/

Nursing and Midwifery Council. (2004). *Standards of proficiency
for specialist community public health nurses*. https://www.
nmc.org.uk/globalassets/sitedocuments/standards/nmc-
standards-of-proficiency-for-specialist-community-public-
health-nurses.pdf

Nursing and Midwifery Council. (2006). *Specialist Community
Public Health Nursing (SCPHN) – requirements for education and training in a differing 'field of specialist community
public health nursing practice'*. https://www.nmc.org.uk/
globalassets/sitedocuments/circulars/2006circulars/nmc-
circular-26_2006.pdf

Nursing and Midwifery Council. (2022). *Standards of proficiency
for specialist community public health nurses*. https://
www.nmc.org.uk/globalassets/sitedocuments/standards/

post-reg-standards/nmc_standards_of_proficiency_for_spe-
cialist_community_public_health_nurses_scphn.pdf

Peckover, S., Shearn, K., Wood, D., Frankland, S., & Day, P.
(2020). Extending the scope of health visiting and school
nursing practice within a 0–19 service. *Journal of Health
Visiting, 8*(10), 426–434. https://doi.org/10.12968/
johv.2020.8.10.426

Public Health England. (2016). *Guidance to support the commissioning of the healthy child programme 0 to 19: Health
visiting and school nursing services*. https://www.gov.uk/
government/publications/healthy-child-programme-0-to-
19-health-visitor-and-school-nurse-commissioning

Public Health England. (2021, May 19). *Health visiting and school nursing service delivery model*.
https://www.gov.uk/government/publications/
commissioning-of-public-health-services-for-children/
health-visiting-and-school-nursing-service-delivery-model

School and Public Health Nurses Association. (2021). *School
Nursing: Creating a healthy world in which children can thrive.
A Service Fit for the Future*. https://saphna.co/wp-content/
uploads/2021/10/SAPHNA-VISION-FOR-SCHOOL-NURSING.pdf

Schwab, N. C., & Gelfman, M. H. B. (2005). *Legal issues in school
health services: A resource for school administrators, school
attorneys, school nurses*. Lincoln, NE: iUniverse.

Seaman, H.E. (2021). *Health visitors' professional identity
and their lived experience of service change* [Doctorate in
Education thesis, University of Hertfordshire].

Shaw S., Rosen R. & Rumbold B. (2011). *What is Integrated
Care? An Overview of Integrated Care in the NHS*. London:
Nuffield Trust.

Thorstensen-Woll, C., Wellings, D., Crump, H., & Graham, C.
(2021). *Understanding integration: How to listen to
and learn from people and communities*. The King's
Fund. https://www.kingsfund.org.uk/publications/
understanding-integration-listen-people-communities

Wheeler, B. A. (2017). A new way forward: a look at one school
nursing team's innovative service model. *British Journal of
School Nursing, 12*(9), 452–454. https://doi.org/10.12968/
bjsn.2017.12.9.452

Further Reading

Institute of Health Visiting (iHV). (2020). *Health visiting in
England: State of health visiting in England*. https://ihv.org.
uk/wp-content/uploads/2020/02/State-of-Health-Visiting-
survey-FINAL-VERSION-18.2.20.pdf

Public Health England. (2021, May 21). *Health visiting and school nursing service delivery model*.
https://www.gov.uk/government/publications/
commissioning-of-public-health-services-for-children/
health-visiting-and-school-nursing-service-delivery-model

School and Public Health Nurses Association (SAPHNA). (2021).
*School Nursing: Creating a healthy world in which children
can thrive. A Service Fit for the Future*. https://saphna.
co/wp-content/uploads/2021/10/SAPHNA-VISION-FOR-
SCHOOL-NURSING.pdf

31

End-of-Life Care Within an Integrated Care Context

Dr Julie Alexandra Lawrence

'We cannot defeat death. However, we can change the way we talk about dying, death and bereavement and prepare, plan, care and support those who are dying and the people who are close to them. We must strengthen and improve our ability to provide care whatever the circumstances of our dying.'

(Ambitions for palliative and end of life care: A national framework for local action 2021-2026, p 9)

KEY CONCEPTS

- Caring for the dying is a lottery
- End-of-life care is a human right
- Palliative care
- Hospice UK
- Leeds Palliative Care Network

INTRODUCTION

Many people fear dying, which is associated with pain and indignity. In England, care of the dying remains a lottery in many cases (Deloitte Centre for Health Solutions, 2014). There is wide variation in quality, and meeting people's preferences for their place of death is often not possible. This situation is further exacerbated by the demise of the extended family network, and an expanding ageing population which increases the pressure to provide effective integrated services on behalf of the dying. During an average year, 500,000 people (aged over 75 years) die in England. The COVID-19 pandemic (2020–2022) added to these figures (182,609) (Gov.UK, 2022). End-of-life can mean any period between the last years of life to the last hours or days of life (Deloitte Centre for Health Solutions, 2014). As Fig. 31.1 illustrates, people in their last phase of life often require a holistic approach from a mixture of family, carers, and specialist services (such as palliative care) to address their health and social care needs.

The subject of death also remains taboo, especially when associated within our multicultural society; factors such as religion and cultural values need to be acknowledged: 'death is an inevitable part of life that no one can avoid. Yet, for too many, it is still a taboo subject.' (Deloitte Centre for Health Solutions, 2014). Meeting people's needs towards the end of their lives depends upon the identified partners (as illustrated in Fig. 31.1) to communicate effectively and work collaboratively for the benefit of those nearing end-of-life. Improved delivery of services will also need more effective commissioning and partnership working between the NHS, social services, and the voluntary sector. End-of-life care has seen significant innovation in recent years (Paget & Wood, 2013). However, professionals involved must be trained to ensure that an integrated and comprehensive approach to end-of-life care is paramount in order to facilitate 'a good death'. As Paul Woodward states:

'At Sue Ryder we approach care from the perspective of the individual receiving it. We are passionate about providing the care that people want. We don't just ask professionals for their expertise, we also ask the people we care for and their families how they would like to be cared for and supported'.

(Paget & Wood, 2013)

PALLIATIVE CARE

Palliative care is a holistic approach to pain relief and support, which can be used for people with serious illness. It is usually delivered by a multidisciplinary team, reflecting the concern with physical, emotional, and spiritual needs of the individual and their family to improve overall well-being. It is most often true that palliative care begins where 'curative' treatment leaves off, but this is not always the case; a cancer patient may begin to use hospice outpatient services while still undergoing chemotherapy, for example. In the UK, the boundary is more fluid than in other countries such as the United States, where patients may only become eligible to receive palliative care when they have ceased curative treatment (Paget & Wood, 2013).

IMPACT ON PEOPLE

Hospice UK is the national charity working for those experiencing dying, death, and bereavement. Team members work for the benefit of people affected by death and dying, collaborating with hospice members and other partners who work in end-of-life care. The charity believes:

CASE STUDY   Mary Caring for Her Younger Sister Lottie Within a Hospital and Palliative Care Setting in England

Lottie (a White Irish woman) was in her early 50 s. She was complaining of back pain for a number of years and visited her GP on a regular basis. The GP asked her to lose weight as he thought this was the cause of the continual back pain Lottie was experiencing. Other tests were not requested via the GP. However, after one particularly severe episode of pain, she was admitted to an acute hospital located some miles away from her home. Subsequently, she was diagnosed with ovarian cancer. Mary and other relatives were very shocked to hear the news. Mary commented that the care Lottie received within the oncology ward was excellent. For example, she had a very sympathetic consultant who listened to her and her symptoms. Accordingly, her care and treatment plan was created and personalised, which also recognised the importance of her sister, Mary, as she had supported Lottie when in pain. As her personalised treatment plan was now set up, she was transferred to her local hospital whereby her care could continue. However, Mary confirmed that Lottie remained in continuous pain over the next 8 weeks. At the time, there was no specific consultant to oversee her care and treatment plan. Lottie mentioned to Mary that the nursing staff were too busy to spend any time with her and felt she was causing 'an unnecessary fuss'. Once Lottie did speak to a consultant, she burst into tears about the high level of pain she was experiencing throughout her body. The consultant acknowledged that she needed additional support and therefore referred Lottie to the local hospice and palliative care service. She remained in the hospice for the following 2 months. The hospice's integrated care team (medical, nursing, and social work) worked in liaison with Lottie, Mary, and other family members to ensure that she had a co-ordinated approach to her ongoing medical and social care needs. Once the wider family members (including Mary) knew that end-of-life for Lottie was approaching, the family decided to care for her at home. Mary discussed how the palliative care team offered a robust service to Lottie and stressed 'how good and caring they were.' Lottie received specialist palliative care products to

enable her to live her remaining days in dignity. She did mention that the taboo subject of approaching the end-of-life to Lottie was 'off limits' as she never accepted that she was dying. She commented that, even as an experienced nurse herself, she found it difficult to broach the subject. However, she did explain to Lottie that she would receive a better integrated service, being placed within a hospice and palliative care setting. For example, the palliative community team explained about the services they would provide and what they would be doing on an ongoing basis considering the fact Lottie was nearing the end of life. Mary confirmed that Lottie did die at home and when the time came, the hospice team members left so that it was a private and dignified ending between family members, to celebrate a life once lived.

Discussion: Reflections Upon the Case Study
This case study is a sad example which begs the question: could Lottie have lived a better quality of life if her genuine health needs had been addressed earlier? Upon her initial visit to the GP, she was asked to lose weight as this was associated with her continuous back pain. It wasn't until she had a severe attack of pain that she was admitted to a hospital some distance away from home, which resulted in a later diagnosis of ovarian cancer.

At the time there was an obvious need for empathetic and competent healthcare staff to look beyond the stated obvious (back pain) which may have avoided the later diagnosis and early death. More recently, a broad partnership of national organisations working in England, discussed the inequalities which are present amongst socioeconomic groups and in particular women's health needs ('good care is often patchy when it must be universal'; Ambitions for palliative and end of life care: A national framework for local action 2021-2026 (NHS, 2021), p.7). National organisations such as NHS England, National Voices, and National Bereavement Alliance state that a personalised care plan for everyone is a positive step forward. However, in this (hospital) scenario, Lottie did have a care plan. The issue for Lottie and the professionals involved was that

(Continued)

an integrated and coordinated approach about her needs was absent. Clearly, shared records (with Lottie's consent) could have improved her overall experiences in the longer term. This included ensuring that Lottie received the right treatment and support when needed. Consequently, Lottie felt responsible for her pain when revealing her thoughts to her sister, Mary. The experience of continuous pain can also exacerbate emotional anguish or spiritual distress, as revealed by Lottie. In addition, the importance of support for family members such as Mary and other relatives should encompass good bereavement care to those who are facing loss and grief. Such care includes supporting them in their own preparation for bereavement.

Currow et al. (2020) outlined the needs of end-of-life cancer patients in Australia, and that patient-defined factors are important. These included being physically independent for as long as possible, in terms of being well enough to spend quality time with friends and family and to deal with unfinished business and finalise any legacy issues.

Hospice care adds to the quality of care and (as in Lottie's case) she was a priority for treatment and support in the last weeks and days of life. Currow et al. (2020) also stated that further integration of cancer services with hospice care would help to provide more seamless care for patients and supporting family members during their caregiving period and after the death of a loved one.

'That everyone, no matter who they are, where they are or why they are ill, should receive the best possible care at the end of their life'.

(Woking & Sam Beare Hospice and Wellbeing Care, 2022)

The charity is well aware of the NHS Long Term Plan about the importance of integrated care systems. The (Hospice UK Future Vision Programme, 2020) states that 'local Hospices can become more engaged as part of the wider system and work more closely with local healthcare partners'.

The programme outlined how there was broad agreement from a number of stakeholders (hospice leaders, service users, and primary care providers) that a successful integrated care service needed to begin with the primary care multidisciplinary team. Team members are then in a position to offer clarity about their roles and which services will be provided for someone at the end of life. As illustrated within the presented case study, relationships between individuals and professional staff within the palliative care service were a key enabler to greater levels of integration. As expected, forming trusting relationships often takes time, but where they are established, hospices overall found that they had a greater influence over service provision. The impact of COVID-19 had intensified the necessity to work within a collaborative context between health and social care services as a matter of urgency and to meet the demands of sick individuals. Consequently, traditional barriers between professionals and services (such as psychosocial perspectives as distinct from a biomedical orientation to care) were overcome more quickly to meet the serious health needs of patients.

One good example of integrated working is the Leeds Palliative Care Network. It was formed in 2016 between all palliative care providers in Leeds. The network includes representation from hospices, acute hospital trusts, community providers, the local authority, commissioners, and a wider range of voluntary sector organisations. The purpose of the Leeds Palliative Care Network, 2022 is to help organisations work together to plan and deliver care in the best possible way for palliative and end-of-life care patients, their families, and carers. The aim is to make sure that patients, families, and carers feel that:
- Each person is seen as an individual
- Each person gets fair access to care
- A patient's comfort and wellbeing is as great as it can be
- Care is co-ordinated
- All staff are prepared to care
- Each community is prepared to care

The aim of the network is to work jointly to improve services for adults approaching the end of their life, providing the right care, at the right time, in the right place. Recurrent funding has been secured from local commissioners and the network is now seen as the key forum for delivering system wide change and transformation. Key successes of the group include ensuring end-of-life care is a core component of the Leeds plan for health and care, supporting the development of the Leeds Care Record (a single citywide joined-up digital care record) and driving standardisation and consistency (e.g., in advanced care planning and education) (Woking & Sam Beare Hospice and Wellbeing Care, 2020).

As mentioned at the beginning of this chapter, the demand for palliative and end-of-life care continues to intensify. Our society is ageing and care needs are becoming increasingly challenging. The need for palliative care

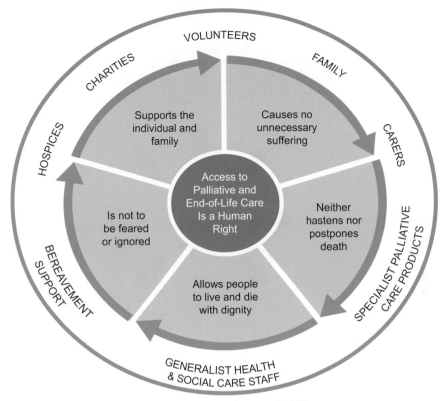

Fig. 31.1 A holistic and integrated approach to end-of-life care. (Hughes-Hallett et al., 2013).

is set to increase by 42% by 2040 (Woking & Sam Beare Hospice and Wellbeing Care, 2020). Alongside rising demand in population groups currently receiving end-of-life care, concerns have been raised that hospices may only offer services to a minority of people living with life-shortening conditions. There are growing levels of unmet demand among individuals and families from different racial groups (i.e., Black Caribbean, Chinese, Eritrean, and Roma). Hospices will need to find ways to reach greater numbers of people with limited resource. As illustrated in Fig. 31.2, hospices can influence a range of potential stakeholders to improve engagement and delivery of high-quality end-of-life care.

As noted from the case study, Mary was very influential in terms of supporting Lottie and also acted as the conduit between family members and professionals. Therefore there is merit in upskilling family members to ensure they are empowered to contribute towards decision-making when an important family member is near to end-of-life. Working alongside citizen-led care can also help to avoid crisis and best meet someone's needs.

CONCLUSION

This chapter has focused upon the importance of person-centred care which makes a positive difference to individuals who are near the end of life. There has also been a paradigm shift in attitudes towards those who are dying. This entails moving from a position of death and dying being a somewhat taboo subject to a more positive position whereby death and dying issues are discussed as part of our mortality. Organisations such as Hospice UK and the Leeds Palliative Care Network are at the forefront in advocating an encouraging approach towards discussions regarding 'dying matters'. Both organisations offer a plethora of information, advice, and support to those who need it.

In addition, an integrated care context can support families during this difficult life phase. Everyone deserves personal dignity when death is imminent. What matters most to people is that effective and compassionate care is paramount at a time when everyone involved is experiencing loss and bereavement. In terms of health and social care professionals, developing trusting and collaborative partnerships are paramount to deliver palliative and end-of-life services. Collaboration can help to define

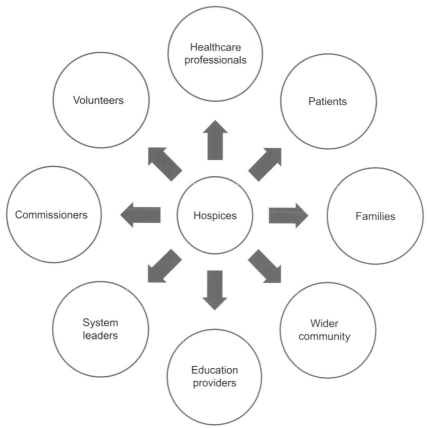

Fig. 31.2 Hospices and potential stakeholders. (Hospice UK Future Vision Programme, 2020).

a suitable integrated care model and therefore encourage funding from community trusts, primary care providers, and acute trusts, supporting hospice-at-home services alongside social care provision.

References

Currow, D., Agar, M., & Phillips, J. (2020). Role of hospice care at the end of life for people with cancer. *Journal of Clinical Oncology*, *38*(9), 937–943. https://doi.org/10.1200/jco.18.02235

Deloitte Centre for Health Solutions. (2014). *Transforming care at the end-of-life: Dying well matters*. London: Deloitte Centre for Health Solutions.

Gov.U.K. (2022). *Coronavirus (COVID-19) in the UK*. https://coronavirus.data.gov.uk/ [Accessed March 7, 2022].

Hospice UK https://www.hospiceuk.org/

Hospice UK Future Vision Programme- Discovery Phase, (2020). https://hukstage-bucket.s3.eu-west-2.amazonaws.com/s3fs-public/2021-10/ hospice-uk-future-vision-programme-discovery-phase-final-report.pdf

Hughes-Hallett, T., Murray, S.A., Cleary, J., Grant, L., Harding, R., Jadad, A., Steedman, M., & Taylor, K. (2013). *Dying healed: Transforming end-of-life care through innovation*. World Innovation Summit for Health, Doha, Qatar, December 10–11, 2013.

National Bereavement Alliance https://nationalbereavemental-liance.org.uk/

National Voices https://www.nationalvoices.org.uk/

NHS England https://www.england.nhs.uk/

NHS England. (2021). Ambitions for palliative and end of life care: A national framework for local action 2021-2026. https://www.england.nhs.uk/wp-content/uploads/2022/02/ambitions-for-palliative-and-end-of-life-care-2nd-edition.pdf

Leeds Palliative Care Network. (2022). Leeds Palliative care network news. https://leedspalliativecare.org.uk

Paget, A., & Wood, C. (2013). *'People's final journey must be one of their choosing…': Ways and Means*. London: Demos.

Woking & Sam Beare Hospice and Wellbeing Care. (2022). *Our vision for the future: Strategic Framework 2021/2023*. https://www.wsbhospices.co.uk/wp-content/uploads/2022/04/Strategic-Framework-2021-23.pdf

Further Reading

Gallagher, R., & Krawczyk, M. (2013). Family members' perceptions of end of life are across diverse location of care. *BMC Palliative Care*, *12*(1), 25. https://doi.org/10.1186/1472-684x-12-25

Moon, F., Fraser, L., & McDermott, F. (2019). Sitting with silence: hospital social work interventions for dying patients and their families. *Social Work in Healthcare*, *58*(5), 444–458. https://doi.org/10.1080/00981389.2019.1586027

Wain, L. M. (2020). Does integrated health and care in the community deliver its vision? A workforce perspective. *Journal of Integrated Care*, *29*(2), 170–184. https://doi.org/10.1108/JICA-10-2020-0061

INDEX

Note: Page numbers followed by *f* indicate figures, *t* indicate tables, and *b* indicate boxes.